"I was pleasantly surprised by the abundance of information regarding wellness, nutrition, and exercise. The author shows the importance of understanding one's own chemistry and how nutrition plays a vital role in dealing with health issues. This also plays an important role in mental health. This book has so many foundational pillars surrounding wellness and nutrition which makes for a great learning resource. As a mental health professional, I will definitely endorse this project and its positive impact on mental health!"

—*Anthony L. Hines, RN-BC, PMHNP-BC, PHN, psychiatric mental health nurse practitioner*

"*The Lifestyle Medicine Toolbox* is a ground-breaking book that equips healthcare and wellness professionals with essential knowledge and tools to seamlessly integrate lifestyle medicine into patient care. This comprehensive resource not only provides evidence-based strategies to enhance patient care for optimal health but also emphasizes self-care practices. I highly recommend this book to every healthcare and wellness professional, as it revolutionizes patient care and transforms the way we view our own well-being. This book is a call to action for a more enlightened and compassionate approach to healthcare—a must-read for anyone committed to making a genuine difference in our patients' lives."

—*Wendy Farnen Price, PT, DPT, MS, NBC-HWC, DipACLM, FACLM, owner of Healthcore Lifestyle Medicine*

"We can all classify ourselves as caregivers, whether we are focused on helping others or finding tools and strategies to help ourselves stay active and healthy. Ziya Altug presents both scientifically supported lifestyle medicine guidelines as well as feasible daily practices to keep a sharp focus on well-being. The user-friendly self-care handouts are great conversation starters for your patients/clients and offer a gentle reminder that you also have to 'take care of yourself before you can care for others.' As a military veteran and physiotherapist, I innately understand the importance of getting back to the basics of healthy food, regular exercise, stress management, good sleep hygiene, and nurturing strong social connections. What I appreciate about this book is the introduction to new topics (to me) of nature-based therapies such as natural light, soothing sounds, and nature walks, together with expressive therapies and healing arts. Ziya provides holistic, inclusive, and accessible lifestyle medicine approaches for health recovery and growth that do not involve medication or surgery. *The Lifestyle Medicine Toolbox* is a must-have book on your shelf if you are serious about sustainable health."

—*Amanda L. Ager, MScPT, MSc. Experimental Medicine, former military physiotherapy officer, chair of the Global Health Division of the Canadian Physiotherapy Association (CPA), Doctoral candidate, Ghent University, Belgium*

"What sets this book apart is the author's dedicated exploration of often overlooked areas in rehabilitation and patient management. He not only highlights their significance but also provides clear guidance on the integration into patient-centered care. The book offers practical examples that can be applied immediately, offering an abundance of options and ideas for tailoring prescriptions to each patient's unique needs, interests, availability, and resources. Whether you're a newcomer to lifestyle medicine or a seasoned practitioner seeking fresh ideas to enrich your toolkit, this book is an invaluable resource. It's a must-read that will leave you equipped to make a positive impact on both your own life and the lives of your patients."

—Tarina van der Stockt, PT, DPT, physical therapist

"Modern healthcare can feel like a fast-paced, numbers-driven pursuit where the patient/provider relationship and quality of care is an afterthought. This book not only provides an alternative approach to patient care but challenges us as healthcare providers to be more mindful and purposeful in our interactions with our patients and more caring toward ourselves. The Lifestyle Medicine Toolbox provides all health and wellness providers with a beautiful set of practical tools and clinical wisdom to enhance our practice. In this era of medical productivity, Ziya Altug's book is a breath of fresh air, which trumpets humble yet effective strategies to treat the entire person using approachable, heart-lead, and evidence-based information. This is the skillset modern healthcare needs to bring about true and honest healing to our patients and the healthcare system as a whole."

—Stacy Schiurring PT, DPT, CSRS, CCVR, physical therapist

"From the minute I picked up this book, I knew it was the perfect addition to my library of lifestyle medicine texts. Just scanning the contents section impressed me— the logical outline, superb organization, and actual tools to use with patients or clients in real time! This book fills a gap not only for clinicians providing lifestyle and integrative medicine but also for the patients and clients on the receiving end. It is a comprehensive text, yet distills important information into key concepts, clinical tips, and self-care patient handouts. I love the incorporation of mind-body practices and expanding concepts within lifestyle medicine such as culinary medicine and, my personal favorite, nature-based therapies. This is an essential evidence-based text for any healthcare clinician's bookshelf!"

—Susan Spell, FNP-BC, DipACLM, lifestyle medicine and holistic health coach, nurse practitioner

The Lifestyle Medicine Toolbox

of related interest

Integrative Rehabilitation Practice
The Foundations of Whole-Person Care for Health Professionals
Matt Erb and Arlene A. Schmid
ISBN 978 1 78775 150 7
eISBN 978 1 78775 151 4

Integrative Wellness Coaching
A Handbook for Therapists and Counsellors
Laurel Alexander
ISBN 978 1 83997 089 4
eISBN 978 1 83997 090 0

Case Studies in Personalized Nutrition
Edited by Angela Walker
ISBN 978 1 84819 394 9
eISBN 978 0 85701 351 4

Nature-Based Allied Health Practice
Creative and Evidence-Based Strategies
Amy Wagenfeld and Shannon Marder
ISBN 978 1 80501 008 1
eISBN 978 1 80501 009 8

THE LIFESTYLE MEDICINE TOOLBOX

Mind-Body Approaches for Health Promotion

Z. ALTUG

Foreword by Dr. Melissa Sundermann

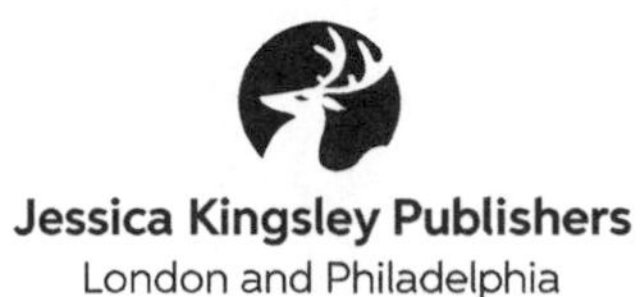

Jessica Kingsley Publishers
London and Philadelphia

First published in Great Britain in 2024 by Jessica Kingsley Publishers
An imprint of John Murray Press
1

Front cover image source: Shutterstock®. The cover image is for illustrative purposes only, and any person featuring is a model.

A CIP catalogue record for this title is available from the British Library and the Library of Congress

ISBN 978 1 83997 908 8
eISBN 978 1 83997 909 5

Printed and bound in Great Britain by CPI Group

Jessica Kingsley Publishers' policy is to use papers that are natural, renewable and recyclable products and made from wood grown in sustainable forests. The logging and manufacturing processes are expected to conform to the environmental regulations of the country of origin.

Jessica Kingsley Publishers
Carmelite House
50 Victoria Embankment
London EC4Y 0DZ

www.jkp.com

John Murray Press
Part of Hodder & Stoughton Ltd
An Hachette Company

Disclaimer

I dedicate this book to my patients and clients,
and to medical researchers around the globe.

Contents

APPENDICES

Foreword

In the ever-evolving realm of healthcare, the search for optimal well-being has led us down numerous avenues, each offering its own perspective on achieving health. However, a fundamental truth has become increasingly evident: our lifestyles are the cornerstone of our well-being. As healthcare professionals, we bear a profound responsibility to guide our patients and clients toward lifestyles that nurture health rather than undermine it. This is precisely where *The Lifestyle Medicine Toolbox*, authored by the esteemed Ziya Altug, PT, DPT, MS, emerges as a beacon of knowledge and practical wisdom.

Throughout my journey as a lifestyle medicine physician, affectionately known as "Doctor Outdoors" by some, I have witnessed the transformative potential of lifestyle choices in the lives of countless individuals. Ziya Altug's new book, *The Lifestyle Medicine Toolbox*, not only reaffirms the significance of these choices, but also equips healthcare professionals with essential tools to effectively promote healthier living. In this book, Ziya Altug adeptly lays out the foundational principles of lifestyle medicine, offering us a compass to navigate the intricate landscape of modern healthcare.

One of the pillars of lifestyle medicine that Ziya passionately explores in this book is the concept of "nature as medicine." In a world where many have become disconnected from the natural world, and where lifestyles often revolve around urban environments rather than the beauty of nature, the importance of rekindling this connection cannot be overstated. As someone who has long advocated for the healing power of the outdoors, I applaud Ziya's inclusion of this critical aspect of lifestyle medicine. In *The Lifestyle Medicine Toolbox*, he not only emphasizes the benefits of nature as medicine but also provides practical strategies for healthcare professionals to integrate this concept into their practice.

The core of this book lies in its comprehensive exploration of the pillars of lifestyle medicine. Ziya Altug takes us on a journey through these pillars, illuminating key concepts, providing invaluable clinical tools, and offering self-care handouts that bridge the gap between knowledge and action. Let's delve into these pillars briefly to understand the depth and breadth of this transformative work.

Healthy Eating: The Foundation of Wellness

Lifestyle medicine emphasizes the power of nutrition as a foundational pillar of health. Ziya Altug's book does not merely touch the surface of this vital concept, but delves deep into the principles of healthy eating. He provides evidence-based guidance on nutrition and offers practical tools for healthcare professionals to assist their patients and clients in making healthier dietary choices. Diet is at the core of wellness, and Ziya's comprehensive approach empowers us to make informed choices that align with our patient's unique needs.

Physical Activity: The Joy of Movement

Physical activity is another cornerstone of lifestyle medicine, and in this book Ziya Altug does an outstanding job of making exercise approachable and enjoyable. He highlights the importance of incorporating movement into our daily lives, irrespective of age or fitness level, and provides healthcare professionals with tools to inspire and motivate their patients toward a more active lifestyle. His emphasis on the joy of movement reminds us that exercise should be something we look forward to, not dread.

Stress Management: Nurturing Mind and Spirit

The modern world is fraught with stressors, and their impact on health cannot be underestimated. Ziya's insights on stress management are a timely and much-needed addition to this book. He guides us through techniques and strategies to foster resilience, mental well-being, and emotional balance. Stress is an ubiquitous presence in our lives, and Ziya Altug's work equips us with the tools to navigate its challenges with grace.

Quality Sleep: The Essential Reset Button

In our fast-paced society, sleep often takes a backseat to other pursuits. However, the importance of quality sleep in maintaining health cannot be overstated. Ziya's exploration of this pillar provides a deep understanding of sleep's role in overall wellness. His practical recommendations for improving sleep hygiene and establishing healthy sleep patterns are invaluable, both for healthcare professionals and their patients.

Avoidance of Risky Substances: The Path to Freedom

The detrimental effects of tobacco, alcohol, and other risky substances are well-documented. Ziya Altug's approach to this pillar is not about judgment or condemnation, but about empowering individuals to make choices that align with their health goals. He provides resources on addiction management and strategies for healthcare professionals to support their patients in breaking free from the grip of harmful substances.

Connection and Community: The Power of Relationships

Human beings are inherently social creatures, and the quality of our relationships profoundly impacts our well-being. Ziya recognizes this truth and explores the importance of connection and community in lifestyle medicine. He provides guidance on building supportive social networks and fostering meaningful relationships, acknowledging that a sense of belonging is essential for holistic health.

Nature as Medicine: Reconnecting with Our Roots

In a world where many of us spend the majority of our lives indoors, the concept of "nature as medicine" has taken on new significance. Ziya Altug's passionate exploration of this pillar underscores the healing power of the natural world. He provides compelling evidence of the physical and psychological benefits of spending time in nature, backed by scientific research. Moreover, he offers practical strategies for incorporating nature into our daily lives, and encourages healthcare professionals to prescribe "doses" of nature as a part of their treatment plans. As "Doctor Outdoors," I wholeheartedly endorse this approach, and am delighted to see it featured prominently in this book.

What sets *The Lifestyle Medicine Toolbox* apart is its practicality. Ziya Altug understands that knowledge, without actionable steps, is of limited value. Therefore, for each pillar of lifestyle medicine he provides concrete clinical tools that healthcare professionals can implement immediately in their practice. These tools range from dietary guidelines and exercise regimens to stress management techniques and sleep hygiene recommendations. They empower us to not only understand the importance of these lifestyle choices but also to guide our patients and clients effectively toward healthier lives.

Furthermore, Ziya goes the extra mile by including self-care handouts. These resources are invaluable for healthcare professionals to share with their patients and clients, ensuring that the journey toward optimal health is a collaborative effort. These handouts simplify complex concepts, making it easier for individuals to grasp the principles of lifestyle medicine and take practical steps toward improving their well-being.

As a lifestyle medicine physician, I understand the profound impact that lifestyle choices can have on health outcomes. I have witnessed individuals transform their lives through simple but meaningful changes in diet, exercise, stress management, and other lifestyle factors. *The Lifestyle Medicine Toolbox* not only reinforces the importance of these choices but also equips healthcare professionals with the knowledge and tools they need to effect positive change in the lives of their patients.

But this book is not just a valuable resource for healthcare professionals; it is also a gift to our patients and clients. It empowers them to take charge of their health, providing them with the information and tools to make informed decisions and adopt healthier lifestyles. In a world where the burden of chronic disease is escalating, this book serves as a beacon of hope and a roadmap to wellness.

In conclusion, I wholeheartedly endorse *The Lifestyle Medicine Toolbox* by Ziya Altug, PT, DPT, MS. It is a comprehensive, practical, and transformative guide to lifestyle medicine. Ziya's work is a testament to his dedication to improving the well-being of individuals and communities. May this book inspire and guide you, as it has inspired and guided me,

Melissa Sundermann, DO, FACOI, FACLM, DipABLM

Acknowledgements

First, I thank the entire Jessica Kingsley Publishers team who helped develop this book. A special thanks to Sarah Hamlin, Senior Commissioning Editor. I am very grateful for her guidance and encouragement. I also thank Masooma Malik, Editorial Assistant; Simon Levy, Cover Designer; Carys Homer, Senior Production Editor; Giuliana di Mitrio, Senior Production Controller; Megan Donny, Marketing Executive; Bonnie Craig, Copy Editor; Colin Wood, Proofreader; and the rest of the team for their effort and support. Thank you to Jessica Kingsley for founding Jessica Kingsley Publishers in 1987 with the mission of empowering individuals to change society through information and knowledge.

I express my sincere appreciation to the following professionals for their contributions:

- Stacy Barrows, PT, DPT, GCFP, NCPT
- Margarita Chamlaian, MA, BCBA, LMFT
- Deepa Deshmukh, MPH, RDN, CDE, BC-ADM
- Tracy Gensler, MS, RD
- Rekha Lund, DAOM, MPT, Dipl.O.M., LAc.
- Julie Shelton, M.AmSAT, CEAS

I would like to extend a special thanks to Juan Cifuentes for his wonderful photos and Lilian Cifuentes for serving as the model for many of the exercise photos in the book. The photo shoots were professional and fun!

A special thanks to my brother Aykut "Ike" Altug for all his support and encouragement.

Finally, I thank Mom and Dad for preparing me for my journey in life. I am grateful for their practical introduction to lifestyle medicine and wellness principles at a very young age.

Preface

The purpose of this book is to offer healthcare providers, health/fitness professionals, and caregivers a workbook on integrative and lifestyle medicine, with a focus on nonpharmacological and nonsurgical approaches. *The Lifestyle Medicine Toolbox* serves as a complement to other integrative and lifestyle medicine texts on the market. It aims to provide practical strategies for selecting self-care programs for patients/clients, as well as serve as a self-care guide for professionals to prevent burnout and reduce stress and anxiety.

The book uses a clinical, evidence-based approach to explore the six primary factors of lifestyle medicine: nutrition, physical activity/exercise, sleep, stress, risky substances/addiction, and social connectedness. It also reviews concepts such as nature-based outdoor activities, expressive therapies, and self-care strategies, with an emphasis on low back pain as a practical application of the approach. However, it should be noted that the lifestyle medicine approach can be applied to a range of medical conditions, including Alzheimer's disease, anxiety, asthma, cancer, chronic pain, diabetes, depression, fibromyalgia, headaches, multiple sclerosis, obesity, osteoarthritis, osteoporosis, Parkinson's, and stroke.

I want to emphasize one key point. The content I am presenting is "a" way of approaching the material and not "the" way or the "only" way. There are many clinical interpretations of the content being presented.

My personal journey into wellness and lifestyle medicine started at a very young age. My father was a physician specializing in internal medicine. I was fascinated by all the anatomy and physiology books throughout our house. Dad routinely talked about the importance of sleep, stress management, wholesome nutrition, and physical activity to stay sharp and fit. He told me he emphasized these areas to his patients so they could recover and heal faster. Mom focused on the practical aspects of wellness. She prepared healthful foods and even taught me how to cook many wonderful Mediterranean dishes when I was in junior high school. Little did I know that my cooking skills would lead me to my current fascination with culinary medicine. When Mom washed our laundry, she added tiny slivers of lavender soap to make the clothes smell great and keep the family calm and relaxed. Even before it became a popular topic, she understood the benefits of aromatherapy. Ever since I was a child, I enjoyed being outdoors building forts, splashing around in the rain, and playing a variety of outdoor and indoor sports. To this day, nature and outdoor activities are a part of my personal self-care routine. I enjoy nature walks and hiking, weight training, basketball, volleyball, pickleball, qigong, and a variety of other activities and sports in an outdoor environment.

Prior to entering the physical therapy, I obtained degrees in physical education and exercise science, where I learned about fitness, health, and coaching. In my professional career, I have practiced primarily in an outpatient rehabilitation setting since graduating from the University of Pittsburgh Department of Physical Therapy program. I have attended numerous continuing education courses and workshops that include orthopedic physical therapy, sports medicine, sports conditioning, wellness, fitness, yoga, tai chi, qigong, Pilates, Feldenkrais Method, and the Alexander Technique.

In my clinical practice, I have routinely emphasized that my patients undergoing rehabilitation include proper sleep, stress management, wholesome foods, avoidance of smoking and other risky substances, and outdoor physical activities as a part of their recovery program. I would have never predicted that what I learned from my parents and in my physical education and exercise science college programs about health and wellness would eventually become an organization emphasizing healthy lifestyle choices.

I have been a member of the American Physical Therapy Association for nearly 30 years and a member of the American College of Lifestyle Medicine since 2017. My writing journey includes publishing health and wellness-related books, articles, blogs, and a newspaper column. I have taught several elective wellness and integrative pain management courses at university level for several semesters. Currently, I provide continuing education courses and webinars for several platforms where I emphasize the integrative and lifestyle medicine approach from the physical therapy and rehabilitation perspective.

So many therapeutic choices and so little time. This is the dilemma many healthcare and health/fitness professionals face daily in their work environment. For the past 30-plus years, I have used many of the self-care strategies outlined in this book. It is my hope that this resource toolbox provides you, the reader, with an easy-to-use and evidence-informed guide for clinical and practical use.

Ziya "Z" Altug

About the Author

Ziya "Z" Altug, PT, DPT, MS, is a doctor of physical therapy with 32 years of clinical experience in treating musculoskeletal conditions. He currently treats patients in Los Angeles and provides webinars and continuing education courses to an international audience. Ziya uses integrative and lifestyle medicine to help patients/clients to improve their well-being and manage pain.

Ziya is the author of three books: *Integrative Healing: Developing Wellness in the Mind and Body* (2018), *The Anti-Aging Fitness Prescription* (2006), and *Manual of Clinical Exercise Testing, Prescription, and Rehabilitation* (1993). Recently, he wrote the chapter "Exercise, Dance, Tai Chi, Pilates and Alexander Technique" in *The Handbook of Wellness Medicine* (2020). Also, in July 2021, he published "Lifestyle Medicine for Chronic Lower Back Pain: An Evidence-Based Approach" in the *American Journal of Lifestyle Medicine*. Additionally, Ziya published two case reports on constipation and back pain (2016), and thoracic outlet syndrome (2015) in *Orthopaedic Physical Therapy Practice*, and a review article on resistance exercise and cognitive function (2014) in the *Strength and Conditioning Journal*. Finally, Ziya published the unique *2012 Healthy Lifestyle Wall Calendar* with a calendar publisher and co-authored the fitness column "Ask the Fitness Pros" in the *Pittsburgh Post-Gazette* from 1987 to 1988.

Ziya received his bachelor's degree in physical therapy at the University of Pittsburgh, his master's degree in sport and exercise studies and a bachelor's degree in physical education from West Virginia University, and a doctor of physical therapy (DPT) degree from the College of St. Scholastica. Ziya is a long-standing member of the American Physical Therapy Association and has been a member of the American College of Lifestyle Medicine since 2017.

LinkedIn: www.linkedin.com/in/zaltug

Contributors

Stacy Barrows, PT, DPT, GCFP, NCPT
Physical Therapist/Feldenkrais Practitioner
Los Angeles, California

Margarita Chamlaian, MA, BCBA, LMFT
Behavior Analyst and Marriage and Family Therapist
Los Angeles, California

Juan Cifuentes
Photographer
Los Angeles, California

Lilian Cifuentes
Graphic Designer/Exercise Model
Los Angeles, California

Deepa Deshmukh, MPH, RDN, CDE, BC-ADM
Registered Dietitian
Greater Chicago Area, Illinois

Tracy Gensler, MS, RD
Registered Dietitian
Chevy Chase, Maryland

Rekha Lund, DAOM, MPT, Dipl.O.M., LAc.
Physical Therapist/Acupuncturist
Los Angeles, California

Julie Shelton, M.AmSAT, CEAS
Alexander Technique Practitioner
Los Angeles, California

How to Use This Book

This book is designed as a workbook to supplement clinical and fitness/wellness coaching practice and other lifestyle medicine textbooks. The content is intended to provide healthcare providers, health/fitness professionals, and caregivers with necessary evidence-based resources. The book also provides practical tools, strategies, and techniques that may help healthcare and fitness professionals create personalized educational handouts and design effective home programs.

The book contains 12 chapters; ideally, the first two chapters should be read first to obtain an overview of lifestyle medicine. The remaining chapters may be read in any order depending on which content is needed for patient/client care or the student and instructor's needs.

Students in healthcare and fitness professions can use the book to explore topics in greater detail and create educational content for their patients/clients. Instructors may use the book to design practical lesson plans and lab activities for their students.

The self-care handouts in this book, indicated by ★, include ready-made practices that you can share with your patients/clients. Each self-care handout is available to download from https://library.jkp.com/redeem using the code TTMJUJG. The sample exercises in Appendix C are also available to download from this link.

Many of the chapters in this toolbox-approach book provide the following key features to help readers develop practical lifestyle medicine programs and prescriptions:

- Learning objectives to understand what is being covered in the chapter
- Chapter highlights to provide a quick overview
- A basic introduction to the topic
- Bullet points and lists that help the reader quickly identify the evidence
- Clinical tips
- Featured topics
- Self-care education guides, strategies, and techniques
- Self-management activities that help the reader discover online resources to manage stress and anxiety by exploring various fun topics

- Classroom and lab activities that may be used to create engaging lab activities for students
- Useful problem-solving clinical resources for additional research and learning
- Research cited in the chapter
- Additional reading to help the reader explore the topic in greater detail

The Appendices section provides the following:

- A list of suggested clinical practice guidelines
- A checklist for creating an effective home program for patients/clients
- A sample exercise selection guide to create a home program for patients/clients

Finally, the index provides a quick way to search for topics and help the reader narrow their search.

I hope this book provides a useful guide to help treat patients and manage client health and wellness.

Further updates about the book can be found at www.linkedin.com/in/zaltug.

CHAPTER 1

Introduction to Lifestyle Medicine

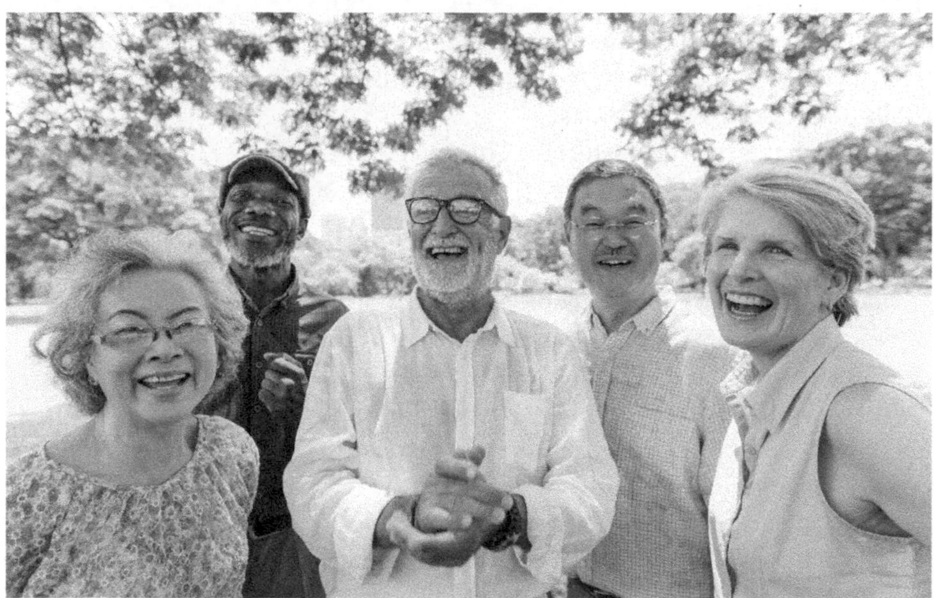

Laughter is medicine

Learning Objectives

- Understand the essential research for integrative and lifestyle medicine.
- Discuss the benefits of integrative and lifestyle medicine.

Chapter Highlights

- Key Concept: Daily Habits and Actions
- Clinical Tip: Static Versus Dynamic Meditation
- Self-Care Handout 1.1: Anti-Inflammatory Lifestyle

- Self-Care Handout 1.2: Personal Health and Safety Checklist
- Self-Management Activities
- Classroom and Lab Activities
- Useful Clinical Resources
- References
- Additional Reading

Lifestyle Matters: *Feeling well is rarely a random event.*

Introduction

There are many excellent books covering the unique field of lifestyle medicine. As mentioned in the Preface, the purpose of this manual is to serve as a practical toolbox for the other textbooks.

First, what is lifestyle medicine? The American College of Lifestyle Medicine (ACLM) (Clayton and Bonnet 2023, p.2) defines lifestyle medicine as:

> ...a medical specialty that uses therapeutic lifestyle interventions as a primary modality to treat chronic conditions including, but not limited to, cardiovascular diseases, type 2 diabetes, and obesity. Lifestyle medicine certified clinicians are trained to apply evidence-based, whole-person, prescriptive lifestyle change to treat and, when used intensively, often reverse such conditions. Applying the six pillars of lifestyle medicine—a whole-food and plant-predominant eating pattern, physical activity, restorative sleep, stress management, avoidance of risky substances, and positive social connections—also provides effective prevention for these conditions.

The ACLM (Clayton and Bonnet 2023, p.2) goes on to state in a clarifying note for the definition that "A whole-food plant-based dietary pattern consists of mostly food from plants (such as whole grains, vegetables, fruits, beans, and legumes) with little to no animal products (such as dairy, meat, or eggs)."

The *Foundations of Lifestyle Medicine: Board Review Manual* (Clayton and Bonnet 2023) indicates that the American College of Lifestyle Medicine organization was founded in 2004 by John Kelly, MD, MPH, and colleagues. According to the *Lifestyle Medicine* book, edited by James M. Rippe, MD, the term "lifestyle medicine" was coined in the first edition published in 1999 (Rippe 2019).

The following figure illustrates the basic pillars of lifestyle medicine. Clinicians may use the pillars to create patient/client-specific prescriptions.

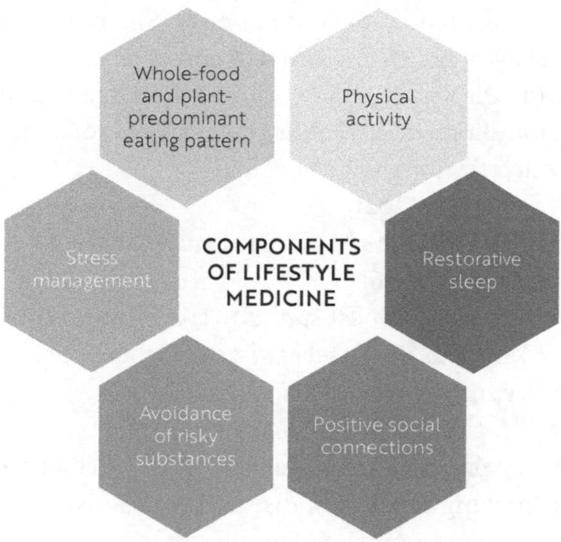

Components of lifestyle medicine

KEY CONCEPT: DAILY HABITS AND ACTIONS

The choices we make today affect everything in our future. In a review article, James Rippe, MD, states, "There is no longer any serious doubt that daily habits and actions profoundly affect both short-term and long-term health and quality of life" (Rippe 2018, p.499).

Why Lifestyle Medicine is Needed

The ACLM (2023) indicates that many chronic diseases today are caused by unhealthy lifestyle choices. Lifestyle medicine interventions may impact chronic disease (Nyberg *et al.* 2020) and medical conditions such as:

- Alzheimer's (Dhana *et al.* 2020)
- back pain (Altug 2021; Bohman *et al.* 2014; Manderlier *et al.* 2022; Moriki *et al.* 2022; Williams *et al.* 2019)
- cancer (Guo *et al.* 2020; Zhang *et al.* 2020)
- cardiovascular disease (Zhang *et al.* 2021)
- chronic pain (Nielsen *et al.* 2021; Nijs *et al.* 2020; Smedbråten *et al.* 2022; Uyeshiro Simon and Collins 2017)
- dementia (Dominguez *et al.* 2021; McMaster *et al.* 2020)
- depression (Bringmann *et al.* 2022; Forsyth *et al.* 2015; Wong *et al.* 2021a; Wong *et al.* 2021b)
- diabetes (Fritsche *et al.* 2021; Kelly *et al.* 2020; Uusitupa *et al.* 2019)

- fibromyalgia (Fernandez-Feijoo *et al.* 2022; Shomer and Roll 2022)
- gastroesophageal reflux disease (Ness-Jensen *et al.* 2016)
- headache (de Oliveira *et al.* 2022; Torres-Ferrus *et al.* 2019)
- hypertension (Blumenthal *et al.* 2021; Paula *et al.* 2015; van Oort *et al.* 2020)
- multiple sclerosis (Johansson *et al.* 2021)
- obesity (Verduci *et al.* 2021)
- osteoarthritis (Gilbert *et al.* 2018; Ho *et al.* 2022)
- osteoporosis (Geyer 2016)
- Parkinson's disease (Advocat *et al.* 2013; Advocat *et al.* 2016)
- rheumatoid arthritis (England *et al.* 2023; Schönenberger *et al.* 2021)
- stroke (Bailey 2016).

In addition to disease prevention and management with lifestyle medicine principles, there is a growing interest in disease reversal using lifestyle medicine (Vodovotz *et al.* 2020). For example, some authors and researchers have explored disease reversal of atrial fibrillation (Chung *et al.* 2020), chronic kidney disease (Díaz-López *et al.* 2021), cognitive decline (Bredesen 2014; Bredesen *et al.* 2016; Rao *et al.* 2023), diabetes (Gregg *et al.* 2012; Kelly *et al.* 2020; Knowler *et al.* 2002; Taylor *et al.* 2019), and heart disease (Marshall *et al.* 2009; Ornish *et al.* 1998).

The following figure outlines some modifiable risk factors affecting various medical conditions such as cardiovascular disease, infectious disease, neurological disorders, diabetes, cancer, obesity, cognitive impairment, anxiety, depression, and musculoskeletal conditions such as back pain. These are areas where medical practitioners and health/fitness professionals can educate their patients/clients to improve medical outcomes.

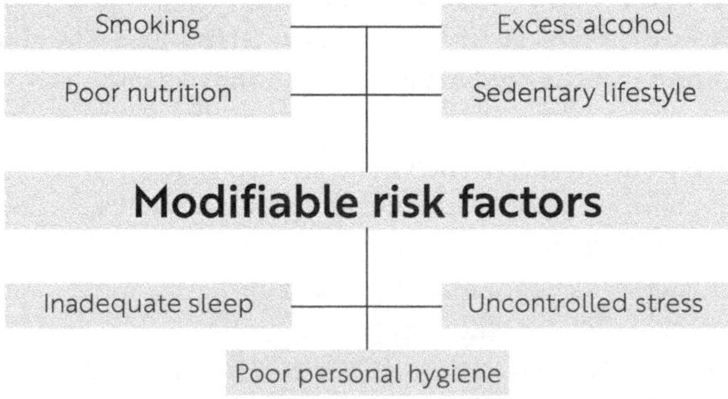

Modifiable risk factors for various medical conditions

CLINICAL TIP: STATIC VERSUS DYNAMIC MEDITATION

Find the best meditation or relaxation routine for your patient/client. For example, static meditation may be useful for individuals who have pain or difficulty with movement or for those who need to focus on calming activities for seated or stationary activities. Dynamic meditation may be useful for individuals who have difficulty focusing in static positions.

- Static meditation—body scan meditation, guided imagery, progressive muscle relaxation, transcendental meditation
- Dynamic meditation—labyrinth walking, mindful or nature walking, qigong, tai chi, yoga

Self-Care Education Guides

See **Self-Care Handout 1.1: Anti-Inflammatory Lifestyle** for evidence-informed strategies to reduce inflammation as a part of a person's life (Alizaei Yousefabadi *et al.* 2021; Chai *et al.* 2019; Chiavaroli *et al.* 2018; Irwin *et al.* 2016; Irwin and Vitiello 2019; Kenđel Jovanović *et al.* 2021; Kiecolt-Glaser *et al.* 2011; Mahdavi-Roshan *et al.* 2022; Melaku *et al.* 2022; Moosavian *et al.* 2020; Morvaridzadeh *et al.* 2020; Puett *et al.* 2019; Rezaie *et al.* 2021; Schell *et al.* 2017; Schönenberger *et al.* 2021; Tibuakuu *et al.* 2017; Tolkien *et al.* 2019; Willcox *et al.* 2014; Wirtz *et al.* 2017).

See **Self-Care Handout 1.2: Personal Health and Safety Checklist** to encourage individuals to live safely.

Self-Care Handout 1.1: Anti-Inflammatory Lifestyle

Foods

- Eat a high-quality anti-inflammatory diet (AID). AID may benefit, for example, sleep apnea, rheumatoid arthritis, obesity, cardiovascular disease, and depression.
- Drink some tart cherry juice.
- Eat some strawberries.
- Use some curcumin, garlic, and ginger in your food.
- Consume probiotics and omega-3-rich foods.

Exercise

- Get enough exercise every day. Consider walking, yoga, tai chi, or qigong.

Stress

- Reduce and control stress. Consider exercise, meditation, and hobbies.

Sleep

- Get adequate sleep every night.

Avoidance of Risky Substances

- Don't smoke.
- Don't consume excess alcohol.

Environment

- Minimize exposure to air pollution (such as traffic).

Self-Care Handout 1.2: Personal Health and Safety Checklist

Medical

- ✓ Get a yearly checkup with your family physician.
- ✓ Get yearly checkups with your dentist and dental hygienist.

Driving

- ✓ Drive cautiously and stay within the speed limit. Whatever is at the end of your journey can wait.
- ✓ Drive courteously to avoid road rage scenarios.
- ✓ Wear your seat belt.
- ✓ Avoid distracted driving (such as while texting and talking on the phone).
- ✓ Never drive under the influence of alcohol or other harmful substances.

Home Safety

- ✓ Make sure you have emergency supplies in the event of a disaster. For example, ensure you have water, blankets, clothes, flashlights, a medical kit, and a radio for news.

Personal Safety

- ✓ Be aware of your surroundings.
- ✓ Wash your hands frequently, especially after work, shopping, or events.

Nutrition

- ✓ To prevent choking, don't talk while you are chewing food.

Exercise

- ✓ Wear protective equipment such as helmets while riding a bike.
- ✓ Avoid exercising in polluted areas.

Stress

- ✓ Find strategies that help you manage stress.
- ✓ Get counseling and medical help if self-care strategies do not help.

Sleep

- ✓ Get restful sleep every night.

Avoidance of Risky Substances

- ✓ Don't smoke, and don't consume excess alcohol.
- ✓ Get counseling and medical help.

Socialization

- ✓ Stay engaged in your community with meaningful and purposeful activities.

Self-Management Activities: Explore Labyrinths

The following resources can help patients/clients, healthcare providers, and health/fitness professionals to manage stress and anxiety by exploring labyrinths:

- The Labyrinth Journey App provides relaxation by using your finger to trace a path: https://labyrinthjourney.app
- The labyrinth tracing/puzzle image below is for relaxation. Start at the perimeter opening on the left side of the labyrinth, trace slowly into the middle, and then trace slowly back to your starting point.

Labyrinth for relaxation

Classroom and Lab Activities

- Perform lifting and carrying activities using different-sized and weighted objects (such as grocery bags, laundry baskets, cases of water, and suitcases). Notice how each person has different body mechanics for lifting and carrying.
- See how you can optimize the lifting and carrying mechanics for each person based on their strength, flexibility, and anatomy (e.g., height, arm length, leg length) to help prevent back pain.

Useful Clinical Resources

Organizations

- Academic Consortium for Integrative Medicine & Health, www.imconsortium.org
- Academy of Aquatic Physical Therapy, https://aquaticpt.org
- Academy of Integrative Health & Medicine, www.aihm.org
- American College of Lifestyle Medicine, www.lifestylemedicine.org
- American College of Sports Medicine, www.acsm.org
- Aquatic Therapy and Rehab Institute, www.atri.org
- Australasian Society of Lifestyle Medicine, www.lifestylemedicine.org.au
- Benson-Henry Institute, https://bensonhenryinstitute.org
- National Center for Complementary and Integrative Health, https://nccih.nih.gov
- UCLA Center for East-West Medicine, https://cewm.med.ucla.edu

Finding Quality Resources

- American Physical Therapy Association—Rehabilitation Reference Center (member access only), www.apta.org
- CINAHL (research tool for nursing and allied health professionals), www.ebsco.com/products/research-databases/cinahl-database
- Cochrane Library, www.cochranelibrary.com
- DiTA (Diagnostic Test Accuracy database), https://dita.org.au
- Google Scholar, https://scholar.google.com
- MedlinePlus (health-related resources), https://medlineplus.gov
- National Library of Medicine (PubMed), https://pubmed.ncbi.nlm.nih.gov
- PEDro (Physiotherapy Evidence Database), https://pedro.org.au
- PubMed Central (free full-text article database), www.ncbi.nlm.nih.gov/pmc

Outcome Measures

- *Tools for the Lifestyle Medicine Team*
  American Academy of Family Physicians, www.aafp.org/dam/AAFP/documents/patient_care/lifestyle-medicine/lifestyle-additional-tools.pdf
- *36-Item Short Form Survey Instrument (SF-36)*
  RAND, www.rand.org/health-care/surveys_tools/mos/36-item-short-form/survey-instrument.html
- *Alcohol Use Disorder Identification Test-Consumption (AUDIT-C)*
  Frank D, DeBenedetti AF, Volk RJ, Williams EC, Kivlahan DR, Bradley KA. Effectiveness of the AUDIT-C as a screening test for alcohol misuse in three race/ethnic groups. *J Gen Intern Med.* 2008;23(6):781–787.
- *Consensus Sleep Diary*
  Carney CE, Buysse DJ, Ancoli-Israel S, *et al.* The consensus sleep diary: standardizing prospective sleep self-monitoring. *Sleep.* 2012;35(2):287–302.
- *International Physical Activity Questionnaire (IPAQ)*
  Craig CL, Marshall AL, Sjostrom M, *et al.* International Physical Activity Questionnaire: 12-country reliability and validity. *Med Sci Sport Exerc.* 2003;35(8):1381–1395.
- *Lifestyle Assessment Short Form*
  Loma Linda University, The American College of Lifestyle Medicine; 2018. https://ihacares.com/assets/pdfs/Lifestyle%20Medicine/ACLM-LLUH_short_form_english_2019.pdf
- *Lifestyle Medicine Assessment*
  Frates B, Bonnet JP, Joseph R, Peterson JA. *Lifestyle Medicine Handbook: An Introduction to the Power of Healthy Habits*, 2nd ed. Monterey, CA: Healthy Learning; 2021.
- *Meaning in Life Questionnaire*
  Steger MF, Frazier P, Oishi S, Kaler M. The Meaning in Life Questionnaire: assessing the presence of and search for meaning in life. *J Couns Psychol.* 2006;53(1):80–93.
- *Mediterranean Diet Adherence Screener (MEDAS)*
  García-Conesa MT, Philippou E, Pafilas C, *et al.* Exploring the validity of the 14-item Mediterranean Diet Adherence Screener (Medas): a cross-national study in seven European countries around the Mediterranean region. *Nutrients.* 2020;12(10):1–18.
- *Patient Health Questionnaire-9 (PHQ-9) and PHQ-2*
  Kroenke K, Spitzer RL, Williams JBW. The PHQ-9: validity of a brief depression severity measure. *J Gen Intern Med.* 2001;16(9):606–613.
  Kroenke K, Spitzer RL, Williams JBW. The patient health questionnaire-2: validity of a two-item depression screener. *Med Care.* 2003;41(11):1284–1292.

- *PAVING Wheel Questionnaire (for well-being and lifestyle medicine)*
  Frates B, Bonnet JP, Joseph R, Peterson JA. *Lifestyle Medicine Handbook: An Introduction to the Power of Healthy Habits*, 2nd ed. Monterey, CA: Healthy Learning; 2021.
- *Physical Activity Readiness Questionnaire for Everyone (PAR-Q+)*
  American College of Sports Medicine. *ACSM's Guidelines for Exercise Testing and Prescription,* 11th ed. Philadelphia, PA: Wolters Kluwer; 2022. http://eparmedx.com/wp-content/uploads/2013/03/January2020PARQPlusFillable.pdf
- *Quality of Life Measures*
  Physiopedia, www.physio-pedia.com/Quality_of_Life
- *Readiness Ruler*
  Indiana University, https://iprc.iu.edu/sbirtapp/mi/ruler.php
- *Screener and Opioid Assessment for Patients with Pain-Revised (SOAPP-R)*
  Butler SF, Fernandez K, Benoit C, Budman SH, Jamison RN. Validation of the revised screener and opioid assessment for patients with pain (SOAPP-R). *J Pain*. 2008;9(4):360–372.
- *Social Needs Screening Tool*
  American Academy of Family Physicians, www.aafp.org/dam/AAFP/documents/patient_care/everyone_project/hops19-physician-form-sdoh.pdf

References

Advocat J, Enticott J, Vandenberg B, Hassed C, Hester J, Russell G. The effects of a mindfulness-based lifestyle program for adults with Parkinson's disease: a mixed methods, wait list controlled randomised control study. *BMC Neurol*. 2016;16(1):166.

Advocat J, Russell G, Enticott J, Hassed C, Hester J, Vandenberg B. The effects of a mindfulness-based lifestyle programme for adults with Parkinson's disease: protocol for a mixed methods, randomised two-group control study. *BMJ Open*. 2013;3(10):e003326.

Alizaei Yousefabadi H, Niyazi A, Alaee S, Fathi M, Mohammad Rahimi GR. Anti-inflammatory effects of exercise on metabolic syndrome patients: a systematic review and meta-analysis. *Biol Res Nurs*. 2021;23(2):280–292.

Altug Z. Lifestyle medicine for chronic lower back pain: an evidence-based approach. *Am J Lifestyle Med*. 2021;15(4):425–433.

American College of Lifestyle Medicine. 2023. https://lifestylemedicine.org

Bailey RR. Lifestyle modification for secondary stroke prevention. *Am J Lifestyle Med*. 2016;12(2):140–147.

Blumenthal JA, Hinderliter AL, Smith PJ, *et al.* Effects of lifestyle modification on patients with resistant hypertension: results of the TRIUMPH randomized clinical trial. *Circulation*. 2021;144(15):1212–1226.

Bohman T, Alfredsson L, Jensen I, Hallqvist J, Vingård E, Skillgate E. Does a healthy lifestyle behaviour influence the prognosis of low back pain among men and women in a general population? A population-based cohort study. *BMJ Open*. 2014;4(12):e005713.

Bredesen DE. Reversal of cognitive decline: a novel therapeutic program. *Aging (Albany NY)*. 2014;6(9):707–717.

Bredesen DE, Amos EC, Canick J, *et al.* Reversal of cognitive decline in Alzheimer's disease. *Aging (Albany NY)*. 2016;8(6):1250–1258.

Bringmann HC, Michalsen A, Jeitler M, *et al.* Meditation-based lifestyle modification in mild to moderate depression: a randomized controlled trial. *Depress Anxiety*. 2022;39(5):363–375.

Chai SC, Davis K, Zhang Z, Zha L, Kirschner KF. Effects of tart cherry juice on biomarkers of inflammation and oxidative stress in older adults. *Nutrients*. 2019;11(2):228.

Chiavaroli L, Nishi SK, Khan TA, *et al.* Portfolio Dietary Pattern and cardiovascular disease: a systematic review and meta-analysis of controlled trials. *Prog Cardiovasc Dis*. 2018;61(1):43–53.

Chung MK, Eckhardt LL, Chen LY, *et al.* Lifestyle and risk factor modification for reduction of atrial fibrillation: a scientific statement from the American Heart Association. *Circulation*. 2020;141(16):e750–e772.

Clayton JS, Bonnet J. *Foundations of Lifestyle Medicine: Board Review Manual*, 4th ed. Chesterfield, MO: American College of Lifestyle Medicine; 2023.

de Oliveira AB, Mercante JPP, Benseñor IM, Goulart AC, Peres MFP. Headache disability, lifestyle factors, health perception, and mental disorder symptoms: a cross-sectional analysis of the 2013 National Health Survey in Brazil. *Neurol Sci*. 2022;43(4):2723–2734.

Dhana K, Evans DA, Rajan KB, Bennett DA, Morris MC. Healthy lifestyle and the risk of Alzheimer dementia: findings from 2 longitudinal studies. *Neurology*. 2020;95(4):e374–e383.

Díaz-López A, Becerra-Tomás N, Ruiz V, *et al.* Effect of an intensive weight-loss lifestyle intervention on kidney function: a randomized controlled trial. *Am J Nephrol*. 2021;52(1):45–58.

Dominguez LJ, Veronese N, Vernuccio L, *et al.* Nutrition, physical activity, and other lifestyle factors in the prevention of cognitive decline and dementia. *Nutrients*. 2021;13(11):4080.

England BR, Smith BJ, Baker NA, *et al.* 2022 American College of Rheumatology Guideline for Exercise, Rehabilitation, Diet, and Additional Integrative Interventions for Rheumatoid Arthritis. *Arthritis Rheumatol*. 2023 May 25. Online ahead of print.

Fernandez-Feijoo F, Samartin-Veiga N, Carrillo-de-la-Peña MT. Quality of life in patients with fibromyalgia: contributions of disease symptoms, lifestyle and multi-medication. *Front Psychol*. 2022;13:924405.

Forsyth A, Deane FP, Williams P. A lifestyle intervention for primary care patients with depression and anxiety: a randomised controlled trial. *Psychiatry Res*. 2015;230(2):537–544.

Fritsche A, Wagner R, Heni M, *et al.* Different effects of lifestyle intervention in high- and low-risk prediabetes: results of the randomized controlled prediabetes lifestyle intervention study (PLIS). *Diabetes*. 2021;70(12):2785–2795.

Geyer C. Postmenopausal osteoporosis: the role of lifestyle in maintaining bone mass and reducing fracture risk. *Am J Lifestyle Med*. 2016;11(2):125–128.

Gilbert AL, Lee J, Ehrlich-Jones L, *et al.* A randomized trial of a motivational interviewing intervention to increase lifestyle physical activity and improve self-reported function in adults with arthritis. *Semin Arthritis Rheum*. 2018;47(5):732–740.

Gregg EW, Chen H, Wagenknecht LE, *et al.* Association of an intensive lifestyle intervention with remission of Type 2 diabetes. *JAMA*. 2012;308(23):2489–2496.

Guo Y, Li ZX, Zhang JY, *et al.* Association between lifestyle factors, vitamin and garlic supplementation, and gastric cancer outcomes: a secondary analysis of a randomized clinical trial. *JAMA Netw Open*. 2020;3(6):e206628.

Ho J, Mak CCH, Sharma V, To K, Khan W. Mendelian randomization studies of lifestyle-related risk factors for osteoarthritis: a PRISMA review and meta-analysis. *Int J Mol Sci*. 2022;23(19):11906.

Irwin MR, Olmstead R, Carroll JE. Sleep disturbance, sleep duration, and inflammation: a systematic review and meta-analysis of cohort studies and experimental sleep deprivation. *Biol Psychiatry*. 2016;80(1):40–52.

Irwin MR, Vitiello MV. Implications of sleep disturbance and inflammation for Alzheimer's disease dementia. *Lancet Neurol*. 2019;18(3):296–306.

Johansson S, Skjerbæk AG, Nørgaard M, Boesen F, Hvid LG, Dalgas U. Associations between fatigue impact and lifestyle factors in people with multiple sclerosis: the Danish MS hospitals rehabilitation study. *Mult Scler Relat Disord*. 2021;50:102799.

Kelly J, Karlsen M, Steinke G. Type 2 diabetes remission and lifestyle medicine: A Position Statement from the American College of Lifestyle Medicine. *Am J Lifestyle Med*. 2020;14(4):406–419.

Kenđel Jovanović G, Mrakovcic-Sutic I, Pavičić Žeželj S, *et al.* Metabolic and hepatic effects of energy-reduced anti-inflammatory diet in younger adults with obesity. *Can J Gastroenterol Hepatol*. 2021:6649142.

Kiecolt-Glaser JK, Belury MA, Andridge R, Malarkey WB, Glaser R. Omega-3 supplementation lowers inflammation and anxiety in medical students: a randomized controlled trial. *Brain Behav Immun*. 2011;25(8):1725–1734.

Knowler WC, Barrett-Connor E, Fowler SE, *et al.* Reduction in the incidence of Type 2 diabetes with lifestyle intervention or metformin. *N Engl J Med*. 2002;346(6):393–403.

Mahdavi-Roshan M, Salari A, Kheirkhah J, Ghorbani Z. The effects of probiotics on inflammation, endothelial dysfunction, and atherosclerosis progression: a mechanistic overview. *Heart Lung Circ.* 2022;31(5):e45–e71.

Manderlier A, de Fooz M, Patris S, Berquin A. Modifiable lifestyle-related prognostic factors for the onset of chronic spinal pain: a systematic review of longitudinal studies. *Ann Phys Rehabil Med.* 2022;65(6):101660.

Marshall DA, Walizer EM, Vernalis MN. Achievement of heart health characteristics through participation in an intensive lifestyle change program (Coronary Artery Disease Reversal Study). *J Cardiopulm Rehabil Prev.* 2009;29(2):84–96.

McMaster M, Kim S, Clare L, *et al.* Lifestyle risk factors and cognitive outcomes from the multidomain dementia risk reduction randomized controlled trial, body brain life for cognitive decline (BBL-CD). *J Am Geriatr Soc.* 2020;68(11):2629–2637.

Melaku YA, Reynolds AC, Appleton S, *et al.* High-quality and anti-inflammatory diets and a healthy lifestyle are associated with lower sleep apnea risk. *J Clin Sleep Med.* 2022;18(6):1667–1679.

Moosavian SP, Paknahad Z, Habibagahi Z, Maracy M. The effects of garlic (Allium sativum) supplementation on inflammatory biomarkers, fatigue, and clinical symptoms in patients with active rheumatoid arthritis: a randomized, double-blind, placebo-controlled trial. *Phytother Res.* 2020;34(11):2953–2962.

Moriki K, Tushima E, Ogihara H, Endo R, Sato T, Ikemoto Y. Combined effects of lifestyle and psychosocial factors on central sensitization in patients with chronic low back pain: a cross-sectional study. *J Orthop Sci.* 2022;27(6):1185–1189.

Morvaridzadeh M, Fazelian S, Agah S, *et al.* Effect of ginger (Zingiber officinale) on inflammatory markers: a systematic review and meta-analysis of randomized controlled trials. *Cytokine.* 2020;135:155224.

Ness-Jensen E, Hveem K, El-Serag H, Lagergren J. Lifestyle intervention in gastroesophageal reflux disease. *Clin Gastroenterol Hepatol.* 2016;14(2):175–182.e823.

Nielsen SS, Christensen JR, Søndergaard J, *et al.* Feasibility assessment of an occupational therapy lifestyle intervention added to multidisciplinary chronic pain treatment at a Danish pain centre: a qualitative evaluation from the perspectives of patients and clinicians. *Int J Qual Stud Health Well-being.* 2021;16(1):1949900.

Nijs J, D'Hondt E, Clarys P, *et al.* Lifestyle and chronic pain across the lifespan: an inconvenient truth? *PM R.* 2020;12(4):410–419.

Nyberg ST, Singh-Manoux A, Pentti J, *et al.* Association of healthy lifestyle with years lived without major chronic diseases. *JAMA Intern Med.* 2020;180(5):760–768.

Ornish D, Scherwitz LW, Billings JH, *et al.* Intensive lifestyle changes for reversal of coronary heart disease [published correction appears in *JAMA.* 1999 Apr 21;281(15):1380]. *JAMA.* 1998;280(23):2001–2007.

Paula TP, Viana LV, Neto AT, Leitão CB, Gross JL, Azevedo MJ. Effects of the DASH Diet and walking on blood pressure in patients with Type 2 diabetes and uncontrolled hypertension: a randomized controlled trial. *J Clin Hypertens (Greenwich).* 2015;17(11):895–901.

Puett RC, Yanosky JD, Mittleman MA, *et al.* Inflammation and acute traffic-related air pollution exposures among a cohort of youth with Type 1 diabetes. *Environ Int.* 2019;132:105064.

Rao RV, Subramaniam KG, Gregory J, *et al.* Rationale for a multi-factorial approach for the reversal of cognitive decline in Alzheimer's disease and MCI: a review. *Int J Mol Sci.* 2023;24(2):1659.

Rezaie S, Askari G, Khorvash F, Tarrahi MJ, Amani R. Effects of curcumin supplementation on clinical features and inflammation, in migraine patients: a double-blind controlled, placebo randomized clinical trial. *Int J Prev Med.* 2021;12:16.

Rippe JM. Lifestyle medicine: the health promoting power of daily habits and practices. *Am J Lifestyle Med.* 2018;12(6):499–512.

Rippe JM, ed. *Lifestyle Medicine*, 3rd ed. Boca Raton, FL: CRC Press; 2019.

Schell J, Scofield RH, Barrett JR, *et al.* Strawberries improve pain and inflammation in obese adults with radiographic evidence of knee osteoarthritis. *Nutrients.* 2017;9(9):949.

Schönenberger KA, Schüpfer AC, Gloy VL, *et al.* Effect of anti-inflammatory diets on pain in rheumatoid arthritis: a systematic review and meta-analysis. *Nutrients.* 2021;13(12):4221.

Shomer L, Roll SC. Lifestyle Redesign® intervention for psychological well-being and function in people with fibromyalgia: a retrospective cohort study. *Am J Occup Ther.* 2022;76(6):7606205060.

Smedbråten K, Grotle M, Jahre H, *et al.* Lifestyle behaviour in adolescence and musculoskeletal pain 11 years later: The Trøndelag Health Study. *Eur J Pain.* 2022;26(9):1910–1922.

Taylor R, Valabhji J, Aveyard P, Paul D. Prevention and reversal of Type 2 diabetes: highlights from a symposium at the 2019 Diabetes UK Annual Professional Conference [published correction appears in *Diabet Med.* 2019 Oct;36(10):1320]. *Diabet Med.* 2019;36(3):359–365.

Tibuakuu M, Kamimura D, Kianoush S, *et al.* The association between cigarette smoking and inflammation: the Genetic Epidemiology Network of Arteriopathy (GENOA) study. *PLoS One.* 2017;12(9):e0184914.

Tolkien K, Bradburn S, Murgatroyd C. An anti-inflammatory diet as a potential intervention for depressive disorders: a systematic review and meta-analysis. *Clin Nutr*. 2019;38(5):2045–2052.

Torres-Ferrus M, Vila-Sala C, Quintana M, *et al.* Headache, comorbidities and lifestyle in an adolescent population (The TEENs Study). *Cephalalgia*. 2019;39(1):91–99.

Uusitupa M, Khan TA, Viguiliouk E, *et al.* Prevention of Type 2 diabetes by lifestyle changes: a systematic review and meta-analysis. *Nutrients*. 2019;11(11):2611.

Uyeshiro Simon A, Collins CER. Lifestyle Redesign® for chronic pain management: a retrospective clinical efficacy study. *Am J Occup Ther*. 2017;71(4):7104190040p1–7104190040p7.

van Oort S, Beulens JWJ, van Ballegooijen AJ, Grobbee DE, Larsson SC. Association of cardiovascular risk factors and lifestyle behaviors with hypertension: a mendelian randomization study. *Hypertension*. 2020;76(6):1971–1979.

Verduci E, Bronsky J, Embleton N, *et al.* Role of dietary factors, food habits, and lifestyle in childhood obesity development: a position paper from the European Society for Paediatric Gastroenterology, Hepatology and Nutrition Committee on Nutrition. *J Pediatr Gastroenterol Nutr*. 2021;72(5):769–783.

Vodovotz Y, Barnard N, Hu FB, *et al.* Prioritized research for the prevention, treatment, and reversal of chronic disease: recommendations from the Lifestyle Medicine Research Summit. *Front Med (Lausanne)*. 2020;7:585744.

Willcox DC, Scapagnini G, Willcox BJ. Healthy aging diets other than the Mediterranean: a focus on the Okinawan diet. *Mech Ageing Dev*. 2014;136–137:148–162.

Williams A, van Dongen JM, Kamper SJ, *et al.* Economic evaluation of a healthy lifestyle intervention for chronic low back pain: a randomized controlled trial. *Eur J Pain*. 2019;23(3):621–634.

Wirtz PH, von Känel R. Psychological stress, inflammation, and coronary heart disease. *Curr Cardiol Rep*. 2017;19(11):111.

Wong VW, Ho FY, Shi NK, Sarris J, Chung KF, Yeung WF. Lifestyle medicine for depression: a meta-analysis of randomized controlled trials [published correction appears in *J Affect Disord*. 2021 Apr 7]. *J Affect Disord*. 2021a;284:203–216.

Wong VW, Ho FY, Shi NK, *et al.* Smartphone-delivered multicomponent lifestyle medicine intervention for depressive symptoms: a randomized controlled trial. *J Consult Clin Psychol*. 2021b;89(12):970–984.

Zhang YB, Pan XF, Chen J, *et al.* Combined lifestyle factors, incident cancer, and cancer mortality: a systematic review and meta-analysis of prospective cohort studies. *Br J Cancer*. 2020;122(7):1085–1093.

Zhang YB, Pan XF, Chen J, *et al.* Combined lifestyle factors, all-cause mortality and cardiovascular disease: a systematic review and meta-analysis of prospective cohort studies. *J Epidemiol Community Health*. 2021;75(1):92–99.

Additional Reading

Carey RM, Moran AE, Whelton PK. Treatment of hypertension: a review. *JAMA*. 2022;328(18): 1849–1861.

Egger G, Binns A, Rossner S, Sagner M, eds. *Lifestyle Medicine: Lifestyle, the Environment and Preventive Medicine in Health and Disease,* 3rd ed. London, United Kingdom: Academic Press; 2017.

Frates B, Bonnet JP, Joseph R, Peterson JA. *Lifestyle Medicine Handbook: An Introduction to the Power of Healthy Habits*, 2nd ed. Monterey, CA: Healthy Learning; 2021.

Garner G, Tatta J, eds. *Integrative and Lifestyle Medicine in Physical Therapy*. Minneapolis, MN: OPTP; 2022.

Mechanick JI, Kushner RF, eds. *Lifestyle Medicine: A Manual for Clinical Practice*. Cham, Switzerland: Springer International Publishing; 2016.

Mechanick JI, Kushner RF, eds. *Creating a Lifestyle Medicine Center: From Concept to Clinical Practice*. Cham, Switzerland: Springer International Publishing; 2020.

Merlo G, Berra K, eds. *Lifestyle Nursing*. Boca Raton, FL: CRC Press; 2023.

Rippe JM. *Manual of Lifestyle Medicine*. Boca Raton, FL: CRC Press; 2021.

Sidossis LS, Kales SN. *Textbook of Lifestyle Medicine*. Hoboken, NJ: John Wiley & Sons; 2022.

US Department of Veteran Affairs. Passport to Whole Health. 2020. www.va.gov/WHOLEHEALTHLIBRARY/docs/Passport_to_Whole-Health_FY2020_508.pdf

CHAPTER 2

Clinical Concepts

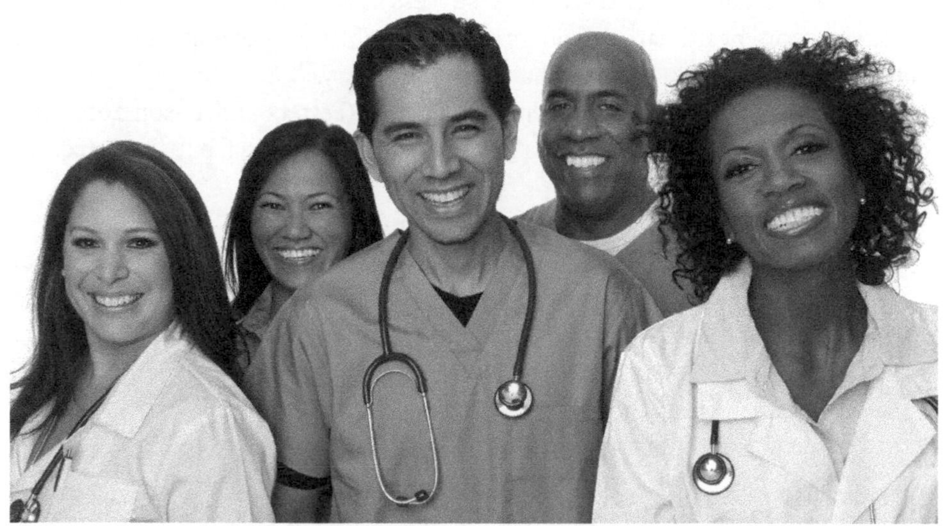

Building rapport is key for success

Learning Objectives

- Understand the basic clinical concepts of lifestyle medicine.
- Discuss the benefits of pain neuroscience education, motivational interviewing, therapeutic alliance, and shared decision-making.

Chapter Highlights

- Key Concept: Building a Strong Therapeutic Alliance as Part of Telehealth
- Clinical Tip: Setting SMART Goals
- Featured Topic 2.1: Cognitive Behavioral Therapy
- Self-Care Handout 2.1: Healthy Lifestyle Prescription
- Self-Management Activities

- Classroom and Lab Activities
- Useful Clinical Resources
- References
- Additional Reading

Lifestyle Matters: *If in doubt, get it checked out.*

Introduction

Teamwork and collaboration are key to success in working with patients/clients. For this reason, healthcare providers and health/fitness professionals should be well versed in techniques that enhance care delivery.

According to *Evidence Based Physical Therapy* (Fetters and Tilson 2019), the following three factors can help practitioners achieve optimal patient outcomes (see the figure below):

- Clinical expertise (e.g., formal academic education, post-professional education, clinical practice)
- Scientific research (e.g., research studies)
- Patient values and circumstances (e.g., patient beliefs, preferences, expectations, cultural identification, access to medical services, family environment)

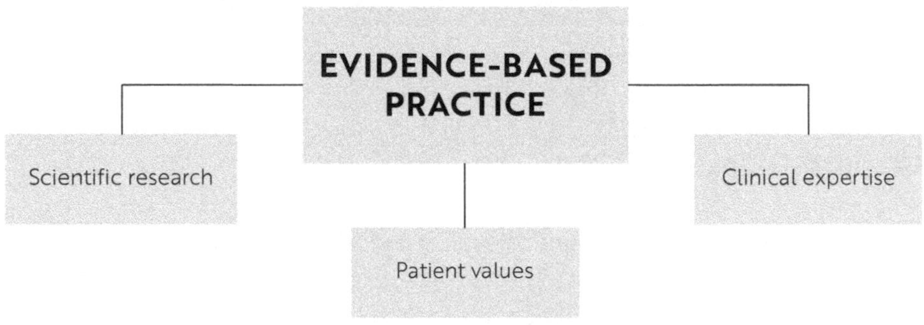

Evidence-based practice

KEY CONCEPT: BUILDING A STRONG THERAPEUTIC ALLIANCE AS PART OF TELEHEALTH

The medical community is moving quickly into the electronic age with courses, conferences, and patient care. To help build a strong therapeutic alliance during telehealth and telerehabilitation virtual visits, consider the following (Tanaka *et al.* 2020; Yedlinsky and Peebles 2021):

- Create a professional and relaxed space for the telehealth meeting that is quiet and without distractions.
- Prepare notes and review any documentation about the patient/client before the meeting.
- At the beginning of the meeting and periodically during the meeting, ask the patient/client if the cameras and sound are working properly.
- Ask if the patient/client needs any assistance with technology in your preliminary phone or email contact.
- Use good lighting in your telehealth space.
- Create a professional background without excess distractions.
- Have all supporting documents at arm's length to avoid excessive movements in front of the camera.
- Maintain eye contact with the camera.
- Lean into the camera periodically to show you are listening.
- Use appropriate facial expressions and voice modulations for the topic being discussed.
- Smile at the beginning and end of meetings.

Biopsychosocial Model of Pain

The following table, an adapted version of the Biopsychosocial Model of Pain (BMP), highlights biological, psychological, behavioral, and sociocultural influences on pain. For this reason, a practitioner's evaluation and treatments need to focus on a multimodal approach. It should be noted that the BMP is only one model for classifying pain.

Biopsychosocial model of pain

Biological Influences	Psychological Influences
• Nociception • Inflammation • Tissue pathology (joint, muscle, organ)	• Coping • Stress • Catastrophizing • Mood and emotions (fear, anger, anxiety)
Behavioral Influences	**Sociocultural Influences**
• Substance use • Exercise • Sleep • Diet	• Social support (family, friends, work) • Education • Income • Occupation • Cultural background

Adapted from Bartley et al. 2017; Engel 1977; Loeser 1982; Sluka 2016.

Pain Neuroscience Education

An article in *Archives of Physical Medicine and Rehabilitation* (Louw *et al.* 2011, p.2041) describes pain neuroscience education as "an educational session or sessions describing the neurobiology and neurophysiology of pain, and pain processing by the nervous system." A review article in the *Journal of Pain* (Moseley and Butler 2015, p.808) indicates that explaining pain "refers to a range of educational interventions that aim to change someone's understanding of what pain actually is, what function it serves, and what biological processes are thought to underpin it." A randomized controlled trial in *JAMA Neurology* (Malfliet *et al.* 2018) found that pain neuroscience education combined with cognition-targeted motor control training appears to be effective for pain and physical function in individuals with chronic spinal pain. Finally, an article in *Physical Therapy* (Nijs *et al.* 2020) provides a practical guide for integrating pain neuroscience education and motivational interviewing to help individuals experiencing chronic pain.

The table below highlights key phrases and terms clinicians may want to consider during patient/client interactions.

Phrases for patient/client interactions

Helpful Clinical Phrases	Potentially Harmful Phrases
• "Motion is lotion." • "Hurt does not equal harm." • "I am sore but I'm safe." • "Movement is medicine." • "You're going to be okay." • "Normal age changes." • "Back pain does not mean your back is damaged—it means it is sensitized." • "Pain with movement does not mean you are doing harm." • "Relaxed movement will help your back settle." • "Let's work out a plan to help you help yourself."	• "Don't lift." • "Don't bend." • "Wear and tear." • "Your back is out." • "Your back is unstable." • "You have a bulging disc." • "Deterioration." • "Collapsing." • "This will be here for the rest of your life."

Adapted from Bedell et al. 2004; Brody and Hall et al. 2018; Louw et al. 2019; Louw 2021; Stewart and Loftus et al. 2018.

Motivational Interviewing

According to *Motivational Interviewing: Helping People Change* (Miller and Rollnick 2013), motivational interviewing (MI) is a collaborative, goal-oriented style of communication that pays attention to the language of change. The authors outline the four basic MI skills:

- Ask open-ended questions.
  Sample question: "How can I help you with...?"
- Affirm (or praise) the person's good intentions and efforts.
  Sample comment: "You did a great job in quitting smoking."
- Use reflective listening.
  Sample comment: "It sounds like..."
- Summarize the person's situation.
  Sample comment: "Here is what I heard you say. Tell me if I missed anything."

CLINICAL TIP: SETTING SMART GOALS

Setting a SMART goal for patients/clients can help them to change unhealthy habits. For example:

- **Specific**: "I will stop consuming soft drinks in seven weeks by eliminating soft drinks one day per week for seven weeks."
- **Measurable**: "I will track my progress on my smartphone calendar to ensure I eliminate soft drinks one day per week for seven weeks."
- **Achievable**: "I will achieve this goal since I know from past experiences I feel much better without soft drinks."
- **Realistic**: "My goal is realistic since I am gradually removing soft drinks from my diet and replacing them with water, tea, or a vegetable juice drink."
- **Timely**: "I will achieve this goal by the end of seven weeks and reward myself with new walking shoes."

Therapeutic Alliance

Improving patient care should be more than selecting interventions or enhancing the delivery of specific interventions. To improve clinical care, a practitioner should focus on better communication skills, teaching, and improved interactions during office visits. For example, an observational study in *Physical Therapy* (Alodaibi *et al.* 2021) showed the importance of physical therapists using therapeutic alliance as a part of therapy for patients with low back pain. Other suggested strategies to improve therapeutic alliance during patient-centered counseling may include using terms such as "healthy eating plan" instead of diet and "physical activity" instead of exercise.

The following list outlines strategies that may be used to improve the therapeutic alliance between the practitioner and patient.

Strategies to Improve Therapeutic Alliance

- Get to know the patient.
- Make eye contact while listening.
- Use a soft smile (when appropriate) during interaction.
- Use different tones of voice to emphasize key subject areas.
- Use the person's name during the interaction.
- Take time to explain tests and treatments.
- Use appropriate body and facial expressions.
- Reassure the patient about pain.
- Provide the patient with feedback on each visit.
- Use visual aids such as handouts and diagrams.
- Work together with the patient toward establishing clear and measurable goals.
- Allow the patient to help set the pace of therapy.
- Make the therapy session highly interactive.
- Approach therapy in a friendly and compassionate manner.
- Allow sufficient time for treatment for empathetic interactions.
- Be attentive and sensitive to the patient's needs.
- Show interest in the patient's life situation.
- Provide a welcoming environment.
- Provide patients with individualized advice, exercises, and supervision.
- Put the needs of the patient first.
- Create a flexible appointment system.
- Reduce patient wait times.
- Create a safe, accessible, and pleasant physical environment in the clinic.
- Collaborate on issues such as discharge planning.
- Use an individualized and collaborative decision-making approach.
- Be punctual, reliable, and dedicated.
- Allow patients to have input into treatment plans and decisions.
- Engage in supportive conversations with patients.
- Use proactive follow-ups with patients for motivation.

Adapted from Babatunde et al. 2017; Fagundes et al. 2017; Hanney et al. 2022.

Shared Decision-Making

An article in the *Journal of Rheumatology* (Toupin-April *et al.* 2015, p.3) defines shared decision-making as "a process in which both the patient and health professional make a decision taking into account the best evidence of available treatment options and the patient's values and preferences."

The following checklist may be used to identify parts of shared decision-making domains:

- ✓ Identify the decision that needs to be made.
- ✓ Provide treatment options and explain the pros and cons.
- ✓ Clarify the patient's views and feelings about the pros and cons of each option.
- ✓ Discuss the feasibility and impact of the options.
- ✓ Make the decision or postpone the decision.

Practitioners may consider the following phrases during an office visit to improve shared decision-making:

- "What if we try...?"
- "What if you do...?"
- "Would you consider trying...?"
- "Would you be open to...?"

Interprofessional Collaboration

The World Health Organization (World Health Organization 2010) indicates that collaborative effort by healthcare providers optimizes health services. A qualitative study in *BMC Musculoskeletal Disorders* (Perreault *et al.* 2014) showed that physical therapists viewed interprofessional practices as being positive when working with adults with low back pain.

The following practical points may help improve interprofessional collaboration among practitioners:

- Attend interprofessional meetings and conferences.
- Promote interdisciplinary rounds.
- Create a monthly meeting in your community with healthcare professionals routinely encountered as part of your patient care.
- Utilize video conferencing with healthcare providers.
- Sign up for e-alerts from journals (typically the journal table of contents) from healthcare professionals routinely encountered as part of your patient care.
- Connect with practitioners from varied healthcare backgrounds on social media sites such as LinkedIn.
- Invite professionals from other professions to provide an educational in-service or "lunch and learn" activity at your facility. In return, offer to speak at other facilities.

- Offer to speak at professional schools to discuss your clinical approach and how collaboration benefits patient care.

Model of Behavior Change

Prochaska and his colleagues (Prochaska *et al.* 1997; Prochaska *et al.* 2007) developed the Transtheoretical Model of Change (TTM). This model may help practitioners with their behavior-change counseling and improve therapeutic outcomes.

The five stages of the TTM based on the American College of Sports Medicine's guidelines (2022) are outlined below:

- Stage 1 is precontemplation, and the patient/client has no intention to take action in the next six months.
- Stage 2 is contemplation, and the patient/client intends to start a healthy behavior in the next six months.
- Stage 3 is preparation, and the patient/client is ready to take action in the next 30 days.
- Stage 4 is action, and the patient/client has changed their behavior.
- Stage 5 is maintenance, and the patient/client has sustained their behavior for more than six months.

Optimizing Clinic Design

A quantitative survey in the *Behavioral Science* journal (Rehn and Schuster 2017) found that the design of rehabilitation facilities may lead patients to have higher degrees of commitment, motivation, and satisfaction.

Some simple changes to optimize medical facilities and clinics without major renovations may include, for example:

- allowing natural light to enter the facility by opening curtains and blinds
- choosing soothing colors for the walls (such as earth-tone colors)
- selecting comfortable furniture
- hanging soothing nature-based art on the walls
- placing a fish tank in the waiting area
- playing relaxing music
- selecting magazines for waiting areas that are comforting and relaxing (such as picture books of scenery)
- having the television tuned to a nature channel showing calming scenery
- having a Zen rock garden in the waiting area or near the checkout.

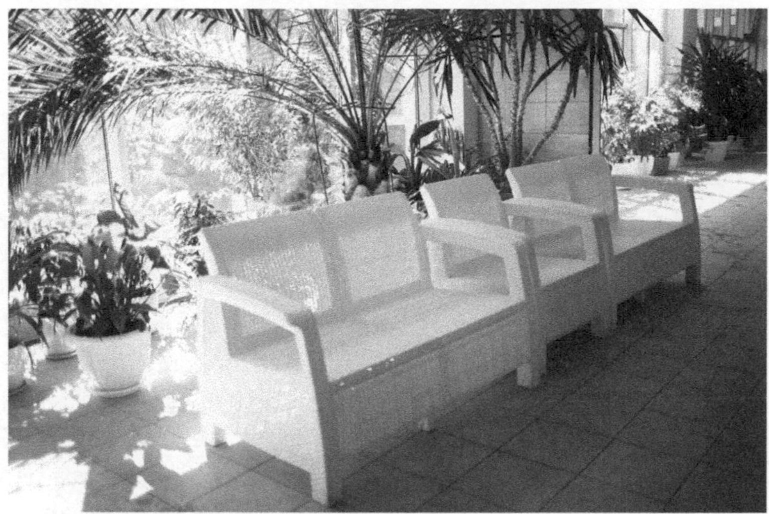

Comforting and relaxing medical waiting area

Strategies to Narrow Treatment Choices

With all the intervention choices in therapy and rehabilitation, sometimes it's challenging to know where to start. Of course, we use facts obtained in our subjective and objective evaluation to determine what type of therapy may be indicated, but sometimes practitioners need additional strategies.

The following questions consider other factors that may be used when deciding which home exercise or self-care strategies may be best for the patient/client.

- What are the person's goals?
- What personal restrictions (e.g., cannot afford a gym or fitness studio membership) or medical restrictions (e.g., cognitive impairment prevents participation in structured classes such as tai chi) does the person have that may prevent participation?
- What activities make the person happy?
- What are the person's past experiences with mind-body medicine?
- Is the person open to trying new ideas?
- Does the person prefer an indoor or outdoor environment? For example, an indoor environment may be needed due to outdoor allergies or sun precaution restrictions.
- Does the person need or prefer socialization?
- Does the person prefer stationary relaxation (e.g., body scan meditation, guided imagery, hypnosis, progressive muscle relaxation) or movement-based mind-body relaxation (e.g., qigong, tai chi, Pilates, yoga)?

■ Featured Topic 2.1: Cognitive Behavioral Therapy

Margarita Chamlaian, MA, BCBA, LMFT

Cognitive behavioral therapy (CBT) is a treatment approach that helps you recognize negative or unhelpful thought and behavior patterns. It combines cognitive and behavioral techniques and is based on the assumption that the individual's way of thinking motivates and affects behavior and emotions. CBT targets maladaptive behaviors and thoughts which identify, challenge, and ultimately change patterns of unhelpful thoughts and behaviors.

Research shows that CBT may be effective for acute and chronic back pain. According to the *Journal of Pain Research* (Sveinsdottir *et al.* 2012), 108 published studies have been evaluated for the effectiveness of CBT for chronic lower back pain. The results demonstrate that CBT is a beneficial treatment for chronic back pain compared to various other approaches. Moreover, multidisciplinary and transdisciplinary interventions that integrate CBT with other approaches with individualized treatment plans are recommended.

Benefits of CBT	Medical Uses of CBT
• Get rid of irrational ideas/thoughts that interfere with the ability to cope that cause pain or excessive emotional reaction. • Challenge automatic thought (rapid self-statements) and track the maladaptive thoughts (identify and be aware of the thought when it occurs) in order to challenge and correct the thoughts and make realistic thoughts about self, others, and the world. These may be pain-related fear or anxiety and anxiety sensitivity (LaRowe *et al.* 2019). • Once you have an awareness of how the thoughts and behaviors interrelate, it makes it easier to change the maladaptive behaviors that correspond to the irrational thoughts.	• Psychoeducation (concept of pain being multifactorial and to correct erroneous pain beliefs, increase knowledge, provide rationale for need to change behavior). • Validation (acknowledge that pain is real). • Lifestyle (look at factors of back pain, diet, inactivity, sleep patterns, and smoking). • Motivation (assess motivation for change and any barriers to lifestyle change). • Goal setting (establish lifestyle goals). • Self-management (use strategies to facilitate self-monitoring behaviors such as keeping diaries for lifestyle and attending follow-up appointments) (Robson *et al.* 2019).

Use of CBT for Smoking Cessation	Methods of Delivering CBT
• Smoking is associated with many painful chronic conditions, such as psoriasis and neuropathic and musculoskeletal pain (including back pain). • Smoking is associated with greater pain intensity. • Smokers with chronic pain showed less motivation to quit since nicotine provides temporary reduction in pain (which creates a cycle of smoking-pain comorbidity). • When smoking and chronic pain co-occur, it is imperative to integrate CBT. Pain-related anxiety makes it difficult to quit smoking as it is maintained by the fear of feeling pain and avoiding pain (LaRowe *et al.* 2019). • When CBT is integrated for pain management and smoking, it can yield clinically meaningful improvement and/or smoking cessation. • CBT strategies that may be utilized: techniques of relaxation, exercise, distraction, pleasant activities, thought restructuring, acknowledging automatic thoughts. • Smoking cessation strategies that may be incorporated: motivation to quit, setting a quit date, preparation to quit activities, nicotine cessation education (Driscoll *et al.* 2018).	• Face-to-face session. • Telehealth (video or telephone).

Created by Margarita Chamlaian, MA, BCBA, LMFT. She is a behavior analyst and marriage and family therapist who practices in Los Angeles, California. Used with permission from Margarita Chamlaian.

Self-Care Education Guide

See **Self-Care Handout 2.1: Healthy Lifestyle Prescription** for a formal healthy lifestyle prescription program that patients/clients can follow.

Self-Care Handout 2.1: Healthy Lifestyle Prescription

Patient/client name: ....

Date: ....

Nutrition Change

- ☐ Drink more water
- ☐ Eat more fruits
- ☐ Eat more veggies
- ☐ Reduce soda
- ☐ Learn to cook
- ☐ ....
- ☐ ....

Physical Activity Change

- ☐ Start walking
- ☐ Train with weights
- ☐ Try dancing
- ☐ Try tai chi, qigong
- ☐ Try yoga
- ☐ ....
- ☐ ....

Socialization Change

- ☐ Join a local center
- ☐ Join a local club
- ☐ Take a class
- ☐ Go to the library
- ☐ Join social media
- ☐ ....
- ☐ ....

Sleep Change

- ☐ Get consistent sleep
- ☐ Create sleep ritual
- ☐ New bed/pillow
- ☐ Less food before bed
- ☐ Less intense night-time television
- ☐ ....
- ☐ ....

Mental Stress Change

- ☐ Create a happy playlist
- ☐ Eat healthily
- ☐ Exercise
- ☐ Find a fun hobby
- ☐ ....
- ☐ ....

Risky Substance Change

- ☐ Stop smoking
- ☐ Reduce alcohol
- ☐ Reduce caffeine
- ☐ Keep a journal
- ☐ Try counseling
- ☐ ....
- ☐ ....

Comments: ....

Signature: ....

Self-Management Activities: Exploring Coloring

The following resources can help patients/clients, healthcare providers, and health/fitness professionals to manage stress and anxiety by exploring coloring.

- Find an adult coloring book that suits the person's interests and needs and ask them to color in the image.

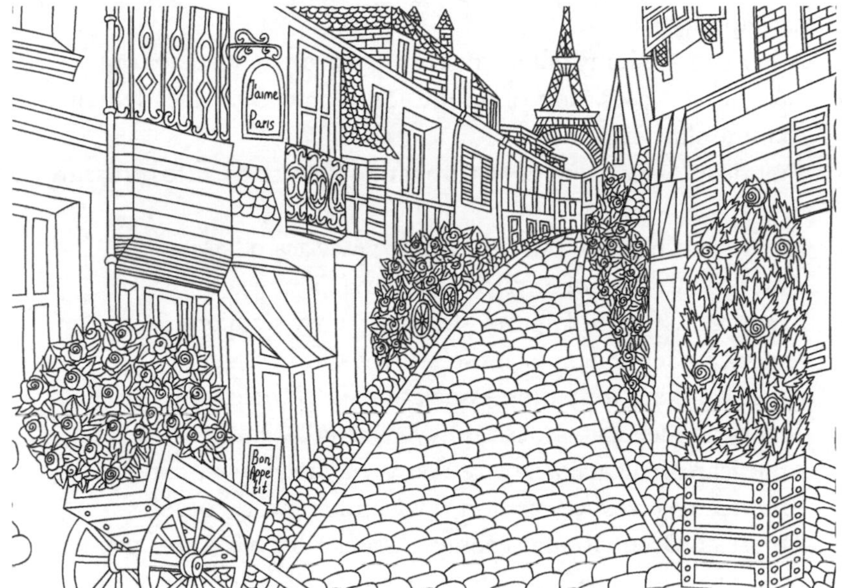

Sample adult coloring page depicting Paris, France

- Coloring apps:
  - The Lake coloring app provides relaxation by using creativity: www.lakecoloring.com
  - The Color Therapy app provides mindfulness art therapy for relaxation: www.colortherapy.app
  - The Pigment app provides various coloring pages for relaxation: www.pixiteapps.com

Classroom and Lab Activities

- What strategies optimize relaxation? Try various relaxation techniques—for example, body scan meditation, progressive muscle relaxation, or guided imagery—in supine, sitting, and standing.
- Does the relaxation position make a difference? Does using a weighted blanket make a difference in the relaxation response?

Useful Clinical Resources
Organizations

- Academy of Nutrition and Dietetics, www.eatright.org
- Academy of Orthopaedic Physical Therapy, www.orthopt.org
- American Academy of Family Physicians, www.aafp.org
- American Academy of Orthopaedic Manual Physical Therapists, https://aaompt.org
- American Academy of Orthopaedic Surgeons, www.aaos.org
- American Association of Acupuncture and Oriental Medicine, www.aaaomonline.org
- American Association of Naturopathic Physicians, https://naturopathic.org
- American Chiropractic Association, www.acatoday.org
- American College of Physicians, www.acponline.org
- American College of Sports Medicine, www.acsm.org
- American Council on Exercise, www.acefitness.org
- American Kinesiotherapy Association, https://akta.org
- American Medical Association, www.ama-assn.org
- American Medical Society for Sports Medicine, www.amssm.org
- American Nurses Association, www.nursingworld.org
- American Occupational Therapy Association, www.aota.org
- American Orthopaedic Society for Sports Medicine, www.sportsmed.org
- American Osteopathic Association, https://osteopathic.org
- American Physical Therapy Association, www.apta.org
- American Psychiatric Association, www.psychiatry.org
- American Psychological Association, http://apa.org
- American Society of Acupuncturists, www.asacu.org
- International Association for the Study of Pain, www.iasp-pain.org
- International Federation of Orthopaedic Manipulative Physical Therapists, www.ifompt.org
- International Society for the Advancement of Spine Surgery, www.isass.org
- Interprofessional Education Collaborative, www.ipecollaborative.org
- Motivational Interviewing Network of Trainers, https://motivationalinterviewing.org
- National Athletic Trainers' Association, www.nata.org
- National Institute for Occupational Safety and Health, www.cdc.gov/niosh/index.htm
- National Strength and Conditioning Association, www.nsca.com
- North American Spine Society, www.spine.org

- Pain Management Collaboratory, https://painmanagementcollaboratory.org
- Physiopedia, www.physio-pedia.com
- Transtheoretical Model and the Stages of Change, www.prochange.com
- Workers Compensation Research Institute, www.wcrinet.org
- World Physiotherapy, https://world.physio

Practitioner Sites

- Communication Regarding Back Pain, https://lowbackpaincommunication.com
- Pain-Ed, www.pain-ed.com

Outcome Measures (For Pain and Back Pain)

- *Back Pain and Body Posture Evaluation Instrument for Adults*
  Candotti CT, Detogni Schmit EF, Pivotto LR, *et al.* Back pain and body posture evaluation instrument for adults: expansion and reproducibility. *Pain Manag Nurs.* 2018;19(4):415–423.
- *Back Pain Functional Scale*
  Stratford PW, Binkley JM, Riddle DL. Development and initial validation of the back pain functional scale. *Spine (Phila Pa 1976).* 2000;25(16):2095–2102.
- *Back Performance Scale*
  Strand LI, Moe-Nilssen R, Ljunggren AE. Back Performance Scale for the assessment of mobility-related activities in people with back pain. *Phys Ther.* 2002;82(12):1213–1223.
- *Beck Anxiety Inventory*
  Beck AT, Epstein N, Brown G, Steer RA. An inventory for measuring clinical anxiety: psychometric properties. *J Consult Clin Psychol.* 1988;56(6):893–897.
- *Central Sensitization Inventory*
  Mayer TG, Neblett R, Cohen H, *et al.* The development and psychometric validation of the central sensitization inventory. *Pain Pract.* 2012;12(4):276–285.
- *Chronic Pain Acceptance Questionnaire*
  McCracken LM, Vowles KE, Eccleston C. Acceptance of chronic pain: component analysis and a revised assessment method. *Pain.* 2004;107(1–2):159–166.
- *Fear Avoidance Beliefs Questionnaire*
  Waddell G, Newton M, Henderson I, Somerville D, Main CJ. A Fear-Avoidance

Beliefs Questionnaire (FABQ) and the role of fear-avoidance beliefs in chronic low back pain and disability. *Pain*. 1993;52(2):157–168.

- *Low Back Pain Rating Scale*
  Manniche C, Asmussen K, Lauritsen B, Vinterberg H, Kreiner S, Jordan A. Low Back Pain Rating scale: validation of a tool for assessment of low back pain. *Pain*. 1994;57(3):317–326.
- *McGill Pain Questionnaire*
  Melzack R. The McGill Pain Questionnaire: major properties and scoring methods. *Pain*. 1975;1(3):277–299.
- *Modified Low Back Disability Questionnaire*
  Fritz JM, Irrgang JJ. A comparison of a modified Oswestry Low Back Pain Disability Questionnaire and the Quebec Back Pain Disability Scale [published correction appears in *Phys Ther*. 2008 Jan;88(1):138–139]. *Phys Ther*. 2001;81(2):776–788.
- *Neuropathic Pain Questionnaire*
  Krause SJ, Backonja MM. Development of a neuropathic pain questionnaire. *Clin J Pain*. 2003;19(5):306–314.
- *Optimal Screening for Prediction of Referral and Outcome*
  George SZ, Beneciuk JM, Bialosky JE, *et al.* Development of a review-of-systems screening tool for orthopaedic physical therapists: results from the Optimal Screening for Prediction of Referral and Outcome (OSPRO) cohort. *J Orthop Sports Phys Ther*. 2015;45(7):512–526.
- *Orebro Musculoskeletal Pain Questionnaire*
  Linton SJ, Halldén K. Can we screen for problematic back pain? A screening questionnaire for predicting outcome in acute and subacute back pain. *Clin J Pain*. 1998;14(3):209–215.
- *Oswestry Disability Index*
  Fairbank JC, Pynsent PB. The Oswestry Disability Index. *Spine (Phila Pa 1976)*. 2000;25(22):2940–2952.
  Fairbank JC, Couper J, Davies JB, O'Brien JP. The Oswestry low back pain disability questionnaire. *Physiotherapy*. 1980;66(8):271–273.
- *Pain Anxiety Symptoms Scale-20*
  McCracken LM, Zayfert C, Gross RT. The Pain Anxiety Symptoms Scale: development and validation of a scale to measure fear of pain. *Pain*. 1992;50(1):67–73.
- *Pain Catastrophizing Scale*
  Sullivan MJL, Bishop SR, Pivik J. The Pain Catastrophizing Scale: development and validation. *Psychol Assess*. 1995;7(4):524–532.
- *Pain Self-Efficacy Questionnaire*
  Nicholas MK. The pain self-efficacy questionnaire: taking pain into account. *Eur J Pain*. 2007;11(2):153–163.

- *Patient Specific Functional Scale*
  Amtmann D, Kim J, Chung H, Askew RL, Park R, Cook KF. Minimally important differences for Patient Reported Outcomes Measurement Information System pain interference for individuals with back pain. *J Pain Res*. 2016;9:251–255.
- *Quebec Back Pain Disability Scale*
  Kopec JA, Esdaile JM, Abrahamowicz M, *et al.* The Quebec Back Pain Disability Scale. Measurement properties. *Spine (Phila Pa 1976)*. 1995;20(3):341–352.
- *Roland-Morris Disability Questionnaire*
  Roland M, Morris R. A study of the natural history of back pain. Part I: development of a reliable and sensitive measure of disability in low-back pain. *Spine (Phila Pa 1976)*. 1983;8(2):141–144.
- *Self-Efficacy for Rehabilitation Outcome Scale*
  Waldrop D, Lightsey OR, Ethington CA, Woemmel CA, Coke AL. Self-efficacy, optimism, health competence, and recovery from orthopedic surgery. *Journal of Counseling Psychology*. 2001;48(2): 233–238.
- *STarT Back Screening Tool*
  Hill JC, Dunn KM, Lewis M, Mullis R, Main CJ, Foster NE. A primary care back pain screening tool: identifying patient subgroups for initial treatment. *Arthritis Rheum*. 2008;59:632–641.
- *State-Trait Anxiety Inventory*
  Spielberger CD, Gorsuch RL, Lushene R, Vagg PR, Jacobs GA. *Manual for the State-Trait Anxiety Inventory*. Palo Alto, CA: Consulting Psychologists Press; 1983.
- *Tampa Scale of Kinesiophobia*
  Miller RP, Kori S, Todd D. The Tampa Scale: a measure of kinesiophobia. *Clin J Pain*. 1991;7(1):51–52.
- *Waddell Disability Index*
  Waddell G, Main CJ. Assessment of severity in low-back disorders. *Spine (Phila Pa 1976)*. 1984;9(2):204–208.

Pain Assessment Scales

- *Color of Pain Description*
  Wylde V, Wells V, Dixon S, Gooberman-Hill R. The colour of pain: can patients use colour to describe osteoarthritis pain? *Musculoskeletal Care*. 2014;12(1):34–46.
- *Coloured Analogue Scale*
  McGrath PA, Seifert CE, Speechley KN, Booth JC, Stitt L, Gibson MC.

A new analogue scale for assessing children's pain: an initial validation study. *Pain.* 1996;64(3):435–443.

- *Numeric Pain Rating Scale*
  Childs JD, Piva SR, Fritz JM. Responsiveness of the numeric pain rating scale in patients with low back pain. *Spine (Phila Pa 1976).* 2005;30(11):1331–1334.
- *Pain Body Diagram*
  Melzack R. The McGill Pain Questionnaire: major properties and scoring methods. *Pain.* 1975;1(3):277–299.
- *Visual Analog Scale*
  Shafshak TS, Elnemr R. The Visual Analogue Scale versus Numerical Rating Scale in measuring pain severity and predicting disability in low back pain. *J Clin Rheumatol.* 2021;27(7):282–285.
- *Wong-Baker FACES Pain Rating Scale*
  Bieri D, Reeve RA, Champion DG, Addicoat L, Ziegler JB. The Faces Pain Scale for the self-assessment of the severity of pain experienced by children: development, initial validation, and preliminary investigation for ratio scale properties. *Pain.* 1990;41(2):139–150.

References

Alodaibi F, Beneciuk J, Holmes R, Kareha S, Hayes D, Fritz J. The relationship of the therapeutic alliance to patient characteristics and functional outcome during an episode of physical therapy care for patients with low back pain: an observational study. *Phys Ther.* 2021;101(4):pzab026.

American College of Sports Medicine. *ACSM's Guidelines for Exercise Testing and Prescription,* 11th ed. Philadelphia, PA: Wolters Kluwer; 2022.

Babatunde F, MacDermid J, MacIntyre N. Characteristics of therapeutic alliance in musculoskeletal physiotherapy and occupational therapy practice: a scoping review of the literature [published correction appears in *BMC Health Serv Res.* 2017 Dec 12;17(1):820]. *BMC Health Serv Res.* 2017;17(1):375.

Bartley EJ, Palit S, Staud R. Predictors of osteoarthritis pain: the importance of resilience. *Curr Rheumatol Rep.* 2017;19(9):57.

Bedell SE, Graboys TB, Bedell E, Lown B. Words that harm, words that heal. *Arch Intern Med.* 2004;164(13):1365–1368.

Brody LT, Hall CM. *Therapeutic Exercise: Moving Toward Function,* 4th ed. Philadelphia, PA: Wolters Kluwer; 2018.

Driscoll MA, Perez E, Edmond SN, *et al.* A brief, integrated, telephone-based intervention for veterans who smoke and have chronic pain: a feasibility study. *Pain Med.* 2018;19(Suppl 1):S84–S92.

Engel GL. The need for a new medical model: a challenge for biomedicine. *Science.* 1977;196(4286):129–136.

Fagundes FR, de Melo do Espírito Santo C, de Luna Teixeira FM, Tonini TV, Cabral CM. Effectiveness of the addition of therapeutic alliance with minimal intervention in the treatment of patients with chronic, nonspecific low back pain and low risk of involvement of psychosocial factors: a study protocol for a randomized controlled trial (TalkBack trial). *Trials.* 2017;18(1):49.

Fetters L, Tilson JK. *Evidence Based Physical Therapy,* 2nd ed. Philadelphia, PA: FA Davis; 2019.

Hanney, WJ, Kolber, MJ, Salamh, PA, Bucci, MJ, Cundiff, MB, Haynes, DP. Development of an effective client-practitioner therapeutic alliance in the management of low back pain. *Strength and Conditioning Journal.* 2022;44(6):9–17.

LaRowe LR, Zvolensky MJ, Ditre JW. The role of anxiety-relevant transdiagnostic factors in comorbid chronic pain and tobacco cigarette smoking. *Cognitive Therapy and Research.* 2019;43(1):102–113.

Loeser JD. Concepts of pain. In: Stanton Hicks M, Boaz R, ed. *Chronic Low Back Pain.* New York, NY: Raven Press; 1982.

Louw A. APTA Centennial Lecture Series: Pain Science and Management. American Physical Therapy Association Learning Center. April 9–10, 2021.

Louw A, Diener I, Butler DS, Puentedura EJ. The effect of neuroscience education on pain, disability, anxiety, and stress in chronic musculoskeletal pain. *Arch Phys Med Rehabil.* 2011;92(12):2041–2056.

Louw A, Puentedura E, Schmidt S, Zimney K. *Integrating Manual Therapy and Pain Neuroscience.* Minneapolis, MN: OPTP; 2019:111–124.

Malfliet A, Kregel J, Coppieters I, *et al.* Effect of pain neuroscience education combined with cognition-targeted motor control training on chronic spinal pain: a randomized clinical trial [published correction appears in *JAMA Neurol.* 2019 Mar 1;76(3):373]. *JAMA Neurol.* 2018;75(7):808–817.

Miller WR, Rollnick S. *Motivational Interviewing: Helping People Change*, 3rd ed. New York, NY: Guilford Press; 2013.

Moseley GL, Butler DS. Fifteen years of explaining pain: the past, present, and future. *J Pain.* 2015;16(9):807–813.

Nijs J, Wijma AJ, Willaert W, *et al.* Integrating motivational interviewing in pain neuroscience education for people with chronic pain: a practical guide for clinicians. *Phys Ther.* 2020;100(5):846–859.

Perreault K, Dionne CE, Rossignol M, Morin D. Interprofessional practices of physiotherapists working with adults with low back pain in Québec's private sector: results of a qualitative study. *BMC Musculoskelet Disord.* 2014;15:160.

Prochaska JO, Norcross JC, DiClemente CC. *Changing for Good.* New York, NY: William Morrow Paperbacks; 2007.

Prochaska JO, Velicer WF. The transtheoretical model of health behavior change. *Am J Health Promot.* 1997;12(1):38–48.

Rehn J, Schuster K. Clinic design as placebo-using design to promote healing and support treatments. *Behav Sci (Basel).* 2017;7(4):77.

Robson EK, Kamper SJ, Davidson S, *et al.* Healthy Lifestyle Program (HeLP) for low back pain: protocol for a randomised controlled trial. *BMJ Open.* 2019;9(9):e029290.

Sluka KA. *Mechanisms and Management of Pain for the Physical Therapist*, 2nd ed. Philadelphia, PA: Wolters Kluwer; 2016.

Stewart M, Loftus S. Sticks and stones: the impact of language in musculoskeletal rehabilitation. *J Orthop Sports Phys Ther.* 2018;48(7):519–522.

Sveinsdottir V, Eriksen HR, Reme SE. Assessing the role of cognitive behavioral therapy in the management of chronic nonspecific back pain. *J Pain Res.* 2012;5:371–380.

Tanaka MJ, Oh LS, Martin SD, Berkson EM. Telemedicine in the era of COVID-19: the virtual orthopaedic examination. *J Bone Joint Surg Am.* 2020;102(12):e57.

Toupin-April K, Barton J, Fraenkel L, *et al.* Development of a draft core set of domains for measuring shared decision making in osteoarthritis: an OMERACT working group on shared decision making. *J Rheumatol.* 2015;42(12):2442–2447.

World Health Organization. *Framework for Action on Interprofessional Education & Collaborative Practice.* Geneva, Switzerland: WHO Press; 2010. https://apps.who.int/iris/handle/10665/70185

Yedlinsky NT, Peebles RL. Telemedicine management of musculoskeletal issues. *Am Fam Physician.* 2021;103(3):147–154.

Additional Reading

Brignardello-Petersen R, Carrasco-Labra A, Guyatt GH. How to interpret and use a clinical practice guideline or recommendation: users' guides to the medical literature. *JAMA.* 2021;326(15):1516–1523.

Cleland JA, Koppenhaver S, Su J. *Netter's Orthopaedic Clinical Examination: An Evidence-Based Approach,* 4th ed. Philadelphia, PA: Elsevier; 2022.

Fritz JM, Lane E, McFadden M, *et al.* Physical therapy referral from primary care for acute back pain with sciatica: a randomized controlled trial. *Ann Intern Med.* 2021;174(1):8–17.

Shepherd M, Courtney C, Wassinger C, Davis DS, Rubine B. *Pain Education Manual: For Physical Therapist Professional Degree Programs.* La Crosse, WI: Academy of Orthopaedic Physical Therapy; 2021. www.orthopt.org/uploads/content_files/files/Pain_Manual_Draft_FINAL_6.25.2021%281%29.pdf

CHAPTER 3

Basics of Culinary Medicine

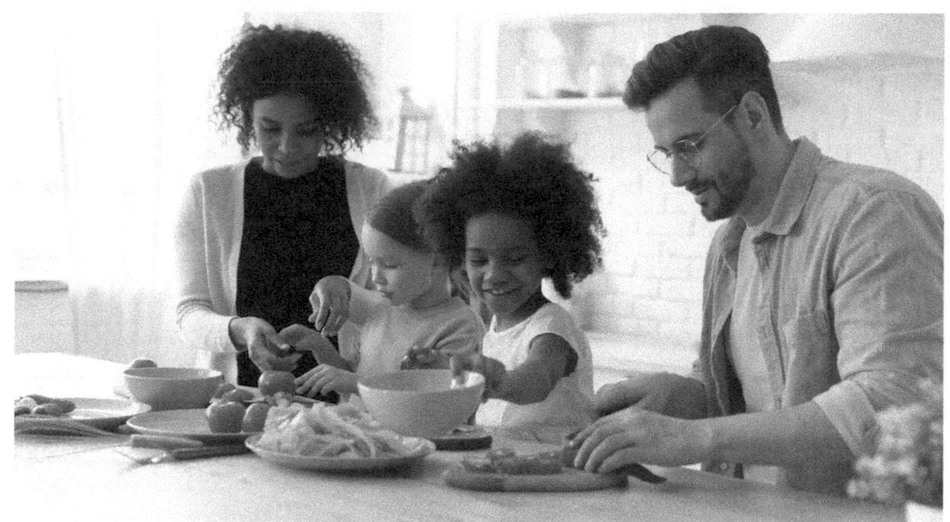

Meal preparation is a key to health

Learning Objectives

- Understand the basics of culinary medicine and anti-inflammatory eating patterns.
- Apply basic nutritional concepts for improving well-being.

Chapter Highlights

- Key Concept: Food for Health and Happiness
- Clinical Tip: The Power of Berries
- Featured Topic 3.1: Healthy Snacks for Peak Performance
- Featured Topic 3.2: National Weight Control Registry
- Sample Recipes
- Self-Care Handout 3.1: Grocery Shopping Guide

- Self-Care Handout 3.2: Components of the Mediterranean Diet
- Self-Management Activities
- Classroom and Lab Activities
- Useful Clinical Resources
- References
- Additional Reading

Lifestyle Matters: *No supplement is going to fix a broken lifestyle or diet.*

Introduction

Greek physician Hippocrates made a great observation when he said, "Let food be thy medicine and medicine be thy food." Food is medicine, and practitioners can fight disease with forks, spoons, and knives. Ideally, prevention is better than intervention.

Nutrition is the utilization of food for growth, repair, and maintenance of activities in the body. Foods include carbohydrates, protein, fats, vitamins, and minerals. Water is also an essential nutrient for health (Venes 2021).

An individual's diet may affect a variety of medical conditions such as anxiety (Richard *et al.* 2022), back pain (Torlak *et al.* 2022), cancer (Castro-Espin and Agudo 2022), cognitive function (Valls-Pedret *et al.* 2015), dementia (Charisis *et al.* 2021), depression (Francis *et al.* 2019), diabetes (Lean *et al.* 2018), fibromyalgia (Silva *et al.* 2022), heart disease (Yubero-Serrano *et al.* 2020), hypertension (Filippou *et al.* 2020), kidney disease (Podadera-Herreros *et al.* 2022), rheumatoid arthritis (Guagnano *et al.* 2021), and sleep apnea (Georgoulis *et al.* 2021). A meta-epidemiological study from the American College of Lifestyle Medicine published in the March 2023 issue of *Advances in Nutrition* (Cara *et al.* 2023) recommends individuals consume a minimally processed plant-predominant diet with limited consumption of alcohol and salt or sodium for preventing and managing or treating major chronic diseases.

KEY CONCEPT: FOOD FOR HEALTH AND HAPPINESS

Eating a healthful diet is one aspect of your health insurance. Also, farmers are an essential part of the healthcare team. For this reason, support farmers and consider going to local farmers' markets for fresh farm-to-table foods.

General

- Choose foods wisely. Select a variety of colorful and predominantly plant-based foods that fit your food preferences and lifestyle.

- Diversify your foods. Humans need to consume a diverse range of foods for optimal health. One way to achieve diversity in the diet is to consume seasonal foods.
- Make small changes. Try to make small changes by adding healthier foods. For example, add more vegetables and/or fruits to each meal.
- Eat mindfully. Take time to eat leisurely to better appreciate the food's shape, texture, smell, and taste.

Home

- Learn how to cook by taking a local or virtual class to prepare nutritious foods. Also see the 'Sample Recipes' section later in this chapter.

Work

- Bring healthful snacks for breaks and lunch. For example, bring fruits, vegetables, nuts, seeds, home-made muffins, a baked potato, and/or smoothie.
- Sit in a quiet, pleasant spot (preferably outdoors or near a window) to enjoy your meal.

Restaurant

- Check online menus before choosing a location to ensure that there are plant-predominant meals, low-salt options, and meals for food sensitivities such as gluten.
- If in doubt, try to choose vegetable-based foods and fresh vegetable dishes.

What is Culinary Medicine?

According to an article in *Critical Care Nursing Clinics in North America* (LeBlanc-Morales 2019, p.109), "Culinary medicine uses what is known about the pharmacologic properties of food to treat, manage, and prevent disease." Furthermore, an article in the *American Journal of Lifestyle Medicine* (La Puma 2020, p.143) defines culinary medicine as "a new evidence-based field in medicine that blends the art of food and cooking with the science of medicine."

Culinary medicine is becoming a part of mainstream medical training and education to provide patient-centered care (D'Adamo *et al.* 2021; Newman *et al.* 2022; Tan *et al.* 2022). For example, a culinary medicine course may benefit medical students by increasing confidence in counseling patients about diseases associated with the diet (Rothman *et al.* 2020) and family medicine residents to recognize the importance of nutrition in clinical care (Johnston *et al.* 2021). In addition, the *Culinary Medicine Curriculum* (Hauser 2019) was published in collaboration with the American College of Lifestyle Medicine as an open-source guide to implementing culinary medicine in training programs (Hauser *et al.* 2020). Also, cooking classes are being offered for children of low-income families (Marshall and Albin 2021), low-income patients with Type 2 diabetes (Sharma *et al.* 2021), and individuals in the community to improve Mediterranean diet adherence (Razavi *et al.* 2021).

Inflammation and the Diet

According to *Taber's Cyclopedic Medical Dictionary* (Venes 2021):

- Inflammation is "an immunological defense against injury, infection, or allergy, marked by increases in regional blood flow, immigration of white blood cells, and release of chemical toxins" (p.1271). Clinical hallmarks of inflammation include pain, swelling, heat, redness, and loss of function of a body part. Systemic inflammation may produce fever, muscle and joint pain, organ dysfunction, weakness, and fatigue.
- Metainflammation is "low-grade, chronic inflammation usually associated with obesity" (p.1536).

Chronic low-grade inflammation may be influenced by diet. The following table shows nutritional factors that may contribute to inflammation.

Nutritional factors and inflammation

Pro-Inflammatory Factors—Increased Risk	Anti-Inflammatory Factors—Decreased Risk
• Westernized diets (such as unhealthy fats, refined grains, sugars, and salt) • Ultra-processed foods • Increased animal protein • Increased red meat • Increased fat • Increased saturated fatty acids • Increased trans fatty acids • Increased glycemic index • Decreased fiber	• Healthy diets (such as the Mediterranean diet and Dietary Approaches to Stop Hypertension [DASH] diet) • Healthful foods (such as vegetables and fruits, legumes, whole grains, fish, olive oil, and green tea) • Vitamins (such as A, D, E, K, B-complex) • Minerals (such as zinc, selenium, magnesium) • Polyphenols (such as resveratrol, quercetin) • Spices (such as cinnamon, garlic, ginger, and turmeric) • Probiotics and prebiotics

Adapted from Ramos-Lopez et al. 2022.

Nutritionist Deepa Deshmukh, MPH, RDN, CDE, BC-ADM indicates that plants provide the following essential nutrients for the whole body (Deshmukh 2023):

- Fruits and vegetables provide antioxidants, polyphenols, and help reduce inflammation.
- Dark greens and beans provide calcium and iron for strong bones, teeth, and vitality.
- Whole grains provide slow-acting carbs for sustained energy.
- Dry beans, lentils, and peas provide plant protein to build muscle and to repair the wear and tear of tissues and cells.
- Herbs and spices have anti-inflammatory, anti-fungal, and anti-bacterial properties.
- Whole plant-based foods are a rich source of prebiotics and feeds the probiotics, helping to maintain good gut health.

Studies show that low-grade inflammation may be reduced by adhering to a Mediterranean diet (Bonaccio *et al.* 2022), and diet can also influence chronic pain (Rondanelli *et al.* 2018). The *Journal of Nutrition* (Cavicchia *et al.* 2009) outlines a Dietary Inflammatory Index (DII) to assess the inflammatory potential of a diet that may influence inflammation-related chronic conditions (Charisis *et al.* 2021; Ruiz-Canela *et al.* 2016; Shivappa *et al.* 2018; Yi *et al.* 2021) such as cardiovascular disease, cancer, dementia, metabolic syndrome, obesity, and Type 2 diabetes.

A retrospective study in the *American Journal of Lifestyle Medicine* (Perzia et al. 2020) found that a Low Inflammatory Foods Everyday (LIFE) diet or smoothie may reduce systemic inflammation. The smoothie in the study consisted of:

- dark green leafy vegetables (e.g., spinach, baby bok choy, or baby kale)
- blueberries
- banana
- unsweetened cocoa powder
- ground flaxseed
- soy milk (plain or vanilla) or unsweetened vanilla almond milk
- water.

There are many diet approaches on the market. However, the key for healthcare and health/fitness professionals is to follow research-based dietary strategies that benefit patients/clients. The Mediterranean diet, for example, has been shown to help cancer (Morze *et al.* 2021), cognitive function (Valls-Pedret *et al.* 2015), coronary heart disease (Jimenez-Torres *et al.* 2021), depression (Parletta *et al.* 2019), diabetes (Esposito *et al.* 2015), and fibromyalgia (Martínez-Rodríguez *et al.* 2020). The Dietary Approaches to Stop Hypertension (DASH) diet has been shown to be beneficial for reducing blood pressure (Filippou *et al.* 2020). Finally, the Mediterranean-DASH Intervention for Neurodegenerative Delay (MIND) diet (which is a hybrid of the Mediterranean and DASH diets) shows benefits for individuals after stroke (Cherian *et al.* 2019), a lower risk of Alzheimer's disease, and less cognitive decline (van den Brink *et al.* 2019).

CLINICAL TIP: THE POWER OF BERRIES

Berries may be small, but they pack a lot of nutritional power. Patients/clients should be encouraged to include more berries, such as blueberries, strawberries, and raspberries, in their diet. For example, berries can be a part of morning oatmeal or cereal, afternoon salads, and/or evening desserts (Agarwal *et al.* 2019; Travica *et al.* 2020).

Nutrition Self-Management Strategies

The following list contains simple self-management steps to help patients/clients improve their health through nutritional strategies:

1. Recommend focusing on a whole food plant-predominant or plant-based approach. The American College of Lifestyle Medicine dietary position statement states (Clayton and Bonnet 2023, p.141): "For the treatment, reversal, and prevention of lifestyle-related chronic disease, the ACLM recommends eating a plant-predominant diet based on a variety of minimally processed vegetables, fruits, whole grains, legumes, nuts, and seeds."
2. Recommend consulting with a registered dietitian (RD) or registered dietitian nutritionist (RDN) to address medical concerns.
   - Physician Committee for Responsible Medicine, www.pcrm.org
   - Plantrician Providers, https://plantrician.org/places
3. Consider the following resources:
   - American College of Lifestyle Medicine, www.lifestylemedpros.org/home
   - Dr. MacDougall, www.drmcdougall.com/recipes
   - Forks Over Knives, www.forksoverknives.com
   - Nutritionist Deepa (for culturally focused nutrition consult), www.nutritionistdeepa.com
4. Encourage taking a cooking class. Consider the following resources:
   - American College of Lifestyle Medicine, Food as Medicine program, https://lifestylemedicine.org
   - Culinary Medicine, https://culinarymedicine.org
   - Teaching Kitchen Collaborative, https://teachingkitchens.org

It is recommended reviewing the following major nutrition studies (partial list provided) to gain a better understanding of the impact nutrition has on chronic diseases and to determine which dietary pattern may be best suited for your patient/client (Clayton and Bonnet 2023):

- *BROAD Study* (Wright *et al.* 2017)
  Aim of the study: Assess the effectiveness of a whole food plant-based diet on body mass index (BMI) and cholesterol.
- *Dietary Approaches to Stop Hypertension Trial (DASH)* (Moore *et al.* 1999)
  Aim of the study: Assess the effect of diet on ambulatory blood pressure.
- *Dietary Portfolio of Cholesterol-Lowering Foods* (Jenkins *et al.* 2006)
  Aim of the study: To assess the effectiveness of consuming a combination of cholesterol-lowering foods (dietary portfolio).
- *European Prospective Investigation into Cancer and Nutrition Oxford Study* (European Prospective Investigation into Cancer and Nutrition Oxford Study 2023)
  Aim of the study: Examine the influence of diet on the risk of cancer and other chronic diseases in the United Kingdom and, later, in ten European countries.
- *Framingham Heart Study* (Framingham Heart Study 2023)
  Aim of the study: Identify factors contributing to cardiovascular disease.
- *Health Professionals Follow-up Study* (Health Professionals Follow-up Study 2023)
  Aim of the study: Evaluate men's health regarding nutritional and lifestyle factors.
- *Lifestyle Heart Trial* (Ornish *et al.* 1990)
  Aim of the study: Assess if lifestyle changes affect coronary atherosclerosis after one year.
- *Lyon Heart Study* (de Lorgeril *et al.* 1999)
  Aim of the study: Assess if a Mediterranean-type diet may reduce the risk of recurrent myocardial infarction.
- *MIND Diet* (Morris *et al.* 2015)
  Aim of the study: Assess the effect of diet on Alzheimer's disease.
- *Multi-Ethnic Study of Atherosclerosis* (Blaha and DeFilippis 2021)
  Aim of the study: Prevalence, progression, and determinants of cardiovascular disease.
- *National Health and Nutrition Examination Survey* (National Health and Nutrition Examination Survey 2023)
  Aim of the survey: To monitor the health and nutritional status of adults and children in the United States.

- *Nurses' Health Study* (Nurses' Health Study 2023)
  Aim of the studies: Impact of various lifestyle factors. Initially, women were enrolled, but later, it included men.
- *OmniHeart Trial* (Appel *et al.* 2005)
  Aim of the study: Assess the effects of three diets on blood pressure and serum lipids.
- *Seventh-Day Adventist Health Study* (Seventh-Day Adventist Health Study 2023)
  Aim of the study: Explore links between lifestyle, diet, and disease.
- *The PREDIMED trial (Prevención con Dieta Mediterránea)* (Estruch *et al.* 2018)
  Aim of the study: Assess the effectiveness of two Mediterranean diets (one supplemented with extra-virgin olive oil and another with nuts and a control group diet with advice on a low-fat diet) on the primary prevention of cardiovascular disease.
- *Women's Health Initiative* (Women's Health Initiative 2023)
  Aim of the study: Long-term study to prevent heart disease, breast and colorectal cancer, and osteoporosis in postmenopausal women.

Featured Topics

Featured Topic 3.1 outlines healthy snacks for peak mental and physical performance at work, school, and athletics.

Featured Topic 3.2 outlines strategies used by National Weight Control Registry members to help keep weight off after a weight loss program.

■ Featured Topic 3.1: Healthy Snacks for Peak Performance

The following are easy-to-eat healthy snacks to consider for work, school, or athletics for peak mental and physical performance:

- A small bag of nuts and seeds.
- A small bag of dried fruits.
- An avocado.
- Gluten-free crackers and bread.
- Celery sticks, carrot sticks, jicama, or snap peas.
- Easy-to-eat fruits such as bananas, kiwis, and oranges.

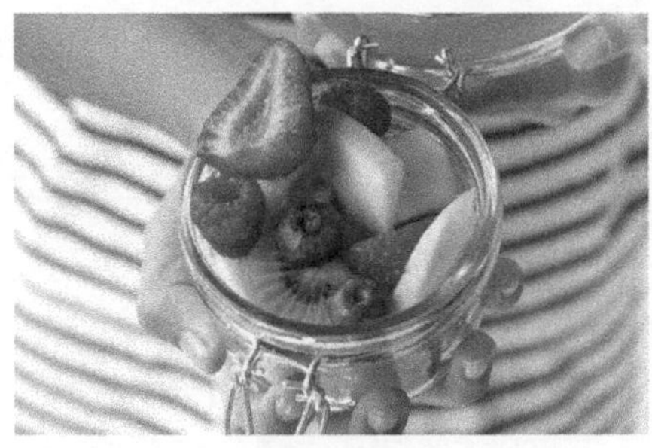

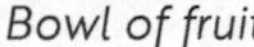
Bowl of fruit

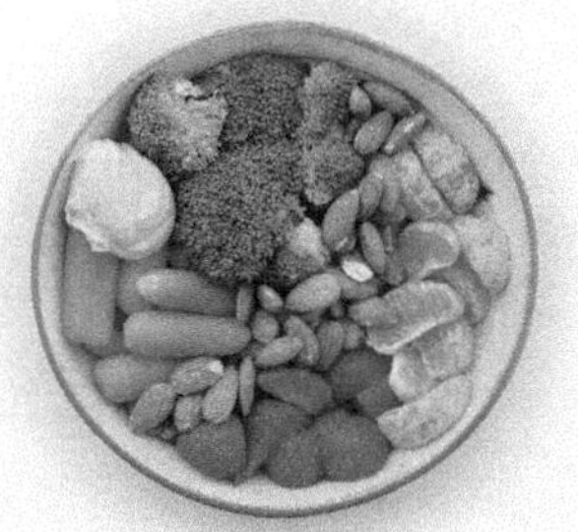
Veggie, fruit, and nut bowl

■ Featured Topic 3.2: National Weight Control Registry

The National Weight Control Registry members say they use the following strategies to keep the weight off:

- 78 percent eat breakfast every day.
- 75 percent weigh themselves at least once a week.
- 62 percent watch less than ten hours of TV per week.
- 90 percent exercise, on average, about one hour per day.

Source: National Weight Control Registry, www.nwcr.ws

Sample Recipes

The following are sample nutritious recipes to consider. Learn more about healthy recipes and culinary medicine from the Academy of Nutrition and Dietetics and the American College of Lifestyle Medicine websites.

Breakfast—Feel Good Chia Pudding

A perfect snack, breakfast, and dessert option.
Serves: 2

Ingredients

- ¼ cup chia seeds
- ⅛ teaspoon ground cardamom (optional)
- ⅛ teaspoon ground nutmeg (optional)
- ⅛ teaspoon cinnamon (to sprinkle on top)
- 2 pitted and diced medjool dates (optional)

- 1 teaspoon pure vanilla extract
- 1 cup unsweetened vanilla plant milk
- ¼ cup papaya (or fresh or frozen fruit)
- 2 tablespoons pumpkin seeds (pepitas) (optional)

Directions

1. Whisk all the ingredients together, except for the fruit and seeds. Let it stand for 15–20 minutes. Top with fresh or frozen fruit and nuts or seeds on top.
2. If you feel that the pudding is too thick, add a little bit of liquid such as water or plant milk. If the pudding feels too thin, then whisk in little bit of chia.

Used with permission from Deepa Deshmukh, MPH, RDN, CDE, BC-ADM (https://dupagedietitians.com and https://nutritionistdeepa.com).

Breakfast—Healthy Overnight Carrot Cake Oats

Quick, easy, and filling breakfast to provide sustained energy throughout the busy morning.
Serves: 4

Ingredients

- 2 cups dry rolled oats
- 4 small carrots (finely grated)
- 1 teaspoon cinnamon (or pie spice)
- 2 teaspoons shredded unsweetened coconut
- 1 tablespoon seedless raisins (or sultanas)
- 1 tablespoon chopped walnuts (optional)
- 2 cups unsweetened vanilla plant milk
- 2 cups hot water
- ½ teaspoon honey or maple syrup (optional)

Directions

1. The night before, divide the ingredients into four wide-mouth jars in a layer. Pour the liquid into each one. Secure the lid. Refrigerate for at least 6 hours (or up to overnight).
2. In the morning, add more liquid if desired. Eat as is or warm in the fall and winter.
3. Drizzle with honey or maple syrup... just a dash for extra flavor.

Used with permission from Deepa Deshmukh, MPH, RDN, CDE, BC-ADM (https://dupagedietitians.com and https://nutritionistdeepa.com).

Lunch or Dinner—Weeknight Veggie Soup

This healthy soup uses protein-rich pasta for a filling, nutrient-dense alternative. A perfect go-to recipe when you have no time to cook!
Serves: 4

Ingredients

- 1 medium yellow onion (chopped)
- 2 cloves garlic (minced)
- 8 ounces red lentil penne pasta (or whole lentils or 4 cups diced potatoes)
- 3 medium carrots (chopped)
- 3 medium celery stalks (chopped)
- 1½ cups frozen vegetable mix (such as corn or zucchini) (chopped)
- 4 cups baby spinach
- 2 cups vegetable stock/broth (no sodium, organic)
- 2 cups hot water
- 1 cup water saved after cooking the pasta
- 1 teaspoon fresh thyme (or herb of choice)
- 1 dash black pepper (freshly ground)
- ½ teaspoon red pepper flakes (optional)
- ½ cup cherry tomatoes (cut into halves)

Directions

1. Cook the pasta per package directions, but avoid overcooking and save some pasta water.
2. Heat a pot over medium heat and gently sauté the onion and garlic until the onion starts to soften.
3. Add in the carrots and celery and continue to cook until carrots start to caramelize. Stir in frozen vegetables. Cook at medium high heat for 3–4 minutes.
4. Add the vegetable broth. Let the soup simmer until the vegetables are tender (about 10 minutes).
5. While the soup is simmering, and when the soup vegetables are tender, stir in the pasta and saved pasta water. Add the herbs, red pepper flakes, and the tomatoes.
6. Add hot water as needed to achieve the desired consistency. Simmer for a couple of minutes. Turn the heat off. Add spinach.
7. Season to taste and serve warm. Leftover soup can be stored in a freezer.

Used with permission from Deepa Deshmukh, MPH, RDN, CDE, BC-ADM (https://dupagedietitians.com and https://nutritionistdeepa.com).

Side Dish—Baked Acorn Squash

Serves: 2

Ingredients

- 1 acorn squash, halved
- 4 teaspoons brown sugar
- 1 teaspoon ground nutmeg
- ⅛ teaspoon ground cinnamon

Directions

1. Preheat the oven to 350 degrees F.
2. Fill a small baking dish with ½ inch water. Scoop out any seeds and place the acorn squash cut side down in the water and bake for 20 minutes.

3. In a small bowl, combine the brown sugar, nutmeg, and cinnamon.
4. Turn the squash over and sprinkle half of the seasoning over each half and continue to bake, cut side up, for another 20 minutes.

From Altug Z and Gensler TO. The Anti-Aging Fitness Prescription. New York, NY: Hatherleigh Press; 2006. Used with permission from Tracy Gensler, MS, RD, registered dietitian.

Self-Care Education Guides

See **Self-Care Handout 3.1: Grocery Shopping Guide** for a simple shopping checklist that may be printed or stored as an electronic document to be used from a phone.

See **Self-Care Handout 3.2: Components of the Mediterranean Diet** to help patients/clients understand the Mediterranean diet and lifestyle approach (Estruch *et al.* 2018; Widmer *et al.* 2015; Willett *et al.* 1995; Yannakoulia *et al.* 2015).

Self-Care Handout 3.1: Grocery Shopping Guide

Select a variety of healthful foods every week for nutritional diversity.

Vegetables (all colors, fresh or frozen)

✓ ....
✓ ....
✓ ....
✓ ....
✓ ....
✓ ....

Beans/Legumes

✓ ....
✓ ....
✓ ....
✓ ....
✓ ....
✓ ....

Nuts/Seeds (limited)

✓ ....
✓ ....
✓ ....
✓ ....

Dairy/Eggs (limited, if any)

✓ ....
✓ ....

Spices , Herbs, Vinegars

✓ ....
✓ ....

Fruits

✓ ....
✓ ....
✓ ....
✓ ....
✓ ....
✓ ....

Grains

✓ ....
✓ ....
✓ ....
✓ ....
✓ ....
✓ ....

Fish/Seafood (limited, if any)

✓ ....
✓ ....
✓ ....
✓ ....

Meats (limited, if any)

✓ ....
✓ ....

Beverages (water, tea, juices)

✓ ....
✓ ....
✓ ....

Self-Care Handout 3.2: Components of the Mediterranean Diet

The Mediterranean diet (MD) is one of the best-studied and researched diets to help prevent and treat a variety of medical conditions. The basic components of the MD include:

- vegetables and fruits
- whole grains
- nuts and legumes
- fish
- olives, olive oil
- limited dairy products (such as yogurt), eggs, and poultry
- low amounts of red meat
- wine in low to moderate amounts.

The Mediterranean lifestyle also includes a way of living consisting of:

- social interaction
- leisure activities
- physical activities
- sleep quality.

Self-Management Activities: Explore Culinary Medicine

The following resources can help patients/clients, healthcare providers, and health/fitness professionals to manage stress and anxiety by exploring nutrition.

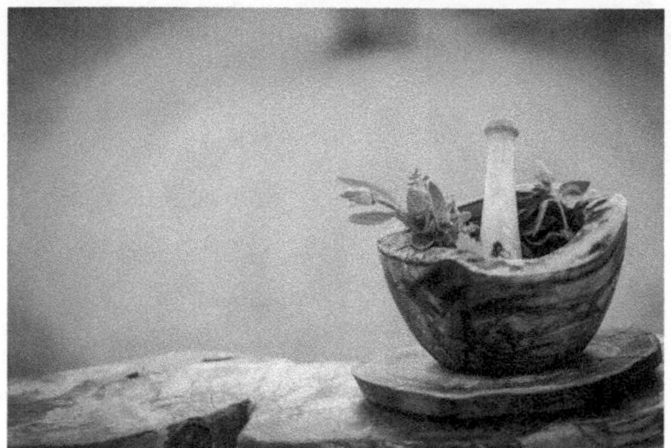

Cooking for health

- Explore nutrition websites and apps:
  - The Academy of Nutrition and Dietetics apps provide nutrition resources: https://apps.apple.com/ml/developer/academy-of-nutrition-and-dietetics/id512279051
  - The Nutrition Source website from the Harvard School of Public Health provides nutrition resources: www.hsph.harvard.edu/nutritionsource
  - The MyFitnessPal app provides a tool to track meals and exercise for weight loss and overall health: www.myfitnesspal.com
- Write out two sample healthy breakfast options:
  - Option 1: ....
  - Option 2: ....
- Write out two sample healthy lunch options:
  - Option 1: ....
  - Option 2: ....
- Write out two sample healthy dinner options:
  - Option 1: ....
  - Option 2: ....

Classroom and Lab Activities

- Become a food detective: Find the best food sources for calcium.
- Become a food researcher: What are alternative foods for a gluten-free diet?

- Become a food analyst: Find and analyze the ingredients in any soft drink. What is the harm caused by each ingredient?

Useful Clinical Resources

Organizations

- Academy of Nutrition and Dietetics, www.eatright.org
- American College of Lifestyle Medicine, Culinary Medicine Curriculum, www.lifestylemedicine.org/culinary-medicine
- American Society for Nutrition, https://nutrition.org
- Blue Zones®, www.bluezones.com (the term Blue Zone® was coined by Dan Buettner, and the original locations include: Okinawa, Japan; Ikaria, Greece; Sardinia, Italy; Nicoya, Costa Rica; Loma Linda, California)
- Cardiovascular Health and Well-Being Dietetic Practice Group, www.cvwell.org
- Consumer Lab, www.consumerlab.com
- Dietary Guidelines for Americans, www.dietaryguidelines.gov
- Dietary Guidelines for Americans—Professional Resources and Handouts, www.dietaryguidelines.gov/professional-resources
- Environmental Working Group, www.ewg.org
- FoodData Central, https://fdc.nal.usda.gov
- Forks Over Knives, www.forksoverknives.com
- Health Meets Food, https://culinarymedicine.org
- Healthy Aging Dietetic Practice Group, www.hadpg.org
- Healthy Grocery Girl, www.healthygrocerygirl.com
- Healthy Kitchens, Healthy Lives, www.healthykitchens.org
- Institute of Culinary Education, www.ice.edu
- Institute of Lifestyle Medicine, www.instituteoflifestylemedicine.org
- International Scientific Association for Probiotics and Prebiotics, https://isappscience.org
- Mediterranean Diet Roundtable (MDR), https://mdrproject.com
- National Institutes of Health (NIH)—New Clinical Digest: Nutritional Approaches for Musculoskeletal Pain and Inflammation, https://content.govdelivery.com/accounts/USNIHNCCIH/bulletins/30ca951
- Nutrition Agricultural Library, www.nal.usda.gov
- Office of Dietary Supplements, https://ods.od.nih.gov
- Physicians Committee for Responsible Medicine, www.pcrm.org/good-nutrition
- Plantrician Providers, https://plantrician.org
- Teaching Kitchen Collaborative, https://teachingkitchens.org

- UnchainedTV, https://unchainedtv.com
- Vegetarian Nutrition Dietetic Practice Group, www.vndpg.org
- World Gastroenterology Organisation, www.worldgastroenterology.org

Outcome Measures

- *Start the Conversation*
  Paxton AE, Strycker LA, Toobert DJ, Ammerman AS, Glasgow RE. Starting the conversation performance of a brief dietary assessment and intervention tool for health professionals. *Am J Prev Med.* 2011;40(1):67–71.
- *Rate Your Plate*
  Gans KM, Sundaram SG, McPhillips JB, Hixson ML, Linnan L, Carleton RA. Rate your plate: an eating pattern assessment and educational tool used at cholesterol screening and education programs. *J Nutr Educ.* 1993;25:29–36.
- *Nutritional Risk Screening*
  Reber E, Gomes F, Vasiloglou MF, Schuetz P, Stanga Z. Nutritional risk screening and assessment. *J Clin Med.* 2019;8(7):1065.
- *Mini Nutrition Assessment-Short Form (MNA-SF)*
  Rubenstein LZ, Harker JO, Salva A, Guigoz Y, Vellas B. Screening for undernutrition in geriatric practice: developing the short-form mini-nutritional assessment (MNA-SF). *J Gerontol A Biol Sci Med Sci.* 2001;56:M366–M372.

References

Agarwal P, Holland TM, Wang Y, Bennett DA, Morris MC. Association of strawberries and anthocyanidin intake with Alzheimer's dementia risk. *Nutrients.* 2019;11(12):3060.

Appel LJ, Sacks FM, Carey VJ, *et al.* Effects of protein, monounsaturated fat, and carbohydrate intake on blood pressure and serum lipids: results of the OmniHeart randomized trial. *JAMA.* 2005;294(19):2455–2464.

Blaha MJ, DeFilippis AP. Multi-ethnic study of atherosclerosis (MESA): JACC Focus Seminar 5/8. *J Am Coll Cardiol.* 2021;77(25):3195–3216.

Bonaccio M, Costanzo S, Di Castelnuovo A, *et al.* Increased adherence to the Mediterranean diet is associated with reduced low-grade inflammation after a 12.7-year period: results from the Moli-sani Study [published online ahead of print, 2022 Dec 19]. *J Acad Nutr Diet.* 2022;S2212-2672(22)01254-0.

Cara KC, Goldman DM, Kollman BK, Amato SS, Tull MD, Karlsen MC. Commonalities among dietary recommendations from 2010–2021 clinical practice guidelines: a meta-epidemiological study from the American College of Lifestyle Medicine [published online ahead of print, 2023 Mar 18]. *Adv Nutr.* 2023;S2161-8313(23)00276-4.

Castro-Espin C, Agudo A. The role of diet in prognosis among cancer survivors: a systematic review and meta-analysis of dietary patterns and diet interventions. *Nutrients.* 2022;14(2):348.

Cavicchia PP, Steck SE, Hurley TG, *et al.* A new dietary inflammatory index predicts interval changes in serum high-sensitivity C-reactive protein. *J Nutr.* 2009;139(12):2365–2372.

Charisis S, Ntanasi E, Yannakoulia M, *et al.* Diet Inflammatory Index and dementia incidence: a population-based study. *Neurology.* 2021;97(24):e2381–e2391.

Cherian L, Wang Y, Fakuda K, Leurgans S, Aggarwal N, Morris M. Mediterranean-Dash Intervention for Neurodegenerative Delay (MIND) diet slows cognitive decline after stroke. *J Prev Alzheimers Dis.* 2019;6(4):267–273.

Clayton JS, Bonnet J. *Foundations of Lifestyle Medicine: Board Review Manual*, 4th ed. Chesterfield,

MO: American College of Lifestyle Medicine; 2023.

Deshmukh Deppa. Nutritionist Deepa. 2023. https://nutritionistdeepa.com

D'Adamo CR, Workman K, Barnabic C, *et al.* Culinary medicine training in core medical school curriculum improved medical student nutrition knowledge and confidence in providing nutrition counseling. *Am J Lifestyle Med.* 2021;16(6):740–752.

de Lorgeril M, Salen P, Martin JL, Monjaud I, Delaye J, Mamelle N. Mediterranean diet, traditional risk factors, and the rate of cardiovascular complications after myocardial infarction: final report of the Lyon Diet Heart Study. *Circulation.* 1999;99(6):779–785.

Esposito K, Maiorino MI, Bellastella G, Chiodini P, Panagiotakos D, Giugliano D. A journey into a Mediterranean diet and Type 2 diabetes: a systematic review with meta-analyses. *BMJ Open.* 2015;5(8):e008222.

Estruch R, Ros E, Salas-Salvadó J, *et al.* Primary prevention of cardiovascular disease with a Mediterranean diet supplemented with extra-virgin olive oil or nuts. *N Engl J Med.* 2018;378(25):e34.

European Prospective Investigation into Cancer and Nutrition Oxford Study. About the study. 2023. www.ceu.ox.ac.uk/research/epic-oxford-1

Filippou CD, Tsioufis CP, Thomopoulos CG, *et al.* Dietary Approaches to Stop Hypertension (DASH) diet and blood pressure reduction in adults with and without hypertension: a systematic review and meta-analysis of randomized controlled trials. *Adv Nutr.* 2020;11(5):1150–1160.

Framingham Heart Study. About the study. 2023. www.framinghamheartstudy.org

Francis HM, Stevenson RJ, Chambers JR, Gupta D, Newey B, Lim CK. A brief diet intervention can reduce symptoms of depression in young adults: a randomised controlled trial. *PLoS One.* 2019;14(10):e0222768.

Georgoulis M, Yiannakouris N, Tenta R, *et al.* A weight-loss Mediterranean diet/lifestyle intervention ameliorates inflammation and oxidative stress in patients with obstructive sleep apnea: results of the "MIMOSA" randomized clinical trial. *Eur J Nutr.* 2021;60(7):3799–3810.

Guagnano MT, D'Angelo C, Caniglia D, *et al.* Improvement of inflammation and pain after three months' exclusion diet in rheumatoid arthritis patients. *Nutrients.* 2021;13(10):3535.

Hauser ME. *Culinary Medicine Curriculum.* St Louis, MO: American College of Lifestyle Medicine; 2019.

Hauser ME, Nordgren JR, Adam M, *et al.* The first, comprehensive, open-source culinary medicine curriculum for health professional training programs: a global reach. *Am J Lifestyle Med.* 2020;14(4):369–373.

Health Professionals Follow-up Study. About the study. 2023. www.hsph.harvard.edu/hpfs

Jenkins DJ, Kendall CW, Faulkner DA, *et al.* Assessment of the longer-term effects of a dietary portfolio of cholesterol-lowering foods in hypercholesterolemia. *Am J Clin Nutr.* 2006;83(3):582–591.

Jimenez-Torres J, Alcalá-Diaz JF, Torres-Peña JD, *et al.* Mediterranean diet reduces atherosclerosis progression in coronary heart disease: an analysis of the CORDIOPREV randomized controlled trial [published correction appears in *Stroke.* 2021 Nov;52(11):e754]. *Stroke.* 2021;52(11):3440–3449.

Johnston EA, Arcot A, Meengs J, Dreibelbis TD, Kris-Etherton PM, Wiedemer JP. Culinary medicine for family medicine residents. *Med Sci Educ.* 2021;31(3):1015–1018.

La Puma J. Culinary medicine and nature: foods that work together. *Am J Lifestyle Med.* 2020;14(2):143–146.

Lean ME, Leslie WS, Barnes AC, *et al.* Primary care-led weight management for remission of Type 2 diabetes (DiRECT): an open-label, cluster-randomised trial. *Lancet.* 2018;391(10120):541–551.

LeBlanc-Morales N. Culinary medicine: patient education for therapeutic lifestyle changes. *Crit Care Nurs Clin North Am.* 2019;31(1):109–123.

Marshall H, Albin J. Food as medicine: a pilot nutrition and cooking curriculum for children of participants in a community-based culinary medicine class. *Matern Child Health J.* 2021;25(1):54–58.

Martínez-Rodríguez A, Rubio-Arias JÁ, Ramos-Campo DJ, Reche-García C, Leyva-Vela B, Nadal-Nicolás Y. Psychological and sleep effects of tryptophan and magnesium-enriched Mediterranean diet in women with fibromyalgia. *Int J Environ Res Public Health.* 2020;17(7):2227.

Moore TJ, Vollmer WM, Appel LJ, *et al.* Effect of dietary patterns on ambulatory blood pressure: results from the Dietary Approaches to Stop *Hypertension* (DASH) Trial. DASH Collaborative Research Group. Hypertension. 1999;34(3):472–477.

Morris MC, Tangney CC, Wang Y, Sacks FM, Bennett DA, Aggarwal NT. MIND diet associated with reduced incidence of Alzheimer's disease. *Alzheimers Dement.* 2015;11(9):1007–1014.

Morze J, Danielewicz A, Przybyłowicz K, Zeng H, Hoffmann G, Schwingshackl L. An updated systematic review and meta-analysis on adherence to Mediterranean diet and risk of cancer. *Eur J Nutr.* 2021;60(3):1561–1586.

National Health and Nutrition Examination Survey. About the study. 2023. www.cdc.gov/nchs/nhanes/index.htm

Newman C, Yan J, Messiah SE, Albin J. Culinary medicine as innovative nutrition education for medical students: a scoping review [published online ahead of print, 2022 Aug 2]. *Acad Med.* 2022;10.1097/ACM.0000000000004895.

Nurse's Health Study. About the study. 2023. https://nurseshealthstudy.org

Ornish D, Brown SE, Scherwitz LW, *et al.* Can lifestyle changes reverse coronary heart disease? The Lifestyle Heart Trial. *Lancet.* 1990;336(8708):129–133.

Parletta N, Zarnowiecki D, Cho J, *et al.* A Mediterranean-style dietary intervention supplemented with fish oil improves diet quality and mental health in people with depression: a randomized controlled trial (HELFIMED). *Nutr Neurosci.* 2019;22(7):474–487.

Perzia B, Ying GS, Dunaief JL, Dunaief DM. Once-daily low inflammatory foods everyday (life) smoothie or the full life diet lowers c-reactive protein and raises plasma beta-carotene in 7 days. *Am J Lifestyle Med.* 2020;16(6):753–764.

Podadera-Herreros A, Alcala-Diaz JF, Gutierrez-Mariscal FM, *et al.* Long-term consumption of a Mediterranean diet or a low-fat diet on kidney function in coronary heart disease patients: the CORDIOPREV randomized controlled trial. *Clin Nutr.* 2022;41(2):552–559.

Ramos-Lopez O, Martinez-Urbistondo D, Vargas-Nuñez JA, Martinez JA. The role of nutrition on meta-inflammation: insights and potential targets in communicable and chronic disease management. *Curr Obes Rep.* 2022;11(4):305–335.

Razavi AC, Sapin A, Monlezun DJ, *et al.* Effect of culinary education curriculum on Mediterranean diet adherence and food cost savings in families: a randomised controlled trial. *Public Health Nutr.* 2021;24(8):2297–2303.

Richard A, Rohrmann S, Pestoni G, *et al.* Associations between anxiety disorders and diet quality in a Swiss cohort study. *Compr Psychiatry.* 2022;118:152344.

Rondanelli M, Faliva MA, Miccono A, *et al.* Food pyramid for subjects with chronic pain: foods and dietary constituents as anti-inflammatory and antioxidant agents. *Nutr Res Rev.* 2018;31(1):131–151.

Rothman JM, Bilici N, Mergler B, *et al.* A culinary medicine elective for clinically experienced medical students: a pilot study. *J Altern Complement Med.* 2020;26(7):636–644.

Ruiz-Canela M, Bes-Rastrollo M, Martínez-González MA. The role of dietary inflammatory index in cardiovascular disease, metabolic syndrome and mortality. *Int J Mol Sci.* 2016;17(8):1265.

Seventh-Day Adventist Health Study. About the study. 2023. https://adventisthealthstudy.org

Sharma SV, McWhorter JW, Chow J, *et al.* Impact of a virtual culinary medicine curriculum on biometric outcomes, dietary habits, and related psychosocial factors among patients with diabetes participating in a food prescription program. *Nutrients.* 2021;13(12):4492.

Shivappa N, Godos J, Hébert JR, *et al.* Dietary Inflammatory Index and cardiovascular risk and mortality: a meta-analysis. *Nutrients.* 2018;10(2):200.

Silva AR, Bernardo A, de Mesquita MF, *et al.* An anti-inflammatory and low fermentable oligo, di, and monosaccharides and polyols diet improved patient reported outcomes in fibromyalgia: a randomized controlled trial. *Front Nutr.* 2022;9:856216.

Tan J, Atamanchuk L, Rao T, Sato K, Crowley J, Ball L. Exploring culinary medicine as a promising method of nutritional education in medical school: a scoping review. *BMC Med Educ.* 2022;22(1):441.

Torlak MS, Bagcaci S, Akpinar E, Okutan O, Nazli MS, Kuccukturk S. The effect of intermittent diet and/or physical therapy in patients with chronic low back pain: a single-blinded randomized controlled trial. *Explore (NY).* 2022;18(1):76–81.

Travica N, D'Cunha NM, Naumovski N, *et al.* The effect of blueberry interventions on cognitive performance and mood: a systematic review of randomized controlled trials. *Brain Behav Immun.* 2020;85:96–105.

Valls-Pedret C, Sala-Vila A, Serra-Mir M, *et al.* Mediterranean diet and age-related cognitive decline: a randomized clinical trial [published correction appears in *JAMA Intern Med.* 2018 Dec 1;178(12):1731–1732]. *JAMA Intern Med.* 2015;175(7):1094–1103.

van den Brink AC, Brouwer-Brolsma EM, Berendsen AAM, van de Rest O. The Mediterranean, Dietary Approaches to Stop Hypertension (DASH), and Mediterranean-DASH Intervention for Neurodegenerative Delay (MIND) Diets are associated with less cognitive decline and a lower risk of Alzheimer's disease—a review. *Adv Nutr.* 2019;10(6):1040–1065.

Venes D, ed. *Taber's Cyclopedic Medical Dictionary,* 24th ed. Philadelphia, PA: FA Davis; 2021.

Widmer RJ, Flammer AJ, Lerman LO, Lerman A. The Mediterranean diet, its components, and cardiovascular disease. *Am J Med.* 2015;128(3):229–238.

Willett WC, Sacks F, Trichopoulou A, *et al.* Mediterranean diet pyramid: a cultural model for healthy eating. *Am J Clin Nutr.* 1995;61(6 Suppl):1402S–1406S.

Women's Health Initiative. About the study. 2023. www.whi.org

Wright N, Wilson L, Smith M, Duncan B, McHugh P. The BROAD study: a randomised controlled

trial using a whole food plant-based diet in the community for obesity, ischaemic heart disease or diabetes. *Nutr Diabetes*. 2017;7(3):e256.
Yannakoulia M, Kontogianni M, Scarmeas N. Cognitive health and Mediterranean diet: just diet or lifestyle pattern? *Ageing Res Rev*. 2015;20:74–78.
Yi Q, Li X, He Y, *et al.* Associations of dietary inflammatory index with metabolic syndrome and its components: a systematic review and meta-analysis. *Public Health Nutr*. 2021;24(16):5463–5470.
Yubero-Serrano EM, Fernandez-Gandara C, Garcia-Rios A, *et al.* Mediterranean diet and endothelial function in patients with coronary heart disease: an analysis of the CORDIOPREV randomized controlled trial. *PLoS Med*. 2020;17(9):e1003282.

Additional Reading

Berner P, Bezner JR, Morris D, Lein DH. Nutrition in physical therapist practice: setting the stage for taking action. *Phys Ther*. 2021;101(5):pzab062.
Berner P, Bezner JR, Morris D, Lein DH. Nutrition in physical therapist practice: tools and strategies to act now. *Phys Ther*. 2021;101(5):pzab061.
Escott-Stump S. *Nutrition and Diagnosis-Related Care,* 8th ed. Philadelphia, PA: Wolters Kluwer; 2015.
Heber D, Li Z. *Primary Care Nutrition: Writing the Nutrition Prescription*. Boca Raton, FL: CRC Press; 2017.
Kesten D, Scherwitz L. *Whole Person Integrative Eating*. Amherst, MA: White River Press; 2020.
La Puma J. What is culinary medicine and what does it do? *Popul Health Manag*. 2016;19(1):1–3.
Raymond J, Morrow K. *Krause and Mahan's Food and the Nutrition Care Process,* 16th ed. St. Louis, MO: Elsevier; 2023.
Saleh H, Williamson TK, Passias PG. Perioperative nutritional supplementation decreases wound healing complications following elective lumbar spine surgery: a randomized controlled trial. *Spine (Phila Pa 1976)*. 2023;48(6):376–383.
Shan Z, Wang F, Li Y, *et al.* Healthy eating patterns and risk of total and cause-specific mortality [published online ahead of print, 2023 Jan 9]. *JAMA Intern Med*. 2023;10.1001/jamainternmed.2022.6117.
Tonelli Enrico V, Hébert JR, Mugford G, *et al.* Assessing diet and musculoskeletal pain in adults: results from a cross-sectional analysis of the National Health and Nutrition Examination Survey (NHANES) [published online ahead of print]. *American Journal of Lifestyle Medicine*. 2023.
Wastyk HC, Fragiadakis GK, Perelman D, *et al.* Gut-microbiota-targeted diets modulate human immune status. *Cell*. 2021;184(16):4137–4153.e14.

CHAPTER 4

Exercise and Physical Activity

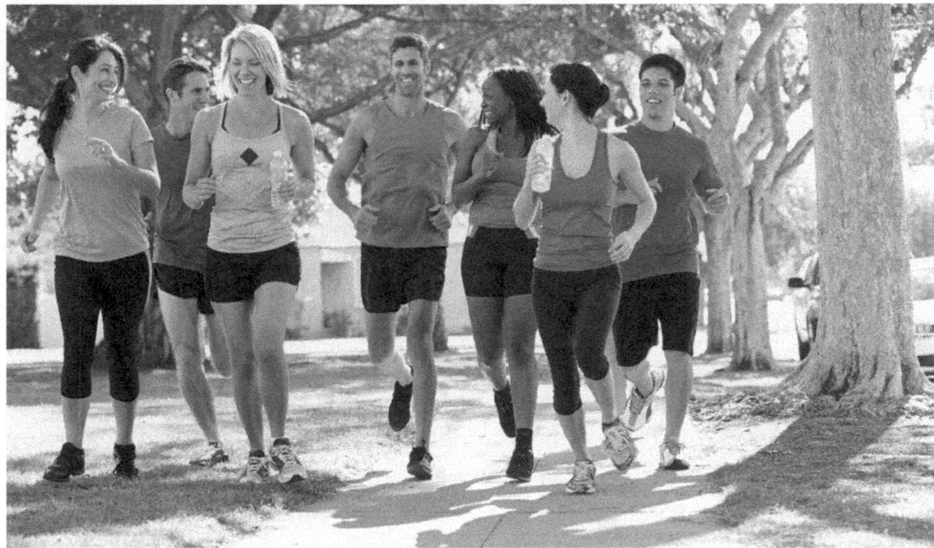

Stay active with friends

Learning Objectives

- Understand the basic research for conventional exercises and physical activity.
- Apply conventional exercises.

Chapter Highlights

- Key Concept: Physical Activity Choices
- Clinical Tip: Table Tennis
- Clinical Tip: Functional Activities
- Featured Topic 4.1: Osteoporosis and Exercise
- Featured Topic 4.2: Elastic Resistance and Bodyweight Exercises

- Featured Topic 4.3: Aquatic Therapy for Pain and Function
- Featured Topic 4.4: Reducing Shoulder Strain During Core Muscle Activation
- Featured Topic 4.5: Fitness Personality
- Featured Topic 4.6: Home Gym Versus Fitness Center
- Featured Topic 4.7: Case Vignette—Intermittent Exercise
- Self-Care Handout 4.1: Weight Management Strategies
- Self-Care Handout 4.2: Core Strengthening Activities and Exercises
- Self-Management Activities
- Classroom and Lab Activities
- Useful Clinical Resources
- References
- Additional Reading

Lifestyle Matters*: Train to sustain.*

Introduction

Exercise and physical activity have many benefits that help individuals improve their quality of life. Perhaps a more user-friendly concept for patients/clients may be that physical activity allows a person to perform necessary daily and functional activities relatively easily and allows for enough reserve for them to pursue leisure activities.

ACSM's Guidelines for Exercise Testing and Prescription (American College of Sports Medicine 2022, p.1) defines physical activity as "any bodily movement produced by the contraction of skeletal muscles that results in an increase in caloric requirements over resting energy expenditure." The book goes on to say that exercise consists of planned movement to improve and/or maintain components of physical fitness.

Exercise and physical activity in general may be helpful for anxiety (Stonerock *et al.* 2015), depressive symptoms (Recchia *et al.* 2022), diabetes (Sampath Kumar *et al.* 2019), fatigue in individuals with multiple sclerosis (Razazian *et al.* 2020), knee osteoarthritis (Ferreira *et al.* 2019), neuropathic pain (Zhang *et al.* 2021), osteoporosis prevention (Pinheiro *et al.* 2020), Parkinson's (Gamborg *et al.* 2022), and other conditions.

KEY CONCEPT: PHYSICAL ACTIVITY CHOICES

The following list presents a variety of strategies for including physical activity in daily life:

- Functional activities (see Clinical Tip: Functional Activities later in this chapter)
- Nature-based activities (such as outdoor walking, gardening, hiking, kayaking, surfing)
- Art-based activities (such as dancing, drama club, music, pottery)
- Sports (such as football or soccer, volleyball, basketball)
- Home gym (such as dumbbells, kettlebells, bodyweight exercises)
- Community center (such as games, classes)
- Fitness centers (such as classes, aerobic and strength equipment)
- Fitness studios (such as yoga, tai chi, martial arts, Pilates)

Basic Components of Physical Activity

This section briefly outlines some of the American College of Sports Medicine (ACSM) health- and skill-related physical fitness components that may be necessary for activities of daily living. The table below lists the components of physical fitness.

A consideration to remember is while the goal is to aim for the physical fitness goals set by the ACSM and other organizations, many patients/clients get frustrated that they cannot meet recommended goals and then avoid exercise altogether. For this reason, we need to understand where patients/clients are in their fitness journey and gradually move them toward standards outlined by leading organizations such as the ACSM.

Components of physical fitness

Health Related	Skill Related
• Cardiorespiratory endurance • Body composition • Muscular strength • Muscular endurance • Flexibility	• Agility • Coordination • Balance • Power • Reaction time • Speed

Adapted from American College of Sports Medicine 2022.

One source, the *Physical Activity Guidelines for Americans* (U.S. Department of Health and Human Services 2018, p.8), recommends the following guidelines that may be used to encourage patient/clients to engage in physical activity to improve and maintain overall health and well-being:

- The key is that any physical activity or exercise is better than none.
- Adults should avoid prolonged sitting and sedentary behavior. For example, adults may aim for 5 minutes of physical activity or exercise (such as

marching in place, shadow boxing, dancing, or walking) for every hour of sitting.

- For health benefits, adults should engage in at least: 150 minutes (2 hours and 30 minutes) to 300 minutes (5 hours) a week of moderate-intensity aerobic physical activity, 75 minutes (1 hour and 15 minutes) to 150 minutes (2 hours and 30 minutes) a week of vigorous-intensity aerobic physical activity, or an equivalent combination of moderate- and vigorous-intensity aerobic physical activity. (Ideally, the 150–300 minutes of aerobic activity should be spread throughout the week).
- For health benefits, adults should also perform muscle-strengthening activities of moderate or greater intensity that include all major muscle groups on two or more days a week. Strengthening exercises may consist of weights (dumbbells or barbells), bodyweight exercises (such as push-ups, pull-ups, or planks), elastic bands, or resistance machines.

Aerobic Activities

Aerobic exercises may include outdoor walking, treadmill walking, hiking, running, outdoor cycling, stationary cycling, stair climber, elliptical apparatus, dancing, swimming, aqua aerobics, cross-country skiing, skating, and various sports activities, such as pickleball, tennis, basketball, volleyball, and soccer. Aerobic training and exercise may be beneficial for anxiety (LeBouthillier and Asmundson 2017), dementia (Bossers *et al.* 2015), depression (Moraes *et al.* 2020), hypertension (Lopes *et al.* 2021), multiple sclerosis (Taul-Madsen *et al.* 2021), osteoarthritis (Rewald *et al.* 2020), pain (Vanti *et al.* 2019), Parkinson's (Johansson *et al.* 2022), and other conditions.

Some practical benefits of aerobic training include:

- fresh air, a little sunshine, and nature exposure (if performed outdoors)
- socialization (if performed in a group)
- improved sleep quality and stress reduction.

Strength Activities

Strength or resistance exercises may include bodyweight exercises (e.g., squats, lunges, push-ups, planks), weight machines, resistance bands, and free weights (e.g., dumbbells, barbells, kettlebells). Resistance training and exercise may, for example, be beneficial for anxiety (Gordon *et al.* 2017), cognitive function (Coelho-Júnior *et al.* 2020), depression (Gordon *et al.* 2017; Gordon *et al.* 2018), osteoarthritis (Turner *et al.* 2020), osteoporosis (Watson *et al.* 2018), and Parkinson's (Ferreira *et al.* 2018).

Some practical benefits of strength training include:

- improved ability to get in and out of chairs and climb stairs
- improved ability to carry groceries and other items
- greater capacity to do chores
- improved sleep quality and stress reduction
- improved posture (if targeting appropriate muscle groups).

Flexibility Activities

Flexibility exercises may include static stretches, dynamic stretching, and proprioceptive neuromuscular facilitation (PNF). Flexibility training and exercise may be beneficial for fibromyalgia (Assumpção *et al.* 2018), improve gait function (Watt *et al.* 2011), pain among office workers (Shariat *et al*. 2018; Tunwattanapong *et al.* 2016), shoulder pain and mobility (Tahran *et al.* 2020), and other conditions.

Some practical benefits of flexibility training include:

- reduced muscle tension
- improved circulation
- improved posture (if targeting appropriate muscle groups)
- improved function for daily tasks such as putting on socks, shoes, and coats (if targeting appropriate muscle groups).

Balance Activities

Balance training exercises may include (Araujo *et al.* 2022; Devasahayam *et al.* 2022):

- static balance such as semi-tandem stance, tandem stance, and single-leg stance
- dynamic balance such as front/back weight shifting, lateral weight shifting, multidirectional stepping, slow marching in place, heel raises, dancing, tai chi, qigong, and yoga
- reactive balance training such as manual perturbations by the clinician (such as pushing or pulling), catch and throw games in the clinic, table tennis, pickleball, and tennis.

Balance training and exercise may, for example, be beneficial for fall prevention (Liu-Ambrose *et al.* 2019), osteoporosis (Halvarsson *et al.* 2015), and Parkinson's (Santos *et al.* 2017).

Some practical benefits of balance training include the:

- ability to walk on uneven surfaces such as old sidewalks or grass
- ability to go up and down curbs and steps in the community when there are no rails
- ability to get in and out of the bathtub
- ability to maintain balance when a person is accidentally bumped in a busy store.

CLINICAL TIP: TABLE TENNIS

Table tennis is a fun and versatile tool that challenges balance and coordination. Table tennis may even help an individual with Parkinson's improve motor symptoms and overall mental well-being (Inoue *et al.* 2020; Olsson *et al.* 2020).

Basic Physical Activity and Exercise Prescription Strategies

The following table outlines the ACSM's (American College of Sports Medicine 2022) physical activity and exercise prescription guidelines for older adults (typically individuals aged 50 to 64 years with physical limitations or clinical conditions, and individuals aged ≥ 65 years), including using the FITT (frequency, intensity, time, type) approach. According to ACSM guidelines, the exercise prescription variables will typically vary for medical conditions such as arthritis, anxiety and depression, cancer, cerebral palsy, cerebrovascular accident, diabetes, fibromyalgia, hypertension, kidney disease, multiple sclerosis, osteoporosis, overweight and obesity, Parkinson's, pulmonary diseases, and spinal cord injury.

Furthermore, physical therapists, occupational therapists, and exercise specialists can design tailored programs to meet the needs of their patients/clients.

Fitness guidelines for older adults

	Aerobic Training	Resistance Training	Flexibility Training	Balance/ Neuromotor Training
Frequency (How Often)	• ≥ 5 days per week for moderate intensity • ≥ 3 days per week for vigorous intensity	≥ 2 days per week	≥ 2 days per week	2–3 days per week
Intensity (How Hard)	Moderate to vigorous	• For beginners, 40–50% of 1 repetition maximum (RM)[1] • Progress to 60% to 80% of 1 RM	Stretch to point of slight discomfort or tightness and tension	(Not identified)
Time (How Long)	• 30 to 60 minutes per day for moderate intensity • 20 to 30 minutes per day for vigorous intensity	• 8–10 exercises covering major muscle groups • Beginners: ≥ 1 set of 10–15 repetitions • Progress to 1–3 sets of 8–12 repetitions	Stretch held for 30 to 60 seconds	(Not identified)
Type (Activity Type)	Walking, aquatic training, and stationary cycling	Weight training (such as bodyweight, elastic, dumbbell, barbell resistance), weight bearing calisthenics	Static stretches for each major muscle group	One-leg stance, semi-tandem stance, tandem stance, toe raises, tandem walk, multidirectional stepping, dancing, tai chi, qigong

Adapted from American College of Sports Medicine 2009; American College of Sports Medicine 2022; Garber et al. 2011.

[1] 1 RM is the maximum amount of weight that a person can lift for one repetition with proper technique for an exercise.

CLINICAL TIP: FUNCTIONAL ACTIVITIES

Functional physical activities count toward overall weekly fitness goals. It's not all about programmed exercise sessions. For this reason, encourage patients/clients to regularly engage in physical activities such as the following:

- Hand-wash the car.
- Park a little distance from the store and carry light to medium-heavy packages back to the car.
- Rake the leaves in the yard.
- Sweep the driveway.
- Take the dog for a long walk.
- Take the stairs at work when possible.
- Take walking meetings at work.
- Work in the garden.

The activity and exercise prescription should consider whether the activity is enjoyable and fun for the individual. Also, the exercise prescription should consider if the program is realistic. For example, a person with financial limitations may be unable to budget for a gym membership. However, a realistic program might be a walking program at a nearby park combined with a simple and sustainable home exercise program for strength, balance, and flexibility.

Modified Exercise Prescription Principles

A typical exercise prescription usually includes frequency, intensity, time, and type of exercise. In this text, enjoyable/engaging and also realistic and substantiable exercise are proposed.

F = frequency
I = intensity
T = time
T = type
E = enjoyable and engaging
R = realistic and sustainable

Practical Training Strategies

Several of the sample exercise programs outlined in this section have been modified from the book *Integrative Healing: Developing Wellness in the Mind and Body* (Altug 2018).

Short-Bout Training

Short-bout training (also known as intermittent training) includes short-duration exercise periods that are accumulated throughout the day (Altug 2018). The exercise bouts may be as short as 8–10 minutes, totaling 30 minutes or more on most days (Jakicic *et al.* 2019). Short bouts of training may, for example, enhance weight loss and exercise adherence (Jakicic *et al.* 1995). Also, a cohort study suggests that 3 to 4 minutes of vigorous intermittent lifestyle physical activity per day may be a feasible option to help reduce cancer risk for individuals unable or unmotivated to exercise (Stamatakis *et al.* 2023).

The potential advantage of short-bout training in rehabilitation and fitness programs may be that it gradually increases activity and exercise capacity. The program may also enhance exercise adherence and improves health outcomes.

Sample Short-Bout Walking Program

- Morning: 10–15-minute walk before work.
- Midday: 10–15-minute walk during lunch break at work.
- Evening: 10–15-minute walk after work.

Exercise Snacks

According to an article in *Exercise and Sport Sciences Reviews* (Islam *et al.* 2022, p.31), "exercise snacks" are "Isolated ≤1-min bouts of vigorous exercise performed periodically throughout the day." Exercise snacks may improve aerobic fitness (Jenkins *et al.* 2019; Little *et al.* 2019; Rafiei 2021) and glycemic control in individuals with insulin resistance (Francois *et al.* 2014).

The potential advantage of "exercise snacks" in rehabilitation and fitness programs may be that it is well tolerated and a time-efficient strategy to improve cardiorespiratory fitness in certain individuals (Islam *et al.* 2022). The key point to keep in mind is that "exercise snacks" are great supplements to boost daily activities, but they do not replace a comprehensive workout or exercise session.

Sample Adapted "Exercise Snack" Program

1. Start: Warm up with multidirectional lunges for 15 seconds.
2. Exercise Snack Routine: 30 seconds marching in place.
3. End: Cool down by walking around for 15 seconds.

   - Bouts per day may include morning, midday, and evening.

- Routine intensity, exercise bouts per day, and exercise selection must be adjusted according to the individual.
- Focus on the safety of the individual.

Interval Training

Interval training is a type of training in which periods of high-intensity exercise intervals (such as fast walking, running, fast cycling) are alternated with low-intensity exercise intervals (such as slow walking, jogging, slow cycling). It can be thought of as alternating between difficult and easy exercise intervals (Altug 2018). Interval training may be used for managing blood pressure (Carpes *et al.* 2022), chronic low back pain (Cerini *et al.* 2022), coronary artery disease (Conraads *et al.* 2015), Type 2 diabetes (Liu *et al.* 2019), and other conditions.

The potential advantage of interval training in rehabilitation and fitness programs may be that it gradually increases activity and exercise capacity. The program may also help with weight loss (if that is a goal), enhance exercise adherence, and prevent boredom.

Sample Interval Walking Program

1. Start: Warm up with mobility exercises for 5 minutes.
2. Normal-paced walk (typically slow) for 5–10 minutes.
3. Fast walk (faster than normal pace) for 1 minute.
4. Normal-paced walk for 5 minutes.
5. Continue with a repetitive cycle of alternating the slow walk (5 minutes) and fast walk (1 minute) for a total of 15–45 minutes, depending on tolerance.
6. End: Cool down with walking and stretching for 3–5 minutes.

Circuit Training

Circuit training involves moving from one activity or exercise to the other with varying amounts of rest or stretching in between (Altug 2018). Circuit training may, for example, be used for improving coronary heart disease (Wu *et al.* 2022), physical performance in older individuals (Marcos-Pardo *et al.* 2019), gait after stroke (task-oriented training) (van de Port *et al.* 2012), and motor performance in Parkinson's (task-oriented training) (Soke *et al.* 2021).

The potential advantage of circuit training in rehabilitation and fitness programs may be that it gradually increases activity and exercise capacity by changing exercises with varying rest periods. The training introduces the person to various movement patterns using different exercise equipment and body-weight exercises. The program may also help with weight loss (if that is a goal), enhance exercise adherence, and prevent boredom.

Sample Home Circuit Strength Program

1. Start: Warm up with mobility exercises for 5 minutes.
2. Walk in place or in your home for 30 seconds to 1 minute.
3. Partial squats for 10–15 repetitions.
4. Walk in place or in your home for 30 seconds to 1 minute.
5. Standing elastic rowing for 10–15 repetitions.
6. Walk in place or in your home for 30 seconds to 1 minute.
7. Supine bridge exercise for 10–15 repetitions.
8. Walk in place or in your home for 30 seconds to 1 minute.
9. Partial push-ups from an elevated surface (such as the bed) for 10–15 repetitions.
10. Walk in place or in your home for 30 seconds to 1 minute.
11. Heel raises for 10 repetitions.
12. End: Cool down by walking and stretching gently for 5 minutes.

Sample Park Circuit Strength Program

1. Start: Warm up with mobility exercises for 5 minutes.
2. Walk outdoors for 5 minutes.
3. Partial squats for 10–15 repetitions.
4. Walk outdoors for 5 minutes.
5. Partial push-ups from an elevated surface (such as a park bench) for 10–15 repetitions.
6. Walk outdoors for 5 minutes.
7. Multidirectional stepping (like tai chi steps) for 1 minute.
8. Walk outdoors for 5 minutes.
9. Slow march in place for 30 seconds.
10. Walk outdoors for 5 minutes.
11. End: Cool down by walking and stretching gently for 5 minutes.

Sample Functional Task Specific Circuit Program

1. Start: Warm up with mobility exercises for 5 minutes.
2. Sit to stand from the dining room chair for 5–15 repetitions.
3. Slow alternate arm overhead reach for 10 repetitions.
4. From standing, lie down on the floor and get back up 1–3 times.
5. Slow alternate arm overhead reach for 10 repetitions.
6. Climb up and down stairs 1–2 times.
7. End: Cool down by walking and stretching gently for 5 minutes.

Sample Mind-Body Fusion Circuit Program at a Park

1. Start: Warm up with slow mindful walking for 5 minutes.
2. Perform tai chi for 5 minutes.
3. Perform qigong Baduanjin for 5 minutes.
4. Perform yoga for 5 minutes.
5. Perform Pilates mat exercises for 5 minutes.
6. Cool down with slow mindful walking for 5 minutes.
7. End: Cool down with gentle stretching for 5 minutes.

Cross-Training

Cross-training has many definitions in the sports world. It may refer to applying several sports, activities, or training techniques to improve a person's performance in their primary sport or activity. In this book, cross-training refers to a "training method in which exercises and activities such as outdoor walking, upper body biking, elliptical training, stair climbing, Tai Chi, dancing, tennis, circuit weight-training, aerobic dance, and calisthenics are varied during the month, week, or even in a single workout session" (Altug 2018, p.158). Cross-training strategies may be used, for example, to improve running performance in high school cross-country runners during early season training (Paquette *et al.* 2018) and as an alternate option to enhance fitness (Grier *et al.* 2015). Cross-training strategies may be adapted for rehabilitation and fitness programs.

The potential advantage of circuit training in rehabilitation and fitness programs may be that it introduces the person to various movement patterns using different exercise equipment, bodyweight exercises, and training approaches. The program may be used during periods of injury and overtraining (Tanaka 1994) and also to enhance exercise adherence and prevent boredom.

The other application of the term cross-training may be seen in stroke rehabilitation. In this case, cross-training is "an indirect intervention to promote muscle activity on the affected side by applying resistance exercise to stronger parts of the body" (Park *et al.* 2021, p.4). A study also showed that cross-training (or unilateral training of the uninjured limb) may be considered after anterior cruciate ligament (ACL) reconstruction (Cuyul-Vásquez *et al.* 2022). However, these topics are beyond the scope of this book.

Sample Weekly Cross-Training Program

- Monday: Outdoor walk for 15–45 minutes.
- Tuesday: Weight-training exercises for 15–45 minutes.
- Wednesday: Outdoor yoga for 15–60 minutes.
- Thursday: Outdoor bike for 15–45 minutes.
- Friday: Weight-training exercises for 15–45 minutes.
- Saturday: Outdoor tai chi for 15–60 minutes.
- Sunday: Outdoor walk for 15–45 minutes.

Sample Single-Session Indoor Cross-Training Program

1. Start: Warm up with mobility exercises for 5 minutes.
2. Walk on an indoor track or treadmill for 10–15 minutes.
3. Exercise on an elliptical machine for 10–15 minutes.
4. Ride a stationary bike for 10–15 minutes.
5. End: Cool down with walking and stretching for 5 minutes.

Sample Single-Session Outdoor Cross-Training Program

1. Start: Warm up with mobility exercises at a park for 5 minutes.
2. Walk at the park for 10–15 minutes.
3. Perform yoga or tai chi at the park for 10–15 minutes.
4. Walk again in the park for another 10–15 minutes.
5. End: Cool down with walking and stretching at the park for 5 minutes.

Featured Topics

Featured Topic 4.1 outlines guidelines for using exercise as a part of managing osteoporosis.

Featured Topic 4.2 outlines some sample elastic resistance and bodyweight exercises.

Featured Topic 4.3 outlines some of the benefits of utilizing aquatic therapy as a part of a rehabilitation program.

Featured Topic 4.4 outlines a simple strategy for reducing shoulder strain during core muscle activation, since many positions use the hands or elbows for front and side planks.

Featured Topic 4.5 outlines some strategies you might use to figure out your fitness personality (Altug and Gensler 2006).

Featured Topic 4.6 outlines the benefits of a home gym versus a fitness center. There is no correct or ideal approach.

Featured Topic 4.7 outlines a case vignette of a sedentary accountant who benefits from an intermittent exercise program.

■ Featured Topic 4.1: Osteoporosis and Exercise

The 2020 Update of the American Association of Clinical Endocrinologists/American College of Endocrinology Clinical Practice Guidelines for the Diagnosis and Treatment of Postmenopausal Osteoporosis (Camacho *et al.* 2020) and other sources (McClung *et al.* 2021; Nikander *et al.* 2009; Zhong *et al.* 2020) recommend the following:

- Maintain an active lifestyle.
- Engage in aerobic exercise—weight-bearing exercises such as walking, jogging, tai chi, stair climbing, or dancing.
- Engage in muscle-strengthening exercises—weight training or other resistance exercises that may include bodyweight exercise, elastic resistance, or dumbbell resistance.
- Engage in balance exercises—tai chi, weight shifting exercises, or single-leg stance exercises.

The following simple multidirectional stepping exercise sequence (as seen in some tai chi routines) may be an effective exercise to improve balance and provide targeted movements for the lower body.

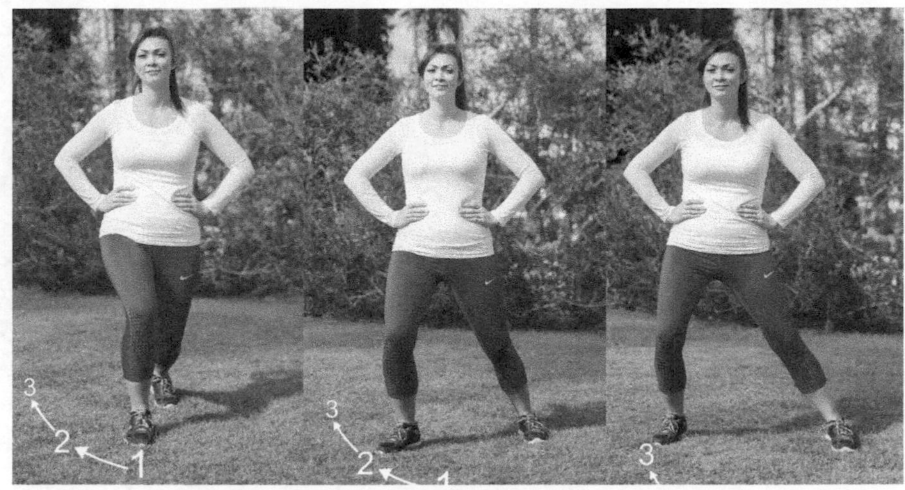

Multidirectional stepping for improving balance

■ Featured Topic 4.2: Elastic Resistance and Bodyweight Exercises

Exercise elastic bands are versatile, inexpensive (compared to gym memberships) tools that are easy to use and transport and may be a part of a rehabilitation or fitness routine. Combined with bodyweight exercises, they can be used to create a variety of fun and effective home exercise programs (Liao *et al.* 2017; Sasaki *et al.* 2023; Stojanović *et al.* 2021).

The following are some example elastic resistance exercises to help improve posture and strengthen the core and upper body.

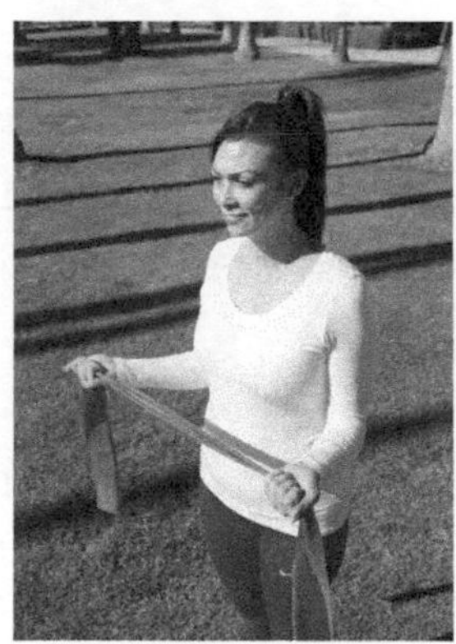

Elastic shoulder external rotation

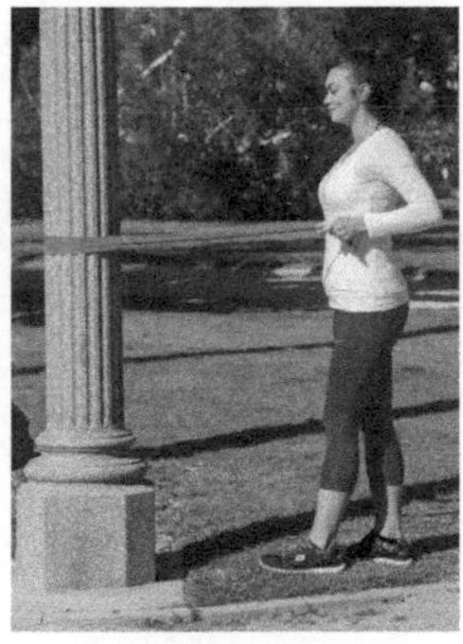

Elastic rowing (high pull)

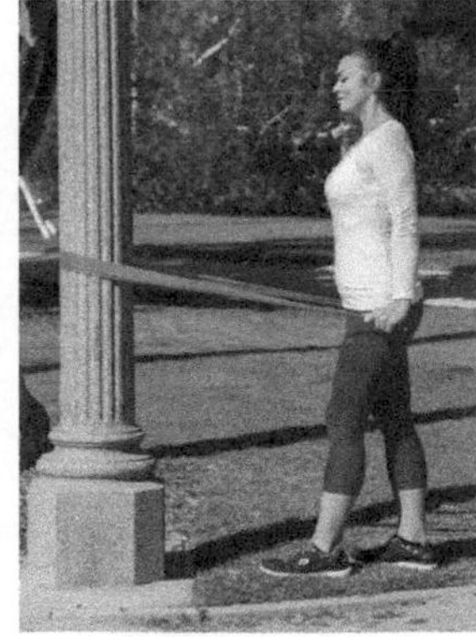

Elastic shoulder extension (low pull)

The following are some example basic bodyweight exercises to help strengthen the lower body, upper body, and core.

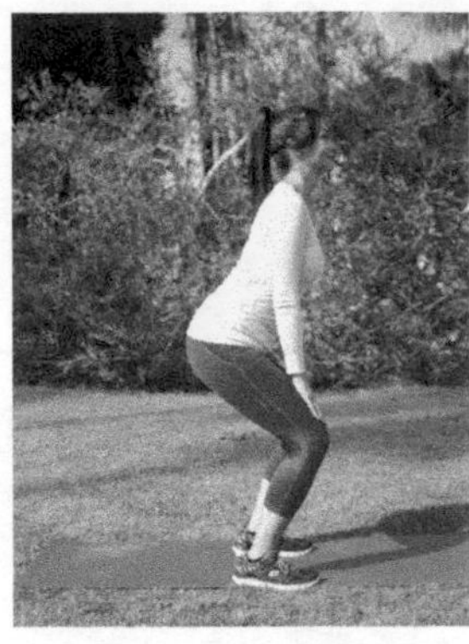

Partial squats

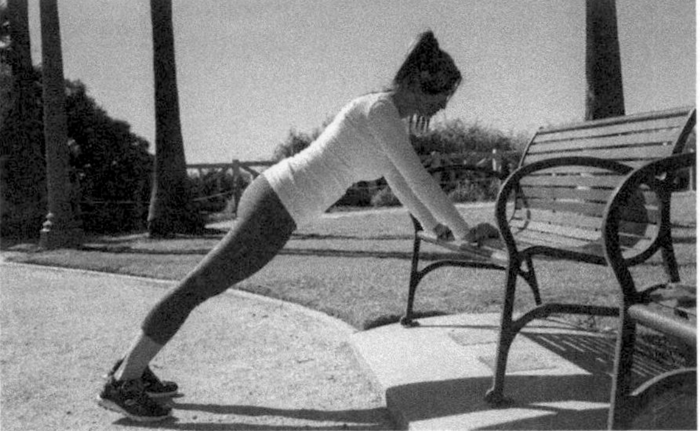

Elevated push-ups

■ Featured Topic 4.3: Aquatic Therapy for Pain and Function

Aquatic therapy may be an effective intervention in rehabilitation (Brody and Geigle 2009). Aquatic therapy may be beneficial for chronic low back pain (Baena-Beato *et al.* 2014; Peng *et al.* 2022; Shi *et al.* 2018), knee osteoarthritis (Rewald *et al.* 2020), multiple sclerosis (Amedoro *et al.* 2020), Parkinson's (Carroll *et al.* 2017; Pérez de la Cruz 2017), and other conditions.

Types of aquatic therapy include Ai Chi (Kurt *et al.* 2018), Bad Ragaz Ring Method (Cha *et al.* 2017), Halliwick Concept (or Halliwick Aquatic Therapy) (Gurpinar *et al.* 2020; Tripp and Krakow 2014), and WATSU™ (water and shiatsu aquatic bodywork and therapy) (Loureiro *et al.* 2022; Pérez Ramírez *et al.* 2019).

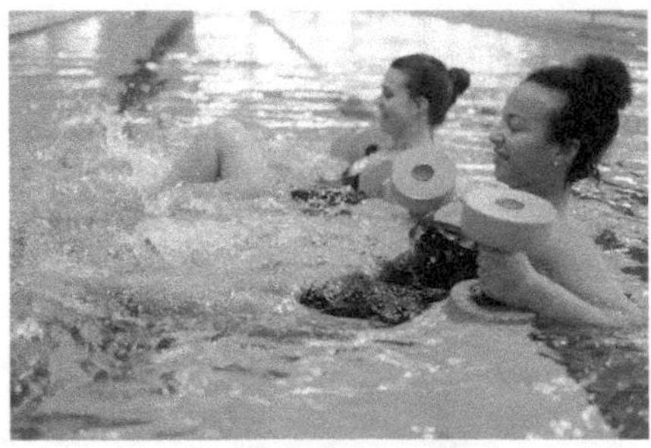

Aquatic therapy

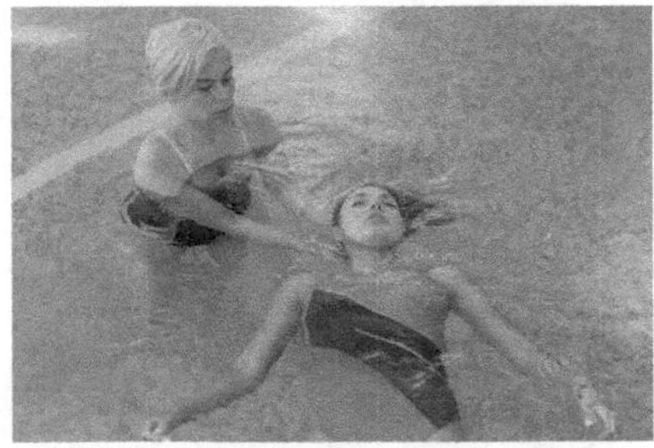

WATSU

■ Featured Topic 4.4: Reducing Shoulder Strain During Core Muscle Activation

Core muscle activation may be achieved in supine, prone, and side positions (Escamilla *et al.* 2016). However, some styles of side planks may be irritating to the shoulders. Consider this side leg lift variation option to engage some of the core muscles without straining the shoulders.

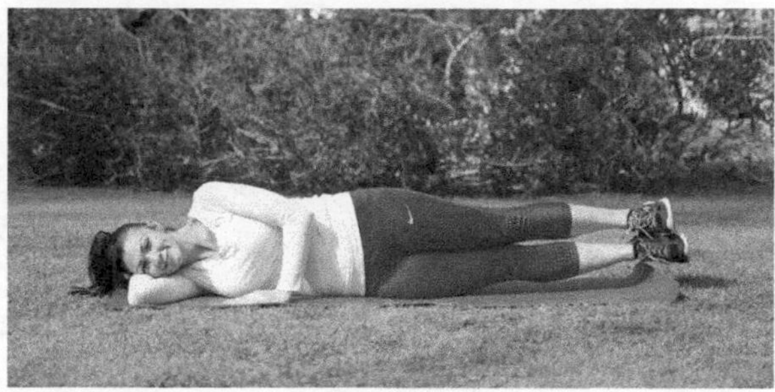

Modified side plank

■ Featured Topic 4.5: Fitness Personality

Read through the following questions and decide which activities best fit your needs:

- Do you want quiet time to be alone with your thoughts?

Consider mindful walking, labyrinth walking, cross-country skiing, or hiking.

- Do you want competition?

Consider sports such as pickleball, tennis, golf, basketball, or volleyball.

- Do you want more social interaction?

Consider activities such as dancing, team sports such as softball, or a fitness center.

- Do you want relaxing activities?

Consider yoga, tai chi, or qigong.

- Do you want intense physical activities?

Consider weight training or martial arts (such as Aikido, Hapkido, Jeet Kune Do, Judo, Jujitsu, Karate, Kung Fu, Taekwondo).

- Do you want more adventure in nature?

Consider activities such as canoeing, cross-country skiing, hiking, horseback riding, kayaking, mountain biking, paddleboarding, rafting, rock climbing, sailing, or windsurfing.

- Do you want easy and fun activities?

Consider rollerblading, ice skating, bowling, or golfing.

Featured Topic 4.6: Home Gym Versus Fitness Center

Home Gym

- No membership fees
- No travel required
- Low risk of exposure to viruses
- Self-selected music
- Self-selected room temperature
- Self-selected gym design

Fitness Center

- Variety of equipment
- Variety of classes
- Expert instruction/coaching
- Social interaction/networking
- Motivation

Featured Topic 4.7: Case Vignette—Intermittent Exercise

Jane, a 50-year-old accountant for a large corporation, has had difficulty exercising due to her knee pain for the past ten years. In this timeframe, she has gained about 40 pounds and recently started to take medications for high blood pressure. During a routine visit with her family physician, the doctor recommends Jane see a physical therapist (PT) for her knee pain. In the consultation with the PT, Jane tells the PT that she does not have time for exercise during the week since her commute is 45 minutes in each direction. The PT and Jane work together to design a program that will fit her needs. Jane's program consists of an intermittent and short-duration walking program at work. Jane takes 10 minutes at work to walk around the corporate grounds after she parks her car in the morning. At lunch, she walks for 10 minutes before she eats. After work, she walks for another 10 minutes as she goes to her car. The intermittent 10-minute program does not result in a flare-up of her knee pain, and the program easily fits into her daily routine. After three months of following this intermittent walking routine, Jane loses about 12 pounds. Encouraged by her success, she adds walking to her routine on the weekend. She also enrolls in a weekend cooking class at a community college to learn how to prepare nutritious foods. Jane maintains periodic communication with her physician and physical therapist via telehealth visits. After nine months, she returns to her family physician for a checkup. Jane and her physician are happy to see she has lost a total of 30 pounds. The physician indicates that she no longer needs the blood pressure medication. Jane's goal for the next year is to see if she can work remotely from her home several days a week. She plans to use the saved commute time to enroll in a yoga program and do two classes a week. Jane also intends to do more gardening for increased interaction with nature for fresh air, sensible sunshine, and outdoor bright light exposure.

Adapted from Altug 2020.

Self-Care Education Guides

See **Self-Care Handout 4.1: Weight Management Strategies** for practical strategies that may be used for weight management (Bonanno *et al.* 2019; Jakicic *et al.* 1995; Kim *et al.* 2020; Mabire *et al.* 2017; Malfliet *et al.* 2021; Perkin *et al.* 2019; Poon *et al.* 2020; Remde *et al.* 2021; Schmidt *et al.* 2001; Seo *et al.* 2019; Siu *et al.* 2021; Spadaro *et al.* 2017). See Appendix B for sample exercises. Weight reduction may be a valuable part of pain management, with benefits such as improved physical functioning (Somers *et al.* 2022), and disease management, with benefits such as improved cardiovascular risk factors (Ge *et al.* 2020).

See **Self-Care Handout 4.2: Core Strengthening Activities and Exercises** to manage back pain and maintain an active lifestyle (Fernández-Rodríguez *et al.* 2022; Hindle *et al.* 2019; Kim and Yim 2020; McGill *et al.* 2009; Salik Sengul *et al.* 2021; Shi *et al.* 2022).

Self-Care Handout 4.1: Weight Management Strategies

Exercise

- Try walking, since it is a simple exercise.
- Try tai chi, yoga, Pilates, or any activity you enjoy.

Nutrition

- Eat a whole food plant-predominant diet.
- Try the Mediterranean diet.

Sleep

- Improve the quality of your sleep and adjust the number of hours you sleep for optimal health (see Chapter 7 for more information on restorative sleep).

Stress

- Try mindfulness meditation or any activity (e.g., hiking, biking, gardening) or hobby (e.g., painting, playing music) that helps control your stress.

Simple Physical Activity Routines

Sample Home Program 1: Short-Bout Bodyweight Training Routine

Duration: approximately 5–10 minutes, 1 set of 10–15 repetitions, 1–2 times a day, performed 2–3 times per week.

- Warm-up exercises: Multidirectional stepping, march in place, and shadow boxing.
- Strength exercises: Squats, push-ups, floor to stand lower and rise, front plank marching, quadruped bird dog.
- Flexibility exercises: Perform two upper-body and two lower-body stretches.

Sample Home Program 2: Short-Bout Resistance Training Routine

Duration: approximately 5–10 minutes, 1 set of 10–15 repetitions, 1–2 times a day, performed 2–3 times per week.

- Warm-up exercises: Multidirectional stepping, march in place, and shadow boxing.
- Strength exercises: Kettlebell floor squats, kettlebell rowing, kettlebell floor to overhead press.
- Flexibility exercises: Perform two upper-body and two lower-body stretches.

Self-Care Handout 4.2: Core Strengthening Activities and Exercises

Keeping your spine healthy and strong is one way to manage back pain and maintain an active lifestyle. Work with your healthcare provider and fitness professional to determine which of the following activities and exercises fit your needs.

Functional Activities

- Sweeping the driveway, patio, or deck (perform on the right and left sides)
- Raking leaves in the yard (perform on the right and left sides)
- Hand-washing the car
- Mopping the floor (perform on the right and left sides)
- Vacuuming (perform on the right and left sides)
- Painting the house or fence
- Carrying groceries with either one or two hands
- Climbing stairs

Mind-Body Training

- Pilates
- Yoga
- Tai chi

Exercises

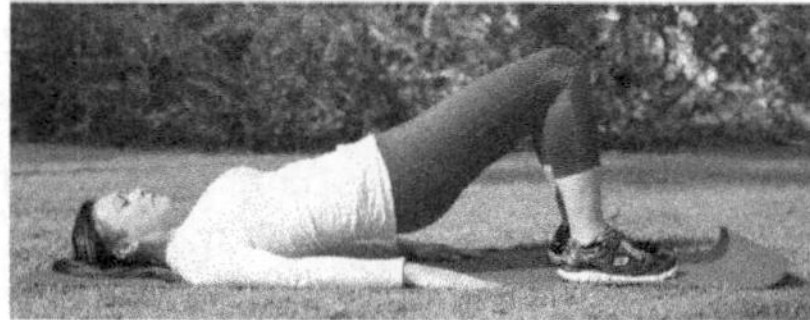

Bridging

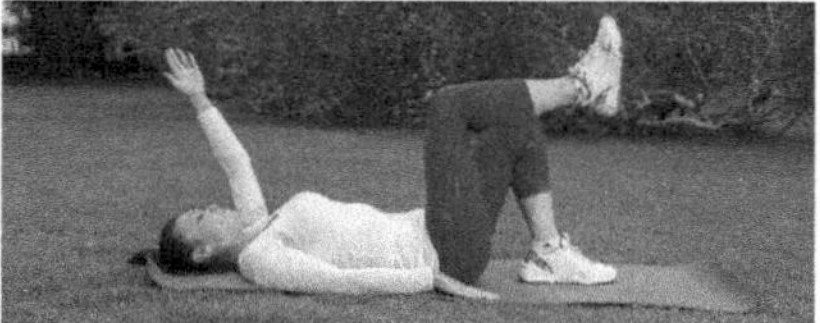

Arm/leg march

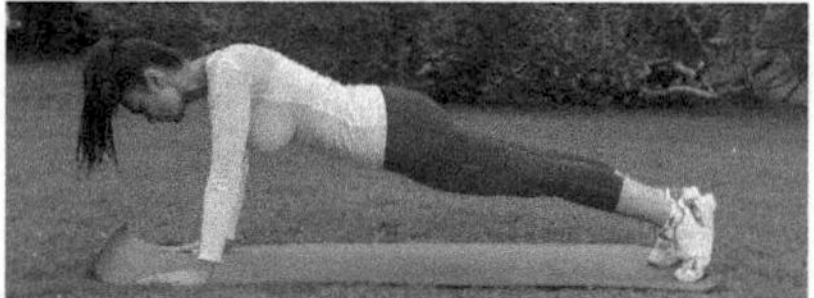

Front plank

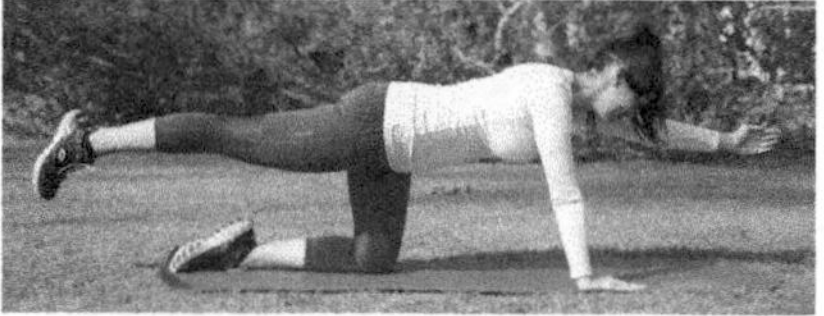

Bird dog

Self-Management Activities: Explore Hiking

The following online resources can help patients/clients, healthcare providers, and health/fitness professionals to manage stress and anxiety by exploring trails and nature.

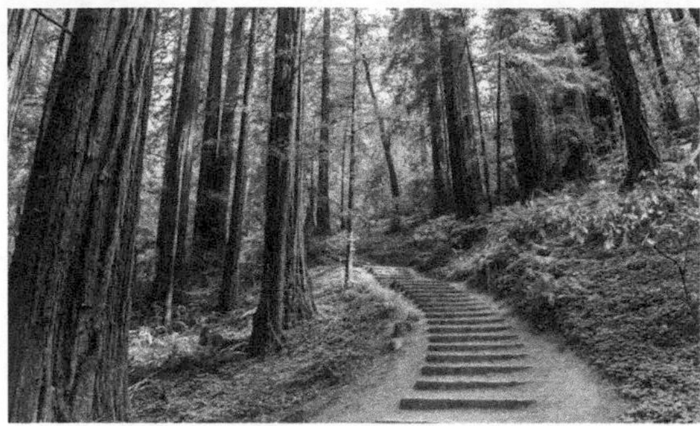

Hiking for happiness

- The AllTrails: Hike, Bike & Run app serves as a companion for outdoor adventure: www.alltrails.com
- The NatureTime app, founded by Iris Rosin, provides a connection with nature to reduce stress and improve overall health: https://naturetimeapp.com

Classroom and Lab Activities

- Identify five simple exercises that can be performed at home and five that can be performed at work.
- Determine the necessary space and tools needed to create a home gym. For example, will the home gym be in the garage, a spare room, or on a patio or balcony? Will the person need an exercise or yoga mat, dumbbells, kettlebell, or elastic resistance bands? Will the fitness space need plants, paintings, and other decorative items such as a wooden table?

Useful Clinical Resources

Organizations

- American College of Sports Medicine, www.acsm.org
- American Council of Exercise, www.acefitness.org
- American Physical Therapy Association, www.apta.org
- Exercise is Medicine, www.exerciseismedicine.org

- National Strength and Conditioning Association, www.nsca.com
- ParkRx, www.parkrx.org
- US Registry of Exercise Professionals, www.usreps.org
- Walk with a DOC, www.walkwithadoc.org

Fitness Equipment Resources

- NordicTrack (treadmills, bikes, ellipticals), www.nordictrack.com
- NuStep Recumbent Cross Trainer, www.nustep.com
- Perform Better (fitness products), www.performbetter.com
- Rogue Fitness (fitness equipment), www.roguefitness.com
- Smovey® Vibroswing, www.smoveynorthamerica.com
- Theraband (resistance bands, rehab products), www.theraband.com
- Trekking Poles (fitness walking poles), www.rei.com/c/trekking-poles

Interactive Fitness Resources

- Fitbit (fitness monitor), www.fitbit.com
- Mirror (home fitness classes), www.mirror.co
- Peloton (home fitness classes), www.onepeloton.com

Activity Questionnaire

- *PAR-Q+ and ePARmed-X+*
  https://eparmedx.com
- *Physical Activity Readiness Questionnaire for Everyone (PAR-Q+)*
  American College of Sports Medicine. *ACSM's Guidelines for Exercise Testing and Prescription,* 11th ed. Philadelphia, PA: Wolters Kluwer; 2022. www.acsm.org/docs/default-source/files-for-resource-library/par-q-acsm.pdf
- *The Physical Activity Vital Sign*
  American College of Sports Medicine. *Exercise is Medicine. Physical Activity Vital Sign*. https://exerciseismedicine.org/wp-content/uploads/2021/04/EIM-Physical-Activity-Vital-Sign.pdf

Physical Performance Tests for Low Back Pain

- *1-minute Stair Climbing, 50-Foot Walk, and Timed Up-and-Go Tests*
  Jakobsson M, Brisby H, Gutke A, Lundberg M, Smeets R. One-minute stair climbing, 50-foot walk, and timed up-and-go were responsive measures for patients with chronic low back pain undergoing lumbar fusion surgery. *BMC Musculoskelet Disord*. 2019;20(1):137.

- *5-Minute Walking, 1-Minute Stair-Climbing, Sit-to-Stand Tests*
  Smeets RJ, Hijdra HJ, Kester AD, Hitters MW, Knottnerus JA. The usability of six physical performance tasks in a rehabilitation population with chronic low back pain. *Clin Rehabil.* 2006;20(11):989–997.

Assessing General Exercise Intensity

- *Exercise Testing Guidelines*
  American College of Sports Medicine. *ACSM's Guidelines for Exercise Testing and Prescription,* 11th ed. Philadelphia, PA: Wolters Kluwer; 2022.
- *Borg Rating of Perceived Exertion Scale*
  Borg GA. *Borg's Perceived Exertion and Pain Scale.* Champaign, IL: Human Kinetics; 1998.
- *OMNI Resistance Exercise Scale of Perceived Exertion*
  Robertson RJ, Goss FL, Rutkowski J, *et al.* Concurrent validation of the OMNI perceived exertion scale for resistance exercise. *Med Sci Sports Exerc.* 2003;35(2):333–341.
- *OMNI-Cycle Scale of Perceived Exertion*
  Robertson RJ, Goss FL, Dube J, *et al.* Validation of the adult OMNI scale of perceived exertion for cycle ergometer exercise. *Med Sci Sports Exerc.* 2004;36(1):102–108.
- *Talk Test*
  Foster C, Porcari JP, Anderson J, Paulson M, Smaczny D, Webber H, Doberstein ST, Udermann B. The talk test as a marker of exercise training intensity. *J Cardiopulm Rehabil Prev.* 2008;28(1):24–30.

Weight Management Resources

- Compendium of Physical Activities (to estimate the energy cost of activities), https://sites.google.com/site/compendiumofphysicalactivities/home
- National Weight Control Registry (long-term successful weight loss maintenance strategies), www.nwcr.ws

References

Altug Z. *Integrative Healing: Developing Wellness in the Mind and Body.* Springville, UT: Cedar Fort, Inc; 2018.

Altug Z. Exercise, dance, tai chi, Pilates, and Alexander technique. In: Ishak WW, ed. *The Handbook of Wellness Medicine.* Cambridge, United Kingdom: Cambridge University Press; 2020.

Altug Z, Gensler TO. *The Anti-Aging Fitness Prescription.* New York, NY: Hatherleigh Press; 2006.

Amedoro A, Berardi A, Conte A, *et al.* The effect of aquatic physical therapy on patients with multiple sclerosis: a systematic review and meta-analysis. *Mult Scler Relat Disord.* 2020;41:102022.

American College of Sports Medicine. *ACSM's Guidelines for Exercise Testing and Prescription,* 11th ed. Philadelphia, PA: Wolters Kluwer; 2022.

American College of Sports Medicine, Chodzko-Zajko WJ, Proctor DN, *et al.* American College of Sports Medicine position stand. Exercise and physical activity for older adults. *Med Sci Sports Exerc.* 2009;41(7):1510–1530.

Araujo CG, de Souza, E Silva CG, Laukkanen JA, *et al.* Successful 10-second one-legged stance performance predicts survival in middle-aged and older individuals. *Br J Sports Med.* 2022;56(17):975–980.

Assumpção A, Matsutani LA, Yuan SL, *et al.* Muscle stretching exercises and resistance training in fibromyalgia: which is better? A three-arm randomized controlled trial. *Eur J Phys Rehabil Med.* 2018;54(5):663–670.

Baena-Beato PÁ, Artero EG, Arroyo-Morales M, Robles-Fuentes A, Gatto-Cardia MC, Delgado-Fernández M. Aquatic therapy improves pain, disability, quality of life, body composition and fitness in sedentary adults with chronic low back pain. A controlled clinical trial. *Clin Rehabil.* 2014;28(4):350–360.

Bonanno L, Metro D, Papa M, *et al.* Assessment of sleep and obesity in adults and children: observational study. *Medicine (Baltimore).* 2019;98(46):e17642.

Bossers WJ, van der Woude LH, Boersma F, Hortobágyi T, Scherder EJ, van Heuvelen MJ. A 9-week aerobic and strength training program improves cognitive and motor function in patients with dementia: a randomized, controlled trial. *Am J Geriatr Psychiatry.* 2015;23(11):1106–1116.

Brody LT, Geigle PR. *Aquatic Exercise for Rehabilitation and Training.* Champaign, IL: Human Kinetics; 2009.

Camacho PM, Petak SM, Binkley N, *et al.* American Association of Clinical Endocrinologists/American College of Endocrinology Clinical Practice Guidelines for the Diagnosis and Treatment of Postmenopausal Osteoporosis—2020 Update. *Endocr Pract.* 2020;26(Suppl 1):1–46.

Carpes L, Costa R, Schaarschmidt B, Reichert T, Ferrari R. High-intensity interval training reduces blood pressure in older adults: a systematic review and meta-analysis. *Exp Gerontol.* 2022;158:111657.

Carroll LM, Volpe D, Morris ME, Saunders J, Clifford AM. Aquatic exercise therapy for people with Parkinson disease: a randomized controlled trial. *Arch Phys Med Rehabil.* 2017;98(4):631–638.

Cerini T, Hilfiker R, Riegler TF, Felsch QTM. 12 weeks high intensity interval training versus moderate intensity continuous training in chronic low back pain subjects: a randomised single-blinded feasibility study. *Arch Physiother.* 2022;12(1):12.

Cha HG, Shin YJ, Kim MK. Effects of the Bad Ragaz Ring Method on muscle activation of the lower limbs and balance ability in chronic stroke: a randomised controlled trial. *Hong Kong Physiother J.* 2017;37:39–45.

Coelho-Júnior HJ, Gonçalves IO, Sampaio RAC, *et al.* Effects of combined resistance and power training on cognitive function in older women: a randomized controlled trial. *Int J Environ Res Public Health.* 2020;17(10):3435.

Conraads VM, Pattyn N, De Maeyer C, *et al.* Aerobic interval training and continuous training equally improve aerobic exercise capacity in patients with coronary artery disease: the SAINTEX-CAD study. *Int J Cardiol.* 2015;179:203–210.

Cuyul-Vásquez I, Álvarez E, Riquelme A, Zimmermann R, Araya-Quintanilla F. Effectiveness of unilateral training of the uninjured limb on muscle strength and knee function of patients with anterior cruciate ligament reconstruction: a systematic review and meta-analysis of cross-education. *J Sport Rehabil.* 2022;31(5):605–616.

Devasahayam AJ, Farwell K, Lim B, *et al.* The effect of reactive balance training on falls in daily life: an updated systematic review and meta-analysis. *Physical Therapy.* 2022;pzac154.

Escamilla RF, Lewis C, Pecson A, Imamura R, Andrews JR. Muscle activation among supine, prone, and side position exercises with and without a Swiss Ball. *Sports Health.* 2016;8(4):372–379.

Fernández-Rodríguez R, Álvarez-Bueno C, Cavero-Redondo I, *et al.* Best exercise options for reducing pain and disability in adults with chronic low back pain: Pilates, strength, core-based, and mind-body. A network meta-analysis. *J Orthop Sports Phys Ther.* 2022;52(8):505–521.

Ferreira RM, Alves WMGDC, de Lima TA, *et al.* The effect of resistance training on the anxiety symptoms and quality of life in elderly people with Parkinson's disease: a randomized controlled trial [published correction appears in *Arq Neuropsiquiatr.* 2018 Dec;76(12):1]. *Arq Neuropsiquiatr.* 2018;76(8):499–506.

Ferreira RM, Torres RT, Duarte JA, Gonçalves RS. Non-pharmacological and non-surgical interventions for knee osteoarthritis: a systematic review and meta-analysis. *Acta Reumatol Port.* 2019;44(3):173–217.

Francois ME, Baldi JC, Manning PJ, *et al.* 'Exercise snacks' before meals: a novel strategy to improve glycaemic control in individuals with insulin resistance. *Diabetologia.* 2014;57(7):1437–1445.

Gamborg M, Hvid LG, Dalgas U, Langeskov-Christensen M. Parkinson's disease and intensive exercise therapy: an updated systematic review and meta-analysis. *Acta Neurol Scand.* 2022;145(5):504–528.

Garber CE, Blissmer B, Deschenes MR, *et al.* American College of Sports Medicine position stand. Quantity and quality of exercise for developing and maintaining cardiorespiratory, musculoskeletal, and neuromotor fitness in apparently healthy adults: guidance for prescribing exercise. *Med Sci Sports Exerc.* 2011;43(7):1334–1359.

Ge L, Sadeghirad B, Ball GDC, *et al.* Comparison of dietary macronutrient patterns of 14 popular named dietary programmes for weight and cardiovascular risk factor reduction in adults: systematic review and network meta-analysis of randomised trials. *BMJ.* 2020 Apr 1;369:m696.

Gordon BR, McDowell CP, Hallgren M, Meyer JD, Lyons M, Herring MP. Association of efficacy of resistance exercise training with depressive symptoms: meta-analysis and meta-regression analysis of randomized clinical trials. *JAMA Psychiatry.* 2018;75(6):566–576.

Gordon BR, McDowell CP, Lyons M, Herring MP. The effects of resistance exercise training on anxiety: a meta-analysis and meta-regression analysis of randomized controlled trials. *Sports Med.* 2017;47(12):2521–2532.

Grier T, Canham-Chervak M, Anderson MK, Bushman TT, Jones BH. The effects of cross-training on fitness and injury in women. *US Army Med Dep J.* 2015;33–41.

Gurpinar B, Kara B, Idiman E. Effects of aquatic exercises on postural control and hand function in multiple sclerosis: Halliwick versus Aquatic Plyometric Exercises: a randomised trial. *J Musculoskelet Neuronal Interact.* 2020;20(2):249–255.

Halvarsson A, Franzén E, Ståhle A. Balance training with multi-task exercises improves fall-related self-efficacy, gait, balance performance and physical function in older adults with osteoporosis: a randomized controlled trial. *Clin Rehabil.* 2015;29(4):365–375.

Hindle BR, Lorimer A, Winwood P, Keogh JWL. The biomechanics and applications of strongman exercises: a systematic review [published correction appears in *Sports Med Open.* 2020 Feb 5;6(1):8]. *Sports Med Open.* 2019;5(1):49.

Inoue K, Fujioka S, Nagaki K, *et al.* Table tennis for patients with Parkinson's disease: a single-center, prospective pilot study. *Clin Park Relat Disord.* 2020;4:100086.

Islam H, Gibala MJ, Little JP. Exercise snacks: a novel strategy to improve cardiometabolic health. *Exerc Sport Sci Rev.* 2022;50(1):31–37.

Jakicic JM, Kraus WE, Powell KE, *et al.* Association between bout duration of physical activity and health: systematic review. *Med Sci Sports Exerc.* 2019;51(6):1213–1219.

Jakicic JM, Wing RR, Butler BA, Robertson RJ. Prescribing exercise in multiple short bouts versus one continuous bout: effects on adherence, cardiorespiratory fitness, and weight loss in overweight women. *Int J Obes Relat Metab Disord.* 1995;19(12):893–901.

Jenkins EM, Nairn LN, Skelly LE, Little JP, Gibala MJ. Do stair climbing exercise "snacks" improve cardiorespiratory fitness? *Appl Physiol Nutr Metab.* 2019;44(6):681–684.

Johansson ME, Cameron IGM, Van der Kolk NM, *et al.* Aerobic exercise alters brain function and structure in Parkinson's disease: a randomized controlled trial. *Ann Neurol.* 2022;91(2):203–216.

Kim B, Yim J. Core stability and hip exercises improve physical function and activity in patients with non-specific low back pain: a randomized controlled trial. *Tohoku J Exp Med.* 2020;251(3):193–206.

Kim H, Reece J, Kang M. Effects of accumulated short bouts of exercise on weight and obesity indices in adults: a meta-analysis. *Am J Health Promot.* 2020;34(1):96–104.

Kurt EE, Büyükturan B, Büyükturan Ö, Erdem HR, Tuncay F. Effects of Ai Chi on balance, quality of life, functional mobility, and motor impairment in patients with Parkinson's disease. *Disabil Rehabil.* 2018;40(7):791–797.

LeBouthillier DM, Asmundson GJG. The efficacy of aerobic exercise and resistance training as transdiagnostic interventions for anxiety-related disorders and constructs: a randomized controlled trial. *J Anxiety Disord.* 2017;52:43–52.

Liao CD, Tsauo JY, Lin LF, *et al.* Effects of elastic resistance exercise on body composition and physical capacity in older women with sarcopenic obesity: a CONSORT-compliant prospective randomized controlled trial. *Medicine (Baltimore).* 2017;96(23):e7115.

Little JP, Langley J, Lee M, *et al.* Sprint exercise snacks: a novel approach to increase aerobic fitness. *Eur J Appl Physiol.* 2019;119(5):1203–1212.

Liu JX, Zhu L, Li PJ, Li N, Xu YB. Effectiveness of high-intensity interval training on glycemic control and cardiorespiratory fitness in patients with Type 2 diabetes: a systematic review and meta-analysis. *Aging Clin Exp Res.* 2019;31(5):575–593.

Liu-Ambrose T, Davis JC, Best JR, *et al.* Effect of a home-based exercise program on subsequent falls among community-dwelling high-risk older adults after a fall: a randomized clinical trial [published correction appears in *JAMA.* 2019 Jul 9;322(2):174]. *JAMA.* 2019;321(21):2092–2100.

Lopes S, Mesquita-Bastos J, Garcia C, *et al.* Effect of exercise training on ambulatory blood pressure among patients with resistant hypertension: a randomized clinical trial. *JAMA Cardiol.* 2021;6(11):1317–1323.

Loureiro APC, Burkot J, Oliveira J, Barbosa JM. WATSU therapy for individuals with Parkinson's disease to improve quality of sleep and quality of life: a randomized controlled study. *Complement Ther Clin Pract.* 2022;46:101523.

Mabire L, Mani R, Liu L, Mulligan H, Baxter D. The influence of age, sex and body mass index on the effectiveness of brisk walking for obesity management in adults: a systematic review and meta-analysis. *J Phys Act Health*. 2017;14(5):389–407.

Malfliet A, Quiroz Marnef A, Nijs J, *et al.* Obesity hurts: the why and how of integrating weight reduction with chronic pain management. *Phys Ther*. 2021;101(11):pzab198.

Marcos-Pardo PJ, Orquin-Castrillón FJ, Gea-García GM, *et al.* Effects of a moderate-to-high intensity resistance circuit training on fat mass, functional capacity, muscular strength, and quality of life in elderly: a randomized controlled trial. *Sci Rep*. 2019;9(1):7830.

McClung MR, Pinkerton JV, Blake J, *et al.* Management of osteoporosis in postmenopausal women: the 2021 position statement of The North American Menopause Society. *Menopause*. 2021;28(9):973–997.

McGill SM, McDermott A, Fenwick CM. Comparison of different strongman events: trunk muscle activation and lumbar spine motion, load, and stiffness. *J Strength Cond Res*. 2009;23(4):1148–1161.

Moraes HS, Silveira HS, Oliveira NA, *et al.* Is strength training as effective as aerobic training for depression in older adults? A randomized controlled trial. *Neuropsychobiology*. 2020;79(2):141–149.

Nikander R, Kannus P, Dastidar P, *et al.* Targeted exercises against hip fragility. *Osteoporos Int*. 2009;20(8):1321–1328.

Olsson K, Franzén E, Johansson A. A pilot study of the feasibility and effects of table tennis training in Parkinson disease. *Arch Rehabil Res Clin Transl*. 2020;2(3):100064.

Paquette MR, Peel SA, Smith RE, Temme M, Dwyer JN. The impact of different cross-training modalities on performance and injury-related variables in high school cross country runners. *J Strength Cond Res*. 2018;32(6):1745–1753.

Park C, Son H, Yeo B. The effects of lower extremity cross-training on gait and balance in stroke patients: a double-blinded randomized controlled trial. *Eur J Phys Rehabil Med*. 2021;57(1):4–12.

Peng MS, Wang R, Wang YZ, *et al.* Efficacy of therapeutic aquatic exercise vs physical therapy modalities for patients with chronic low back pain: a randomized clinical trial. *JAMA Netw Open*. 2022;5(1):e2142069.

Pérez de la Cruz S. Effectiveness of aquatic therapy for the control of pain and increased functionality in people with Parkinson's disease: a randomized clinical trial. *Eur J Phys Rehabil Med*. 2017;53(6):825–832.

Pérez Ramírez N, Nahuelhual Cares P, San Martín Peñailillo P. Efectividad de la terapia Watsu en pacientes con artritis idiopática juvenil. Un ensayo clínico controlado paralelo, aleatorio y simple ciego [Effectiveness of Watsu therapy in patients with juvenile idiopathic arthritis. A parallel, randomized, controlled and single-blind clinical trial]. *Rev Chil Pediatr*. 2019;90(3):283–292.

Perkin OJ, McGuigan PM, Stokes KA. Exercise snacking to improve muscle function in healthy older adults: a pilot study. *J Aging Res*. 2019:7516939.

Pinheiro MB, Oliveira J, Bauman A, Fairhall N, Kwok W, Sherrington C. Evidence on physical activity and osteoporosis prevention for people aged 65+ years: a systematic review to inform the WHO guidelines on physical activity and sedentary behaviour. *Int J Behav Nutr Phys Act*. 2020;17(1):150.

Poon ET, Little JP, Sit CH, Wong SH. The effect of low-volume high-intensity interval training on cardiometabolic health and psychological responses in overweight/obese middle-aged men. *J Sports Sci*. 2020;38(17):1997–2004.

Rafiei H, Omidian K, Myette-Côté É, Little JP. Metabolic effect of breaking up prolonged sitting with stair climbing exercise snacks. *Med Sci Sports Exerc*. 2021;53(1):150–158.

Razazian N, Kazeminia M, Moayedi H, *et al.* The impact of physical exercise on the fatigue symptoms in patients with multiple sclerosis: a systematic review and meta-analysis. *BMC Neurol*. 2020;20(1):93.

Recchia F, Leung CK, Chin EC, *et al.* Comparative effectiveness of exercise, antidepressants and their combination in treating non-severe depression: a systematic review and network meta-analysis of randomised controlled trials. *Br J Sports Med*. 2022;56(23):1375–1380.

Remde A, DeTurk SN, Almardini A, Steiner L, Wojda T. Plant-predominant eating patterns: how effective are they for treating obesity and related cardiometabolic health outcomes? A systematic review [published online ahead of print, 2021 Sep 8]. *Nutr Rev*. 2021;nuab060.

Rewald S, Lenssen AFT, Emans PJ, de Bie RA, van Breukelen G, Mesters I. Aquatic cycling improves knee pain and physical functioning in patients with knee osteoarthritis: a randomized controlled trial. *Arch Phys Med Rehabil*. 2020;101(8):1288–1295.

Salik Sengul Y, Yilmaz A, Kirmizi M, Kahraman T, Kalemci O. Effects of stabilization exercises on disability, pain, and core stability in patients with non-specific low back pain: a randomized controlled trial. *Work*. 2021;70(1):99–107.

Sampath Kumar A, Maiya AG, Shastry BA, *et al.* Exercise and insulin resistance in Type 2 diabetes mellitus: a systematic review and meta-analysis. *Ann Phys Rehabil Med*. 2019;62(2):98–103.

Santos SM, da Silva RA, Terra MB, Almeida IA, de Melo LB, Ferraz HB. Balance versus resistance training on postural control in patients with

Parkinson's disease: a randomized controlled trial. *Eur J Phys Rehabil Med.* 2017;53(2):173–183.

Sasaki M, Sasaki KI, Ishizaki Y, *et al.* Safety and efficacy of a bodyweight exercise training program in symptomatic patients with severe aortic valve stenosis. *Am J Cardiol.* 2023;186:163–169.

Schmidt WD, Biwer CJ, Kalscheuer LK. Effects of long versus short bout exercise on fitness and weight loss in overweight females. *J Am Coll Nutr.* 2001;20(5):494–501.

Seo YG, Noh HM, Kim SY. Weight loss effects of circuit training interventions: a systematic review and meta-analysis. *Obes Rev.* 2019;20(11):1642–1650.

Shariat A, Cleland JA, Danaee M, Kargarfard M, Sangelaji B, Tamrin SBM. Effects of stretching exercise training and ergonomic modifications on musculoskeletal discomforts of office workers: a randomized controlled trial. *Braz J Phys Ther.* 2018;22(2):144–153.

Shi J, Hu ZY, Wen YR, *et al.* Optimal modes of mind-body exercise for treating chronic non-specific low back pain: systematic review and network meta-analysis. *Front Neurosci.* 2022;16:1046518.

Shi Z, Zhou H, Lu L, *et al.* Aquatic exercises in the treatment of low back pain: a systematic review of the literature and meta-analysis of eight studies. *Am J Phys Med Rehabil.* 2018;97(2):116–122.

Siu PM, Yu AP, Chin EC, *et al.* Effects of tai chi or conventional exercise on central obesity in middle-aged and older adults: a three-group randomized controlled trial. *Ann Intern Med.* 2021;174(8):1050–1057.

Soke F, Guclu-Gunduz A, Kocer B, Fidan I, Keskinoglu P. Task-oriented circuit training combined with aerobic training improves motor performance and balance in people with Parkinson's disease. *Acta Neurol Belg.* 2021;121(2):535–543.

Somers TJ, Blumenthal JA, Dorfman CS, *et al.* Effects of a weight and pain management program in patients with rheumatoid arthritis with obesity: a randomized controlled pilot investigation. *J Clin Rheumatol.* 2022;28(1):7–13.

Spadaro KC, Davis KK, Sereika SM, Gibbs BB, Jakicic JM, Cohen SM. Effect of mindfulness meditation on short-term weight loss and eating behaviors in overweight and obese adults: a randomized controlled trial. *J Complement Integr Med.* 2017;15(2):/j/jcim.2018.

Stamatakis E, Ahmadi MN, Friedenreich CM, *et al.* Vigorous intermittent lifestyle physical activity and cancer incidence among nonexercising adults: The UK Biobank Accelerometry Study [published online ahead of print, 2023 Jul 27]. *JAMA Oncol.* 2023;e231830.

Stojanović MDM, Mikić MJ, Milošević Z, Vuković J, Jezdimirović T, Vučetić V. Effects of chair-based, low-load elastic band resistance training on functional fitness and metabolic biomarkers in older women. *J Sports Sci Med.* 2021;20(1):133–141.

Stonerock GL, Hoffman BM, Smith PJ, Blumenthal JA. Exercise as treatment for anxiety: systematic review and analysis. *Ann Behav Med.* 2015;49(4):542–556.

Tahran Ö, Yeşilyaprak SS. Effects of modified posterior shoulder stretching exercises on shoulder mobility, pain, and dysfunction in patients with subacromial impingement syndrome. *Sports Health.* 2020;12(2):139–148.

Tanaka H. Effects of cross-training. Transfer of training effects on VO2max between cycling, running and swimming. *Sports Med.* 1994;18(5):330–339.

Taul-Madsen L, Connolly L, Dennett R, Freeman J, Dalgas U, Hvid LG. Is aerobic or resistance training the most effective exercise modality for improving lower extremity physical function and perceived fatigue in people with multiple sclerosis? A systematic review and meta-analysis. *Arch Phys Med Rehabil.* 2021;102(10):2032–2048.

Tripp F, Krakow K. Effects of an aquatic therapy approach (Halliwick-Therapy) on functional mobility in subacute stroke patients: a randomized controlled trial. *Clin Rehabil.* 2014;28(5):432–439.

Tunwattanapong P, Kongkasuwan R, Kuptniratsaikul V. The effectiveness of a neck and shoulder stretching exercise program among office workers with neck pain: a randomized controlled trial. *Clin Rehabil.* 2016;30(1):64–72.

Turner MN, Hernandez DO, Cade W, Emerson CP, Reynolds JM, Best TM. The role of resistance training dosing on pain and physical function in individuals with knee osteoarthritis: a systematic review. *Sports Health.* 2020;12(2):200–206.

U.S. Department of Health and Human Services. *Physical Activity Guidelines for Americans*, 2nd ed. 2018. https://health.gov/sites/default/files/2019-09/Physical_Activity_Guidelines_2nd_edition.pdf

van de Port IG, Wevers LE, Lindeman E, Kwakkel G. Effects of circuit training as alternative to usual physiotherapy after stroke: randomised controlled trial. *BMJ.* 2012;344:e2672.

Vanti C, Andreatta S, Borghi S, Guccione AA, Pillastrini P, Bertozzi L. The effectiveness of walking versus exercise on pain and function in chronic low back pain: a systematic review and meta-analysis of randomized trials. *Disabil Rehabil.* 2019;41(6):622–632.

Watson SL, Weeks BK, Weis LJ, Harding AT, Horan SA, Beck BR. High-intensity resistance and impact training improves bone mineral density and physical function in postmenopausal women with osteopenia and osteoporosis: the LIFTMOR randomized controlled trial [published correction appears in *J Bone Miner Res.* 2019 Mar;34(3):572]. *J Bone Miner Res.* 2018;33(2):211–220.

Watt JR, Jackson K, Franz JR, Dicharry J, Evans J, Kerrigan DC. Effect of a supervised hip flexor stretching program on gait in elderly individuals. *PM R.* 2011;3(4):324–329.

Wu C, Bu R, Wang Y, *et al.* Rehabilitation effects of circuit resistance training in coronary heart disease patients: a systematic review and meta-analysis. *Clin Cardiol.* 2022;45(8):821–830.

Zhang YH, Hu HY, Xiong YC, *et al.* Exercise for neuropathic pain: a systematic review and expert consensus. *Front Med (Lausanne).* 2021;8:756940.

Zhong D, Xiao Q, Xiao X, *et al.* Tai chi for improving balance and reducing falls: an overview of 14 systematic reviews. *Ann Phys Rehabil Med.* 2020;63(6):505–517.

Additional Reading

Altug Z. Resistance exercise to improve cognitive function. *Strength and Conditioning Journal.* 2014;36(6):46–50.

Bezner JR. Promoting health and wellness: implications for physical therapist practice. *Phys Ther.* 2015;95(10):1433–1444.

Brito LB, Ricardo DR, Araújo DS, Ramos PS, Myers J, Araújo CG. Ability to sit and rise from the floor as a predictor of all-cause mortality. *Eur J Prev Cardiol.* 2014;21(7):892–898.

Dull H, Keating I, eds. *The Heart of WATSU: Therapeutic Applications in Clinical Practice.* London, United Kingdom: Singing Dragon; 2023.

Lundqvist S, Börjesson M, Cider Å, *et al.* Long-term physical activity on prescription intervention for patients with insufficient physical activity level: a randomized controlled trial. *Trials.* 2020;21(1):793.

Paluch AE, Gabriel KP, Fulton JE, *et al.* Steps per day and all-cause mortality in middle-aged adults in the coronary artery risk development in young adults study. *JAMA Netw Open.* 2021;4(9):e2124516.

Stamatakis E, Ahmadi MN, Gill JMR, *et al.* Association of wearable device-measured vigorous intermittent lifestyle physical activity with mortality. *Nat Med.* 2022;28(12):2521–2529.

CHAPTER 5

Mind-Body Movements

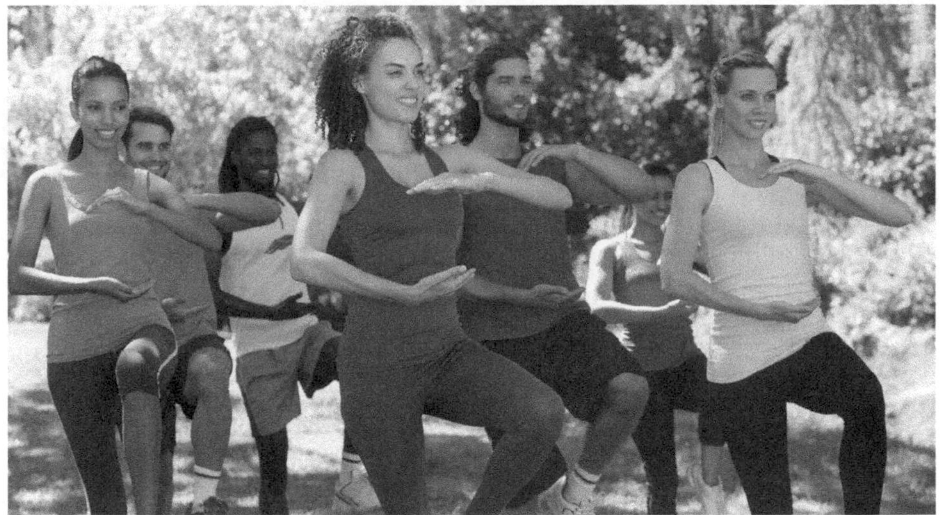

Tai chi for meditation in motion

Learning Objectives

- Understand basic research for using mind-body movements.
- Apply mind-body movements for practical pain management.

Chapter Highlights

- Key Concept: Yin-Yang
- Alexander Technique: Self-Care Lesson
- Feldenkrais Method: Self-Care Lesson
- Clinical Tip: Balance Assessment and Prescription
- Self-Care Handout 5.1: Mindful Walking Routine
- Self-Care Handout 5.2: Qigong Baduanjin Home Routine
- Self-Management Activities

- Classroom and Lab Activities
- Useful Clinical Resources
- References
- Additional Reading

Lifestyle Matters: *Think positive. Your body believes what your brain tells it.*

Introduction

The beauty and elegance of many mind-body movements are that they typically require very little or no equipment. Also, many mind-body movements have roots in Traditional Chinese Medicine and Ayurvedic Medicine. Traditional Chinese Medicine includes acupuncture and acupressure, massage, medicinal herbs, meditative exercise called tai chi, and therapeutic exercise called qigong. On the other hand, Ayurvedic Medicine is practiced in India and other Asian countries and includes massage that may include warm oils and heated herbal pouches, diet modifications, yoga, meditation, and therapeutic detoxification through enemas or nasal lavage.

Mind-body movements may be helpful for pain management and many other medical conditions, such as anxiety, asthma, cognitive impairments, depression, diabetes, multiple sclerosis, osteoarthritis, osteoporosis, and Parkinson's. The following figure outlines various integrative and mind-body movement strategies.

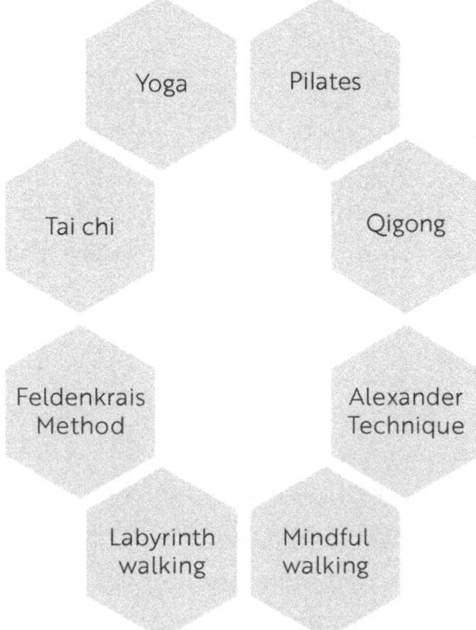

Integrative and mind-body movement strategies

The Merck Manual of Diagnosis and Therapy (Porter and Kaplan 2018, p.3152) indicates that mind-body medicine is "based on the theory that mental and emotional factors regulate physical health through a system of interdependent neuronal, hormonal, and immunologic connections throughout the body." This chapter focuses on mind-body movements such as mindful walking, labyrinth walking, yoga, Pilates, Alexander Technique, the Feldenkrais Method, tai chi, and qigong.

KEY CONCEPT: YIN-YANG

Yin-yang is an ancient Chinese philosophical concept of complementary opposites such as light and dark. The key is maintaining or restoring balance and harmony in mental and physical health (Venes 2021).

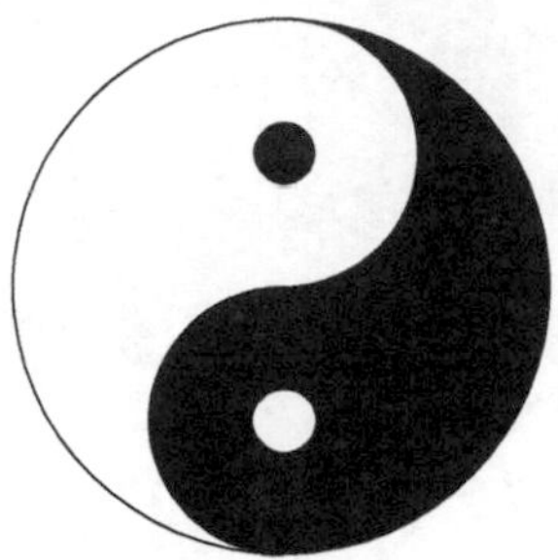

Integrative Movement Strategies

Mindful Walking

According to Kabat-Zinn and colleagues (Kabat-Zinn 1982; Kabat-Zinn *et al.* 1985; Kabat-Zinn *et al.* 1986; Kabat-Zinn *et al.* 1992), mindfulness meditation may help individuals to manage chronic pain and anxiety. A mindful walking program is a movement-based meditation that can help a person become focused on the present. Studies show that an integrated approach of walking meditation may be helpful for back pain (Banth and Ardebil 2015), improve the exercise capacity of individuals with chronic obstructive pulmonary disease (Lin *et al.* 2021), reduce psychological stress (Teut *et al.* 2013), and reduce university students' mood disturbances during a pandemic (Ma *et al.* 2022). Also, a study shows that walking may increase functional connectivity in the brain (Voss *et al.* 2010), and walking in nature can enhance cognitive functioning (Berman *et al.* 2008).

The following images show locations for performing a mindful walking program, and some ways to engage the senses during outdoor mindful walking, hiking, exercises, or physical activities. See Self-Care Handout 5.1 for a mindful walking routine.

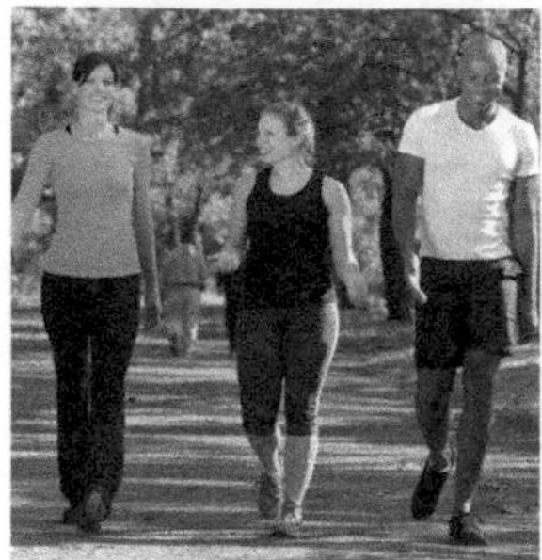

Mindful outdoor walk at a park

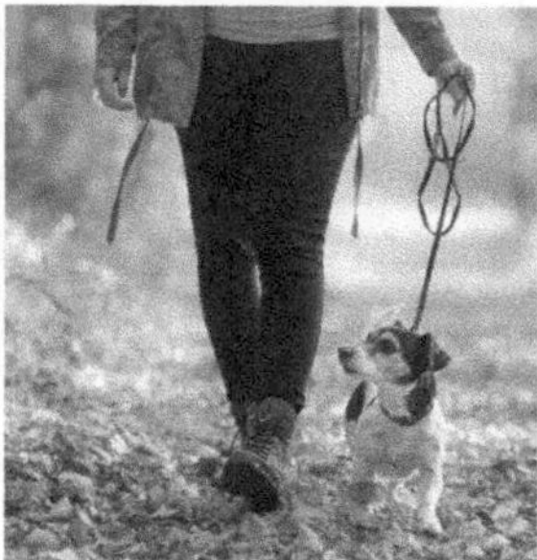

Mindful outdoor walk on a trail

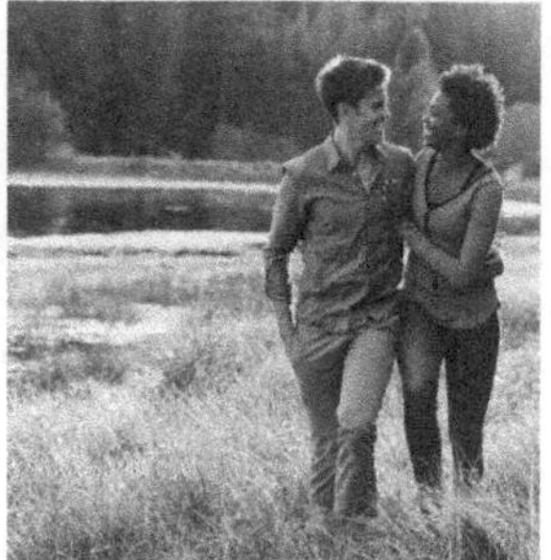

Mindful outdoor walk near a lake

Locations for performing a mindful walking program

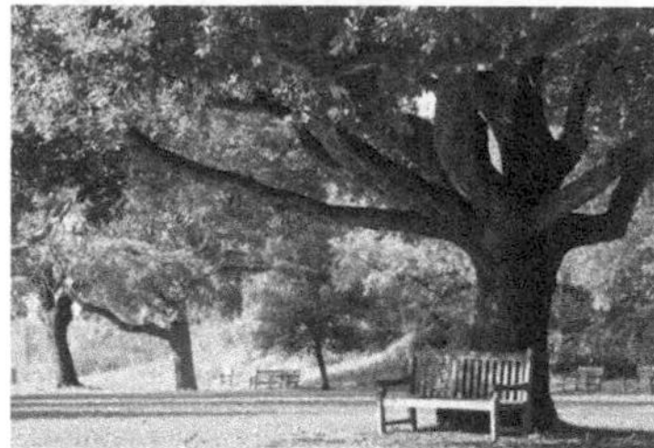

Sight—see the colors of nature

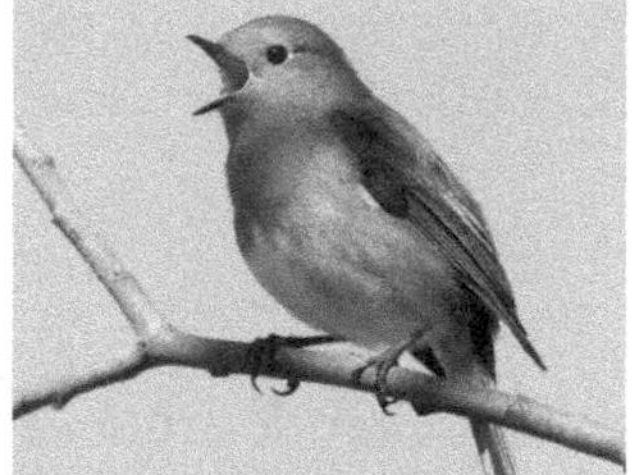

Hearing—hear the birds singing or the wind rustling the leaves

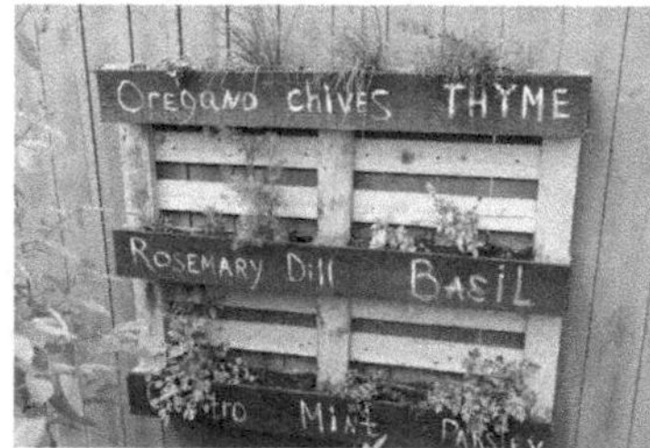

Smell—smell the aroma of the herbs, flowers, trees, lake, or ocean air

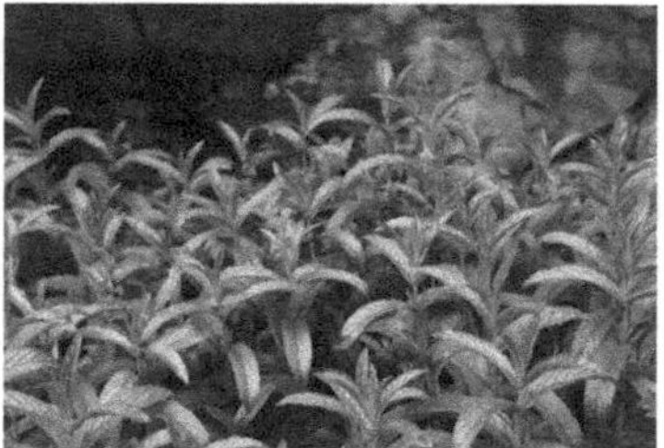

Taste—taste the mint leaves or fruits in a water bottle

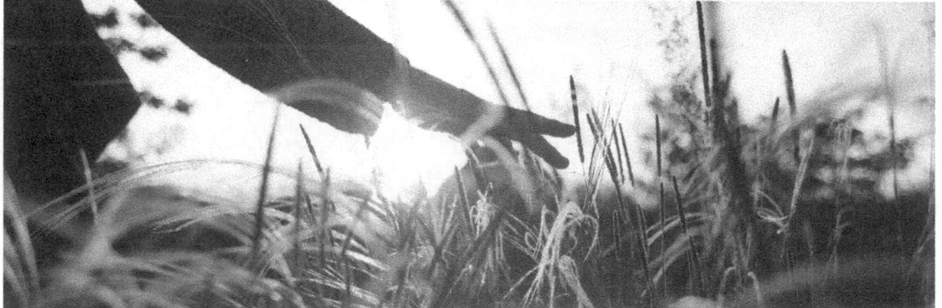

Touch—touch the tall grass during a walk or sense the ground with the feet

Engaging the senses during outdoor activities

Labyrinth Walking

The labyrinth is an ancient meditative tool that may be used for movement-based meditation, relaxation, reflection, stress reduction, and personal wellness (Altug 2018). The labyrinth is unlike a maze, since walking on a labyrinth path brings a person to the center and out again. In contrast, a maze has multiple paths and is designed to make a person lose their way. Some individuals in pain may find that walking in a labyrinth is comforting and helps reduce stress. Also, printing out labyrinth images for clients/patients to trace in clinical waiting areas may help reduce anxiety and stress.

A paper in the *Medicines* journal (Lizier *et al.* 2018) found that walking a labyrinth is a sensory, emotional, and physical experience. A study in the *Cogent Psychology* journal (Behman *et al.* 2018) found that walking a labyrinth path resulted in subjects having self-reported relaxation during and after the labyrinth walk. The following images show an outdoor and finger-tracing labyrinth.

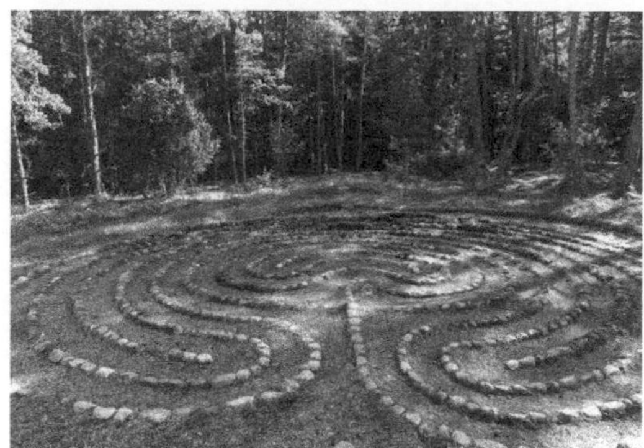

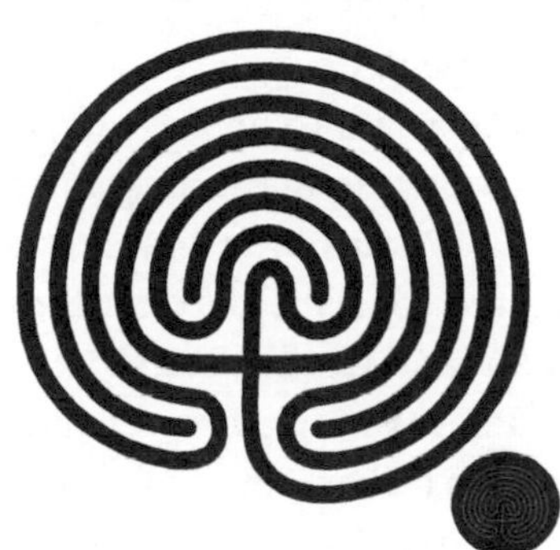

Outdoor and finger-tracing labyrinths

Yoga

According to Venes (2021), yoga is a system of traditional Hindu rituals, beliefs, and activities to help provide self-knowledge and spiritual enlightenment. The dictionary says that yoga is associated with physical postures called asanas and diaphragmatic breathing in the Western world. Yoga may be used to manage pain, insomnia, anxiety, and stress, and improve strength, flexibility, and balance. There are many styles of yoga, such as Restorative yoga, Iyengar yoga, Ashtanga yoga, Kundalini yoga, Bikram yoga, Yin yoga, and Vinyasa Flow.

Yoga may be beneficial for back pain (Aboagye *et al.* 2015; Saper *et al.* 2017), improved balance in postmenopausal osteoporotic women (Solakoglu *et al.* 2022), cancer-related fatigue (Lin *et al.* 2019), depression (de Manincor *et al.* 2016), diabetes (Jayawardena *et al.* 2018; Singh and Khandelwal 2020), hyperkyphosis (Greendale *et al.* 2009), knee osteoarthritis (Kuntz *et al.* 2018), multiple sclerosis (Hao *et al.* 2022), and Parkinson's (Kwok *et al.* 2019). Also, yoga may be helpful for military service members to help manage back pain (Groessl *et al.* 2017) and post-traumatic stress disorder (PTSD) (Bayley *et al.* 2022).

The following figure shows one yoga sequence variation for a Sun Salutation.

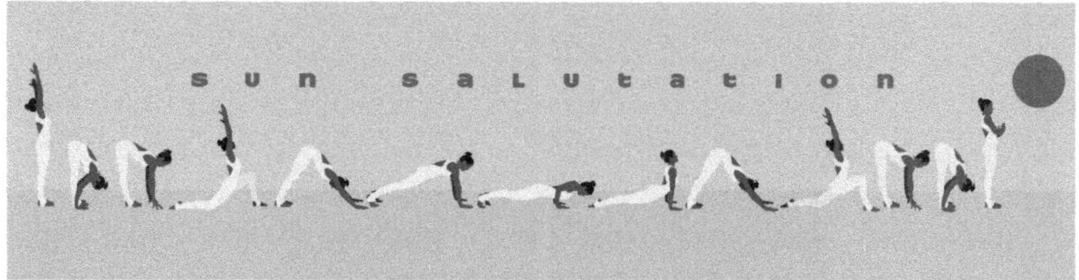

A variation of a yoga sequence

Pilates

Webster's New World College Dictionary (Webster's New World Dictionary 2016) defines Pilates as "an exercise program usually involving the use of special equipment, designed to strengthen the muscles of the abdomen, lower back, and buttocks and to improve overall flexibility and coordination." The method was created by German fitness instructor Joseph H. Pilates (1883–1967) who wrote two books (Pilates 1934; Pilates *et al.* 1945). Pilates designed a mat exercise series and created specialized exercise equipment such as the Reformer, Cadillac, Wunda Chair, and Ladder Barrel.

Pilates may be beneficial for anxiety and depression in postmenopausal women (Aibar-Almazán *et al.* 2019), chronic low back pain (Fernandez-Rodriguez *et al.* 2022; Natour *et al.* 2015), low back pain in pregnant women (Sonmezer *et al.* 2021), fibromyalgia (de Medeiros *et al.* 2020), improving mood disorders in overweight/obese individuals (Vancini *et al.* 2017), multiple sclerosis (Kalron *et al.* 2017), and Parkinson's (Suárez-Iglesias *et al.* 2019). The following images show a sample Pilates mat-based exercise, and a variety of Pilates equipment-based exercises.

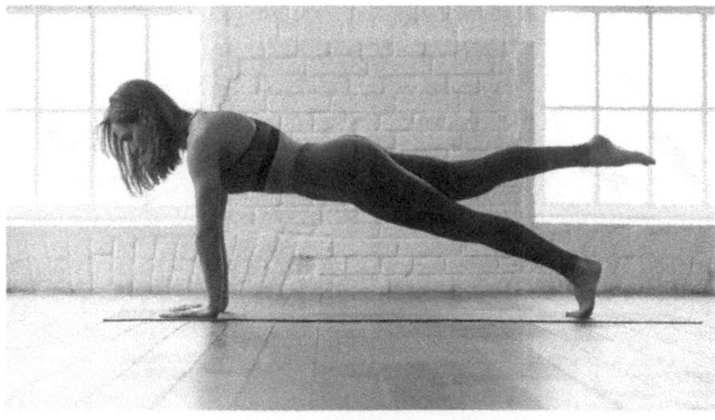

Mat-based Pilates exercise

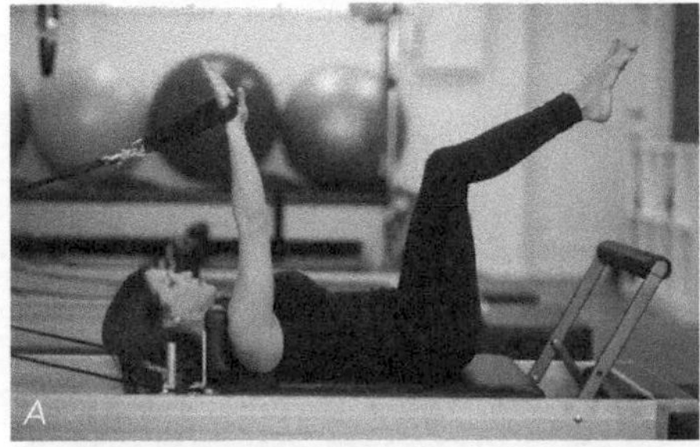

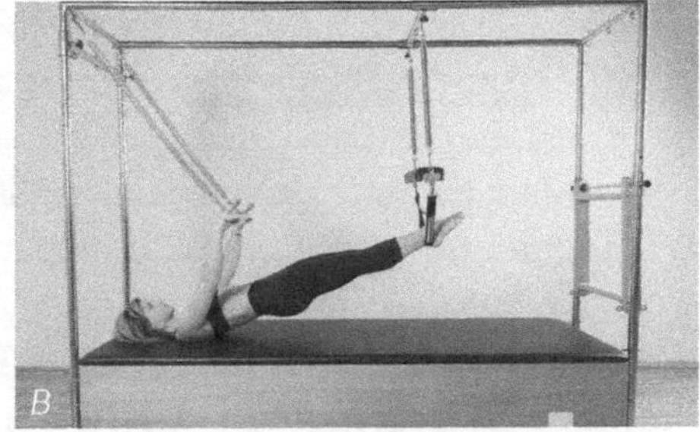

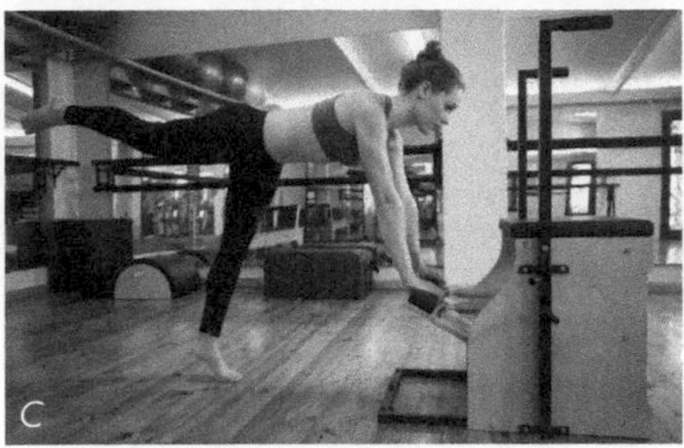

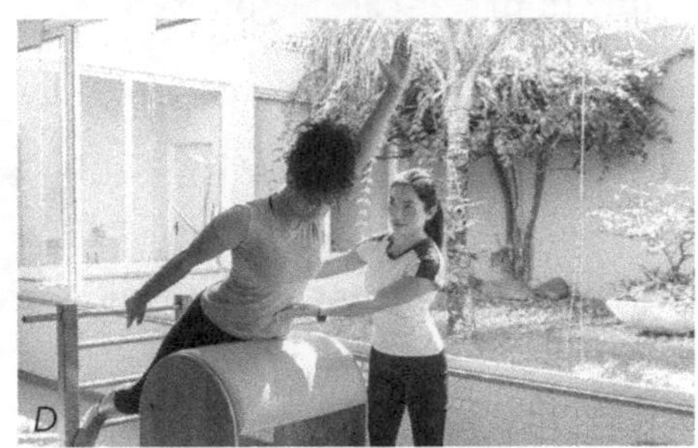

Equipment-based Pilates exercises: A) Reformer apparatus; B) Cadillac apparatus; C) Wunda Chair apparatus; D) Ladder Barrel apparatus

Alexander Technique

According to Venes (2021, p.79), the Alexander Technique (AT) is "A form of bodily training that promotes postural health, especially of the spine, head, and neck." The method was created by Australian actor Frederick Matthias Alexander (1869–1955) who wrote four books (Alexander 1918; 1923; 1932; 1941).

The American Society for the Alexander Technique (2023) states that, "By teaching how to change faulty postural habits, it enables improved mobility, posture, performance and alertness along with the relief of chronic stiffness, tension and stress."

Julie Shelton, M.AmSAT, shares, "The Alexander Technique allows you to open up to new possibilities of awareness in mental and physical well being. It will help you 'undo' unhealthy habits and bring you back to a neutral state. This neutrality will allow you to de-stress and take charge of your inner and physical well being" (Shelton n.d.)

The Alexander Technique is experiential. Typically, an Alexander Teacher accommodates you along your Alexander Technique journey to ensure and enliven your kinesthetic and proprioceptive awareness. Alexander Technique's sophisticated, gentle hands-on teaching approach will guide you to practice awareness, to avoid reacting automatically to the stimulus of life, and to redirect you to efficiently obtain optimal body posture. It is a conscious practice you can use anytime and anywhere.

The Alexander Technique may be beneficial for chronic back pain (Little *et al.* 2008), chronic neck pain (MacPherson *et al.* 2015), enhanced dynamic modulation of postural tone (Cacciatore *et al.* 2011), Parkinson's (Stallibrass *et al.* 2002), and performance anxiety in musicians (Klein *et al.* 2014). Additionally, the Alexander Technique may be useful to help musicians, singers, and performing artists improve posture and performance.

To view a video on the Alexander Technique's scientific model, see: https://youtu.be/YZaUgt8wyoY. The following shows a sample of an Alexander Technique mini self-care lesson.

■ Alexander Technique: Self-Care Lesson

Julie Shelton, M.AmSAT, CEAS

Name of movement: Dynamic Wall Exercise.

Purpose of movement: To gain insight about your back support and how the hips, back, and head can work dynamically with each other. Explore how the three joints in your hips, knees, and ankles work independently from your back.

Technique: Mindfully explore habitual patterns and unhealthy tension and release the patterns to allow you to perform with greater ease and less effort.

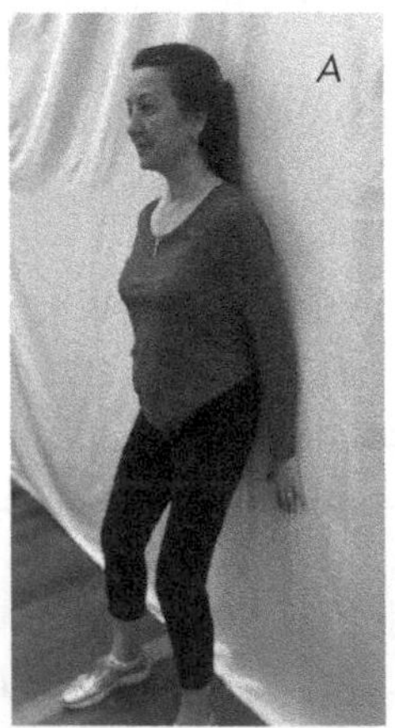

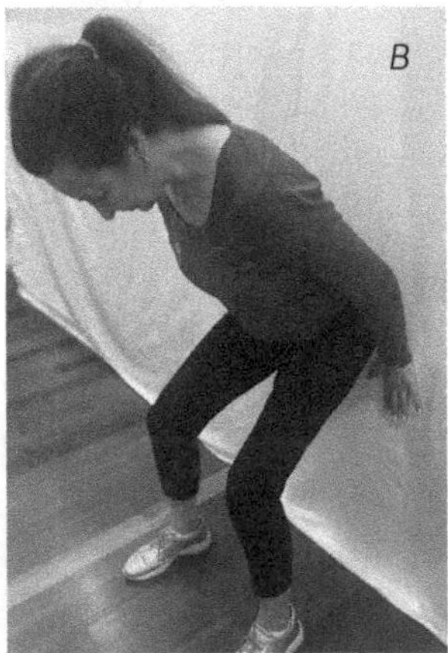

Alexander Technique—Dynamic Wall Exercise

The most basic activities can take us off balance, as we may slouch or over tense. Here's an exercise to go back to balance and promote lengthening of the spine. The pause and releases of the breath will help inhibit any tightening.

The set-up: Stand with your back to a wall, about 5 inches away. Feet are hip-width apart. Head is floating up.

1. Keeping your eyes open, start off with sensing your breath. Where do you notice your breath expanding in your body? Do you notice it at the upper chest, the abdomen, the back, or the side of your ribs? You don't have to do anything. Just notice. Allow the air to *come to you* as you breathe through your nose, in and out for 5 natural breaths.
2. Bring your hands behind you to meet the wall. Pause and release a breath.
3. Slowly bring your whole back to the wall as the heels are releasing down (the head is not touching the wall). Pause and release a breath (see Figure A).
4. Slowly release to bend the hips, knees, and ankles to come down the wall as far as it is comfortable. No need to push to flatten out the back. Allow the lower back to release on its own. Notice your shoulders releasing away from each other. Soft hips release away from each other. Pause and release a breath.
5. Thinking "up" with the head releasing from the hips, hinge over your hip joints leaving your tush on the wall as the back is lengthening (the head is dynamically opposing the tail bone). Think about your heels releasing to the floor. Pause and release a breath (see Figure B).
6. The hands gently guide you to push off the wall as the knees are still bent and come over your feet. The arms now rest to your side. Pause and release a breath.
7. Think about your heels releasing to the floor as your head leads you up to stand. Pause and release a breath.
8. Take a walk. What did you notice? Repeat the exercise 3 times.

This lesson was created by Julie Shelton, M.AmSAT, CEAS. Currently, Julie enjoys teaching at the California Institute of the Arts and Henry Mayo Hospital Educational Center (where she piloted a program for people living with Parkinson's) and teaching private sessions. Along with the Alexander Technique, Julie has a certificate in Primordial Sound Meditation and is an Ergonomic Assessment Specialist. She says, "I've searched for many years to find an intelligent natural approach to well-being and I hope you will find the Alexander Technique as fascinating and helpful as I have." To learn more, visit Julie at www.julieshelton.com or www.ReleaseAndLetGo.com.

Used with permission from Julie Shelton, M.AmSAT, CEAS.

Feldenkrais Method®

According to Venes (2021, p.922), the Feldenkrais Method is "A form of therapy devoted to improving limitations of range of motion, improving poor posture, and relieving stress." The method was created by Ukrainian physicist Dr. Moshe Feldenkrais (1904–1984) who wrote eight books (Feldenkrais 1944; 1949; 1952; 1972; 1977; 1981; 1984; Feldenkrais and Kimmey 1985).

Stacy Barrows, PT, DPT, GCFP, NCPT, a physical therapist and Guild Certified Feldenkrais Practitioner[CM], states that:

> The Feldenkrais Method is a unique body-centered learning process that is acquired through exploration of gentle sequenced movements which came to us naturally as infants. There are two formats that are used to optimize this form of learning. Functional Integration® (FI), often done one on one, uses a gentle informative touch that does not impose, but enlightens the student of ways to learn something different. The other format, Awareness Through Movement® (ATM), is usually taught in a group setting, using verbally guided movement sequences. These sequences provide a space to explore, in a non-dogmatic way, movement that becomes easy, elegant, and natural. (Barrows 2018; Barrows *et al.* 2021).

The Feldenkrais Method may be beneficial for balance (Berland *et al.* 2022; Connors *et al.* 2011), chronic back pain (Ahmadi *et al.* 2020; Paolucci *et al.* 2017), neck pain (Lundqvist *et al.* 2014), Parkinson's (Teixeira-Machado *et al.* 2015), and other conditions. The following shows a sample Feldenkrais Method mini self-care lesson.

■ Feldenkrais Method: Self-Care Lesson

Stacy Barrows, PT, DPT, GCFP, NCPT

Name of movement: Turning with ease.

Purpose of movement: To discover efficient turning without engaging internal resistance.

Technique: This is a short example of an Awareness Through Movement® lesson. This somatic puzzle optimizes the learning process best when used with small, slow, attentive movements while avoiding strain or pain.

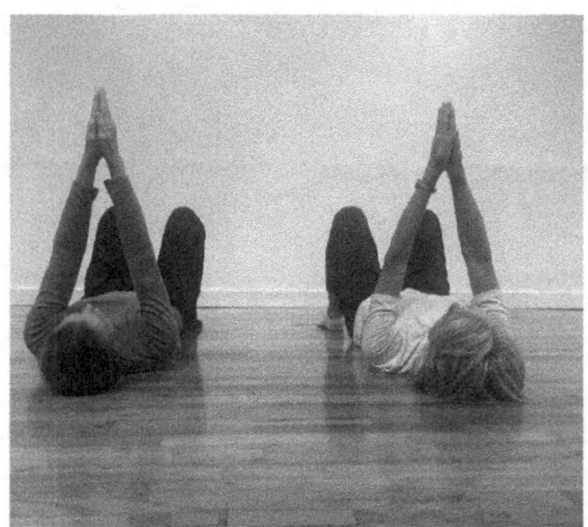

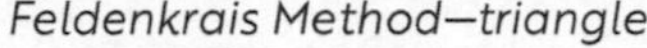

Feldenkrais Method—triangle

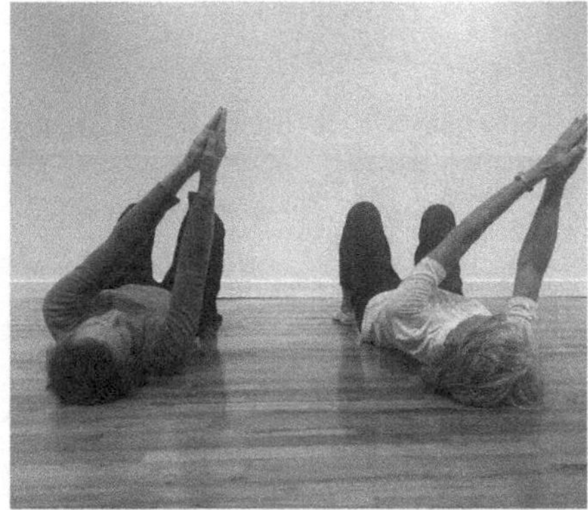

Feldenkrais Method—tilted triangle

1. Bend your knees to easily balance your legs, and roll your head gently side to side; notice the quality (this will be your reference movement).
2. Bring your arms to form a triangle (as seen in the first image above), and without deforming the triangle, or sliding your hands, tilt them side to side. Notice which side is easier, and how you do the movement. Repeat 5 times, each time with more ease. Rest.
3. With your knees still bent, tilt your legs gently side to side, without going to your end range. Again, repeat 5 times to notice the quality, your breath, and differences between the sides. Rest.
4. Bring your arms up into a triangle again. Begin to tilt your arms side to side. What does your head do? Does it stay still, move in the same or opposite direction? Notice first without changing.
5. Continue to tilt the arms side to side, and focus your eyes on something on the ceiling. How has the movement changed? Repeat 5 times. Rest.
6. Bring your arms back into the triangle, and this time allow your head and eyes to go with the movement. Repeat 5 times. Then, very gently, with half as much movement, turn your eyes and head in the opposite direction to the arm movement. Notice and repeat 5 times. Rest.
7. Return to your reference movement; slowly roll your head side to side. Has it changed? The key to improvement is to explore with curiosity, much as we did when we were infants.

This lesson created by Stacy Barrows, PT, DPT, GCFP, NCPT, is derived from lessons Dr. Feldenkrais developed to codify his method. Dr. Barrows combines her knowledge of physical therapy, the Feldenkrais Method, and Pilates to offer an integrative approach for self-care and learning. She patented a tool, the Smartroller®, authored the book *Smartroller Guide to*

Optimal Movement, and contributed to the recently published book *The Feldenkrais Method* on Feldenkrais and Pilates. Her passion is teaching somatic empowerment (embodied learning). To learn more, visit www.smartsomaticsolutions.com or www.smartroller.net.

Used with permission from Stacy Barrows, PT, DPT, GCFP, NCPT.

Tai Chi

Venes (2021) defines tai chi as a type of traditional Chinese martial art where a series of slow and controlled movements are performed to develop mental concentration, balance, coordination, flexibility, and strength. Tai chi involves multidirectional stepping and may help with dual task performance. The short form of tai chi has around 15–60 moves and may be good for individuals with memory impairments who have difficulty remembering too many movements. The long form of tai chi has about 80–130 moves and is good for building endurance. Interestingly, some practitioners use the long form to challenge memory. Finally, it should be noted that tai chi includes the Yang, Chen, Wu, Hao, and Sun styles. Each style emphasizes different movement patterns; some styles are gentle, while other styles are more intense. The key is to find the appropriate style and form for the individual.

Tai chi may be beneficial for anxiety and depression in patients with cancer, stroke, and heart failure (Cai *et al.* 2022), cognitive function (Liu *et al.* 2021a), diabetes (Qin *et al.* 2021), fall prevention (Li *et al.* 2018), fibromyalgia (Wang *et al.* 2018), knee osteoarthritis (Wang *et al.* 2016), low back pain (Qin *et al.* 2019), lung cancer (Cheung *et al.* 2021), multiple sclerosis (Taylor and Taylor-Piliae 2017), Parkinson's (Song *et al.* 2017), and stroke rehabilitation (Song *et al.* 2021). Also, tai chi may be helpful for military veterans to help manage post-traumatic stress symptoms (Niles *et al.* 2016). The following image shows tai chi movement patterns.

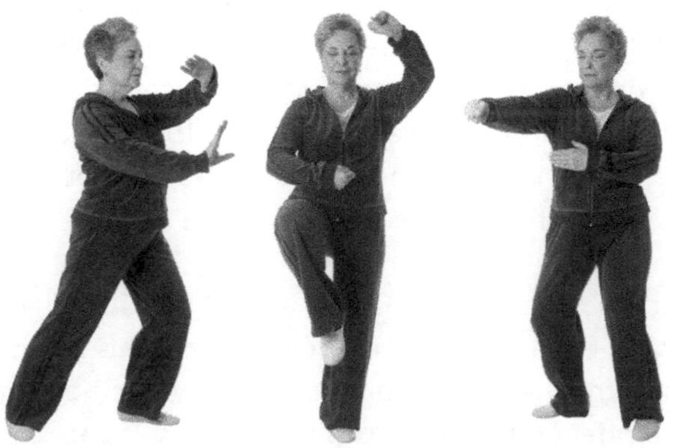

Tai chi movements

CLINICAL TIP: BALANCE ASSESSMENT AND PRESCRIPTION

Include balance assessments in clinical visits (Araujo *et al.* 2022). Balance assessments and balance exercise prescriptions are underutilized aspects of fitness. Include home program activities and single-leg stance exercises that challenge balance, such as:

- tai chi
- yoga Tree Pose
- slow march in place
- standing boxing movements in a step stance
- slow multidirectional stepping
- weight shifting forward and back, side to side
- heel raises
- heel-to-toe walking.

Qigong

Venes (2021) defines qigong (also written as qi gong and chi kung and pronounced as "che goong") as an ancient Chinese practice that combines movement, meditation, breathing exercises, and relaxation. *Qi* (breath, air, spirit) in traditional Chinese medicine means "energy of life" or "vital force." The earliest qigong-like exercises in China are from animal movements. *The Way of Qigong* (Cohen 1997) indicates that many qigong postures have names such as Bathing Duck, Leaping Monkey, Turning Tiger, Coiling Snake, Old Bear in the Woods, and Flying Crane.

There are many forms of qigong, such as:

- Eight Section Brocade Qigong (also known as Eight Strands of Brocade, Eight Pieces of Brocade, Eight Silken Movements, Baduanjin, or Ba Duan Jin) (Chinese Health Qigong Association 2008a; Liu and Perry 1997).
- Six Healing Sounds Qigong (*Liu Zi Jue*) (Chinese Health Qigong Association 2008b)
- Five Animal Qigong (*Wu Qin Xi*) (Chinese Health Qigong Association 2008c)
- Fragrant Qigong
- Guo Lin Qigong (walking qigong)
- Laughing Qigong
- Medical Qigong
- Tai Chi Qigong.

Qigong may be beneficial for back pain (Blödt *et al.* 2015; Li *et al.* 2019; Phattharasupharerk *et al.* 2019), cancer-related fatigue (Kuo *et al.* 2021), cognitive function (Lin *et al.* 2023; Wan *et al.* 2022; Wang *et al.* 2021), Type 2 diabetes (Wen *et al.*

2017), multiple sclerosis (Pan *et al.* 2022), Parkinson's (Lai *et al.* 2022; Zhang *et al.* 2022), and sleep (Chen *et al.* 2012). Also, qigong may be helpful for military service members to improve sleep and reduce stress (Reb *et al.* 2017).

In the form of Chinese qigong called the Six Healing Sounds (known as *Liu Zi Jue*) (Chinese Health Qigong Association 2008c), internal sounds are created by various breathing patterns and vocalizations. The healing sound form of qigong may, for example, be used for improving sleep in breast cancer survivors (Liu *et al.* 2015), reducing stress, and strengthening respiratory muscles (Feng *et al.* 2020), and for shortness of breath in patients with mild COVID-19 (Liu *et al.* 2021b; Qingguang *et al.* 2022). Other external healing sounds may be generated by bells, chimes, drums, flutes, gongs, Tibetan singing bowls (singing bowl meditation) (Goldsby *et al.* 2017), or tingshas (tiny cymbals).

Self-Care Education Guides

See **Self-Care Handout 5.1: Mindful Walking Routine** for a practical dynamic routine that can be performed in nature.

See **Self-Care Handout 5.2: Qigong Baduanjin Home Routine** for a simple mind-body qigong routine that can be used at home, in the garden, at the park or beach, or any location the individual chooses. Depending on the goals of the rehabilitation and wellness program, the following sequence may be performed once all the way through and repeated several times, or the person may perform each exercise several times before moving to the next sequence. The practitioner may also select several poses from the series to address a patient's/client's particular needs. For example, the practitioner may choose the Draw the Bow exercise if a person has limitations in cervical rotation. Also, the practitioner may choose to omit any motion that may increase pain or is not indicated for the patient/client.

For safety and optimal results, the key is to work with a qigong and tai chi professional to fine-tune all movements. The ten steps in this qigong routine were adapted from several sources (Altug 2018; Chinese Health Qigong Association 2008a; Liu *et al.* 1997) to create the home qigong (also known as Baduanjin) routine to help patients/clients manage pain, improve balance, and reduce stress and anxiety.

The purpose of these exercises is defined in terms of Western medicine. However, Traditional Chinese Medicine defines these individual exercises in terms of restoring *Qi* or the "vital force or energy of life" (Venes 2021) for various medical conditions involving circulation, digestion, blood pressure, psychological stress, and pain. Additionally, some pose names, such as Look Back and Let Go, Turn and Release, and Bend a Little, may have positive psychological implications for patients/clients.

Self-Care Handout 5.1: Mindful Walking Routine

The following ten steps may help patients/clients create mindful walking routines to improve endurance and reduce stress, anxiety, and pain.

Step 1: Start by becoming familiar with your walking course, so there will be no need to look at a watch to know how long you have been walking. Prepare a small water bottle flavored with mint or basil leaves (or fruits like blueberries).

Step 2: Take off your watch and turn off your phone before you start the walk.

Step 3: Direct your thoughts away from potential stressors, such as work and bills. Try to make no judgments (about yourself or others), no decisions, and no plans. Just enjoy the walk.

Step 4: Start walking at a pace your body is comfortable with. Remember, this is a walking program for relaxation and not necessarily an intense aerobic program for burning calories.

Step 5: Notice your posture as you walk. Are you tense or relaxed? Make minor adjustments in your body to walk with ease.

Step 6: Focus on your feet. Feel each step for hardness or softness. Make minor adjustments in your walking pattern for ease of movement.

Step 7: Notice your surroundings.

- What colors do you see?
- What shapes do you notice in the trees?
- How does the air smell?
- Do you hear any birds or animals?
- Do you feel the wind on your face?
- How do your clothes feel on your body?
- Take a small sip of your flavored water. How does it taste?

Step 8: Notice your breathing. Is it slow or fast? Make minor adjustments in your breathing pattern to breathe easier.

Step 9: Notice your thoughts. Where does your mind want to drift off to? Explore those feelings. See if you can reframe the experience into something positive.

Step 10: As you near the end of your walk, think about the strongest sensation (color, sound, shape, taste, or feeling) you experienced. Think about the positive aspects of that sensation as you finish your walk.

Self-Care Handout 5.2: Qigong Baduanjin Home Routine

Step 1: Standing Form (Opening Sequence)

Purpose: Help quiet the mind.

Technique: Stand with the feet hip-width apart. Inhale and exhale several times slowly using diaphragmatic breathing. Relax your body and try to quiet the mind.

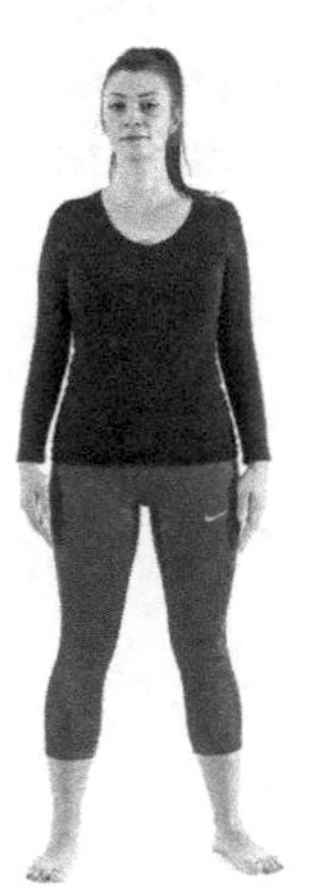

Step 2: Reach for the Sky

Purpose: Help stretch the upper back and improve balance.

Technique: Slowly move your left foot out slightly from the Standing Form position. Inhale as you bring your hands upward to your abdomen with the palms facing upward. Interlace your hands and exhale as you rotate your palms upward as you reach overhead. If you can balance, reach further upward by standing on the balls of your feet. Inhale as you let your arms float down to your midsection. Unlock your hands and exhale as your arms return to your sides.

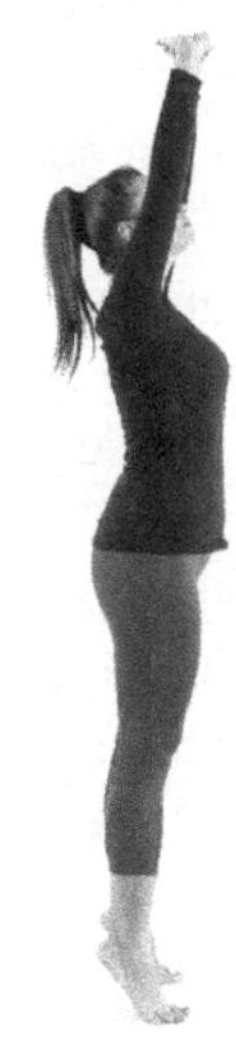

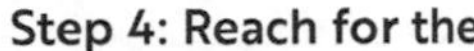

Step 3: Draw the Bow

Purpose: Help improve neck rotation and posture and provide gentle strengthening for the core and lower body.

Technique: Stand with the feet shoulder-width apart. Inhale as you squat partially and bring your arms from your side to a crossed position in front of your chest with your thumbs pointing up. Exhale as you straighten your left arm and turn your head to the left while bending your right arm as if drawing a bow. Pretend you are looking at a target through your extended left hand. Inhale and return to the arms-crossed position. Repeat the same sequence to the right.

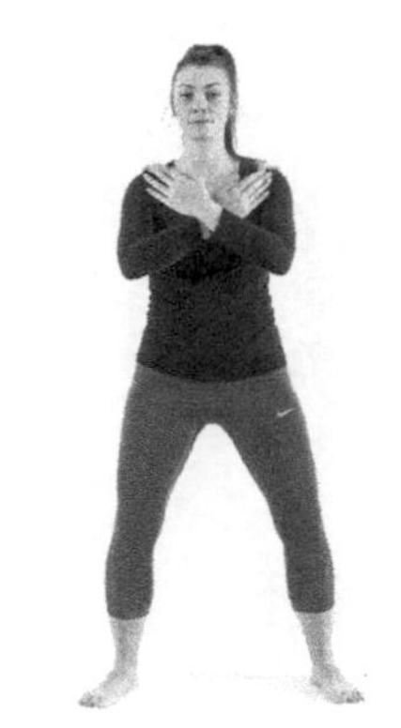

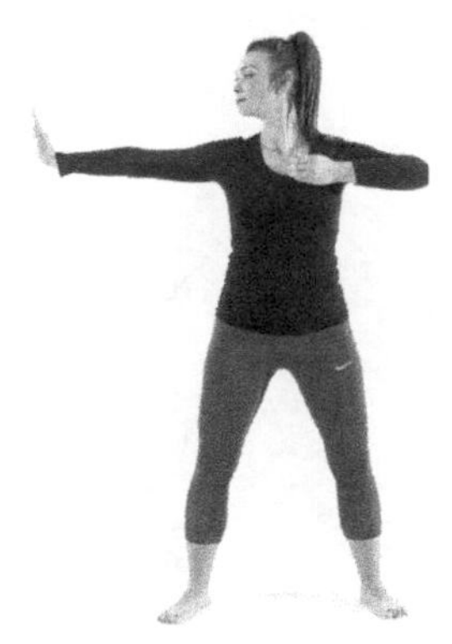

Step 4: Reach for the Sky and Earth

Purpose: Help stretch the upper back and improve balance.

Technique: Stand with the feet shoulder-width apart. Inhale as you bring your hands upward to your abdomen with the palms facing upward. Exhale as you bring your left hand with your palm up overhead and your right hand with your palm down toward the ground. If you can balance, reach further upward by standing on the balls of your feet. Inhale as you let your arms float down to your midsection. Repeat the same sequence on the opposite side.

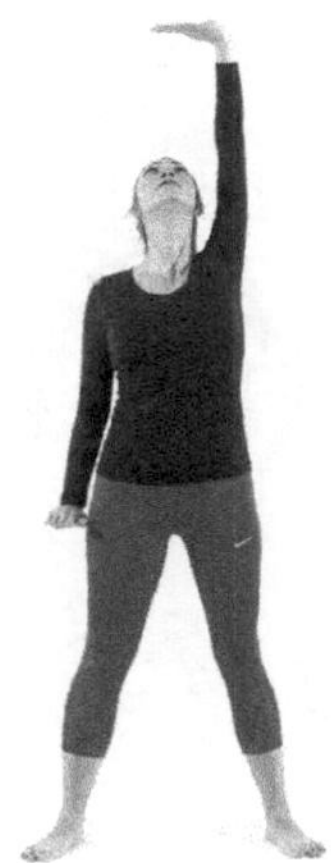

Step 5: Look Back and Let Go

Purpose: Provide gentle trunk and neck rotation and strengthening for the core and lower body.

Technique: Stand with the feet shoulder-width apart. Inhale as you bring your open hands near your hip level with the palms facing down (the thumb and fingers are stretched to make a V). Keep your hands a few inches away from your body. Exhale as you squat partially and distribute your weight evenly across both feet. Inhale as you gently turn your trunk within a comfortable range to the left, and exhale as you return to the center position by straightening your knees. Repeat the same sequence to the right.

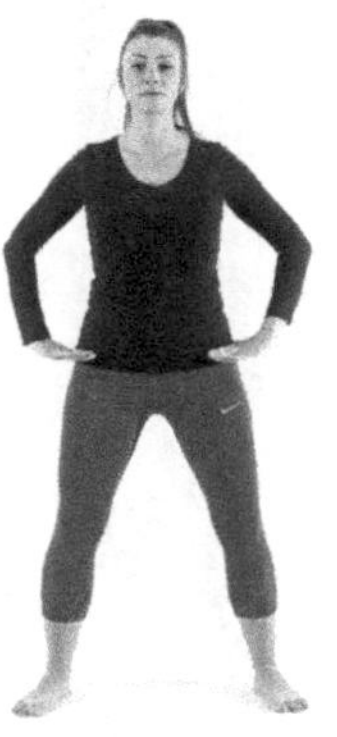

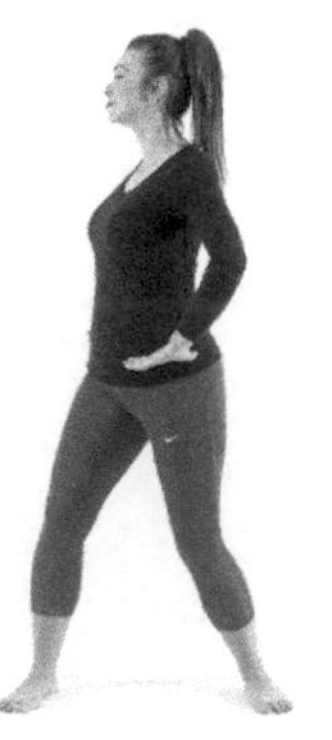

Step 6: Turn and Release

Purpose: Provide gentle trunk and neck rotation, side-bending, and gentle strengthening for the core and lower body.

Technique: Stand with the feet shoulder-width apart. Inhale as you bring your open hands to your upper thighs with the palms facing down (the thumb and fingers are stretched to make a V). Exhale as you squat partially and distribute your weight evenly across both feet. Your hands can lightly touch your upper thighs. Inhale as you gently turn your trunk within a comfortable range to the left by trying to look at your left heel. Then exhale as you return to the center position by straightening your knees. Repeat the same sequence to the right.

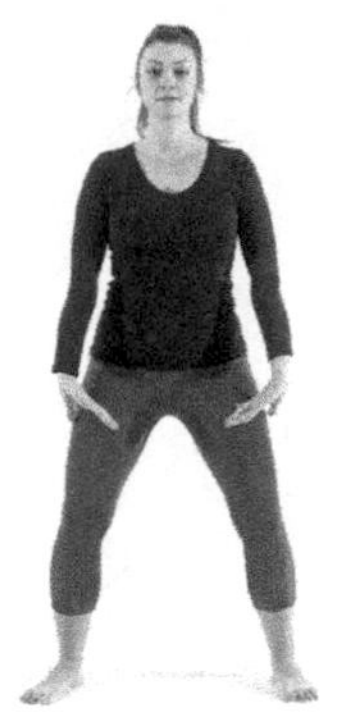

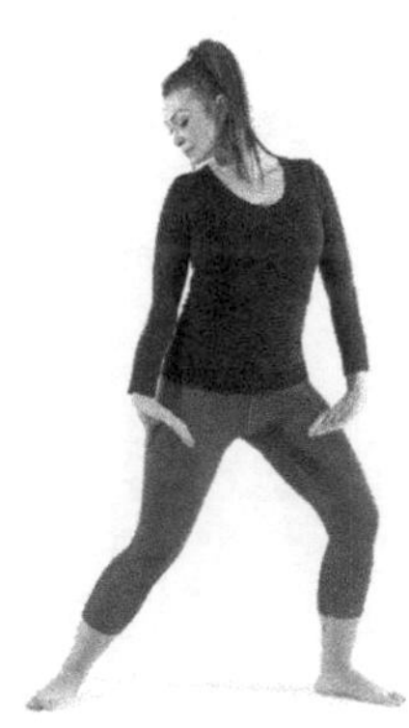

Step 7: Bend a Little

Purpose: Gently improve trunk range and core and strengthening for daily bending-related activities.

Technique: Stand with the feet shoulder-width apart. Inhale and then exhale as you slowly slide your hands down your thighs to either the mid-thigh, knee, or mid-shin level (depending on your ability and pain). Inhale as you return to standing and then place your hands to rest on your lower back as you exhale to straighten to an upright position or bend partially backward (if able or not contraindicated), and inhale by returning to the standing position.

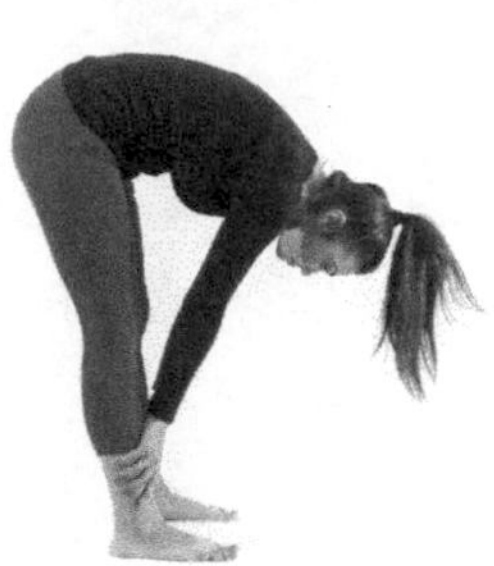

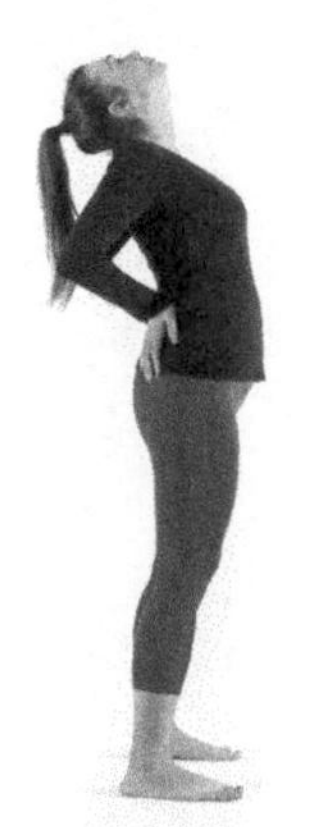

Step 8: Power Punch

Purpose: Increase vitality and confidence.

Technique: Stand with the feet slightly wider than shoulder-width apart. Inhale and exhale as you bend your knees slightly (to what is sometimes called the "horse stance" in martial arts) and bend your elbows with your hands closed in a fist and the palm side facing up. Inhale, and then on the exhale, punch your left fist forward as you rotate your forearm from the palm side up to the palm side down position. Inhale and return the left elbow to the bent position. Repeat on the right side.

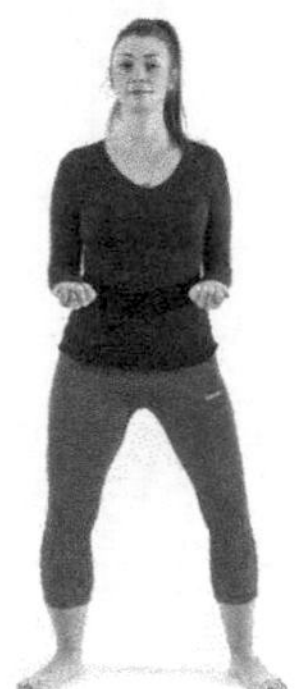

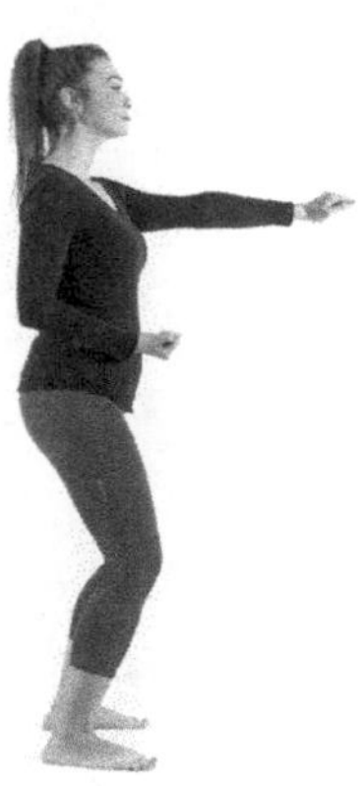

Step 9: Soft Landings

Purpose: Help improve the ability to bend at the knees with control for tasks such as stepping off a curb, walking downstairs, and landing from a jump.

Technique: Stand with the feet hip-width apart. As you inhale, raise up onto the balls of your feet. Exhale as you drop your heels to the ground by bending your knees and ankles to absorb the force.

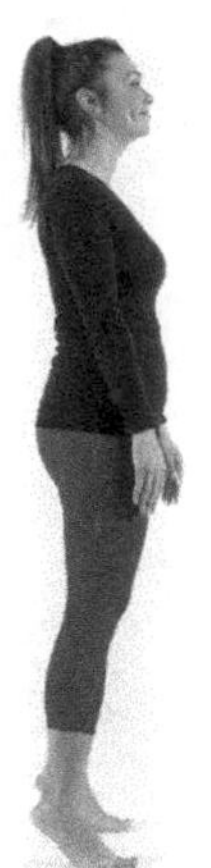

Step 10: Standing Form (Closing Sequence)

Purpose: Help quiet the mind.

Technique: Stand with the feet hip-width apart. Inhale and exhale several times slowly using diaphragmatic breathing. Relax your body and try to quiet the mind.

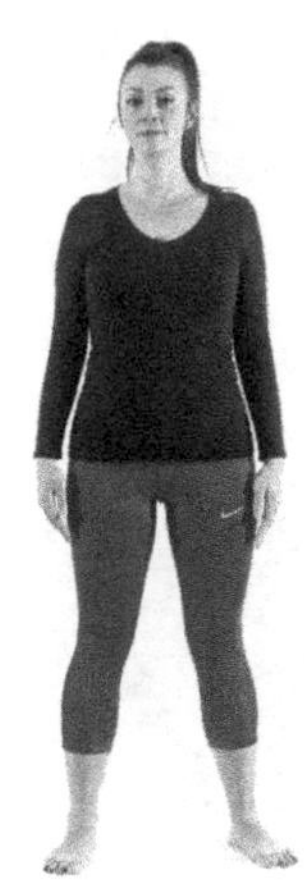

Self-Management Activities: Tai Chi for Health

The following online resources can help patients/clients, healthcare providers, and health/fitness professionals to manage stress and anxiety by exploring tai chi.

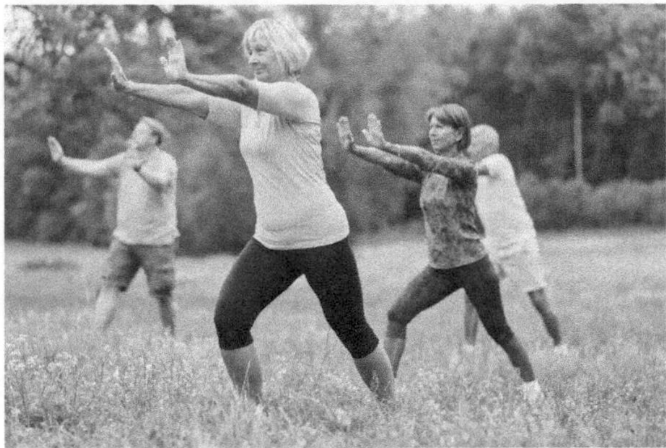

Tai chi for health

- The Tai Chi Productions site by Dr. Paul Lam provides instructional materials for tai chi and qigong: www.taichiproductions.com
- The Yang Tai Chi for Beginners 1 app by Master Yang provides instructions for the Yang-style Tai Chi long form: https://ymaa.com

Classroom and Lab Activities

- Perform various tai chi moves and pay attention to the position of the feet. How may the multidirectional stepping patterns in tai chi be used to create home programs for individuals with a balance dysfunction?
- Notice how a person breathes during tai chi.

Useful Clinical Resources

Alexander Technique

- American Society for the Alexander Technique, www.amsatonline.org
- The Complete Guide to the Alexander Technique, www.alexandertechnique.com

Feldenkrais Method

- Feldenkrais Guild of North America, www.feldenkrais.com

- Feldenkrais Resources, www.feldenkraisresources.com
- International Feldenkrais Federation, https://feldenkrais-method.org
- OpenATM, free online lessons, https://openatm.org

Labyrinth Walking

- Labyrinth Society, https://labyrinthsociety.org
- Labyrinth Locator, https://labyrinthlocator.com
- Veriditas (labyrinth experiences), www.veriditas.org
- Labyrinth Journey app, https://labyrinthjourney.app
- Wooden finger labyrinths, www.bwatsonstudios.com

Mindfulness

- American Mindfulness Research Association, https://goamra.org
- Guided Mindfulness Meditation, Jon Kabat-Zinn, Ph.D., www.mindfulnesscds.com
- Mind & Life Institute, www.mindandlife.org
- Mindful, www.mindful.org
- Mindful Schools, www.mindfulschools.org
- UCLA Mindful Awareness Research Center, www.uclahealth.org/marc

Pilates

- Balanced Body, www.pilates.com
- Pilates Method Alliance, www.pilatesmethodalliance.org
- Polestar Pilates Education, www.polestarpilates.com
- STOTT Pilates, www.merrithew.com/brands/stott-pilates

Tai Chi and Qigong

- American Tai Chi and Qigong Association, www.americantaichi.org
- International Medical Tai Chi Qigong Association, www.imtqa.org
- National Qigong Association, http://nqa.org
- Qigong Institute, www.qigonginstitute.org
- Qigong in Cancer Care, http://theqigongnetwork.com
- QiMaster (Grandmaster Hong Liu), www.qimaster.com
- Tai Chi for Health, http://taichimania.com
- Tai Chi for Health Institute, https://taichiforhealthinstitute.org

Yoga

- International Association of Yoga Therapists, www.iayt.org
- Iyengar Yoga National Association of the United States, https://iynaus.org
- Sit N Fit Chair Yoga, www.sitnfitchairyoga.com
- Yoga Alliance, www.yogaalliance.org

Outcome Measures

- *Five Facet Mindfulness Questionnaire*
  Baer RA, Smith GT, Hopkins J, Krietemeyer J, Toney L. Using self-report assessment methods to explore facets of mindfulness. *Assessment.* 2006;13(1):27–45.
- *Freiburg Mindfulness Inventory*
  Buchheld N, Grossman P, Walach H (2001). Measuring mindfulness in insight meditation (Vipassana) and meditation-based psychotherapy: the development of the Freiburg Mindfulness Inventory. *J Medit Medit Res.* 2001;1:11–34.
- *Mindful Attention Awareness Scale*
  Brown KW, Ryan RM. The benefits of being present: mindfulness and its role in psychological well-being. *J Pers Soc Psychol.* 2003;84(4):822–848.
- *Philadelphia Mindfulness Scale*
  Cardaciotto L, Herbert JD, Forman EM, Moitra E, Farrow V. The assessment of present-moment awareness and acceptance: the Philadelphia Mindfulness Scale. *Assessment.* 2008;15(2):204–223.
- *Scale of Body Connection*
  Price CJ, Thompson EA, Cheng SC. Scale of Body Connection: a multi-sample construct validation study. *PLoS One.* 2017;12(10):e0184757.
  Price CJ, Thompson EA. Measuring dimensions of body connection: body awareness and bodily dissociation. *J Altern Complement Med.* 2007;13(9):945–953.
- *State Mindfulness Scale*
  Tanay G, Bernstein A. State Mindfulness Scale (SMS): development and initial validation. *Psychol Assess.* 2013;25(4):1286–1299.

References

Aboagye E, Karlsson ML, Hagberg J, Jensen I. Cost-effectiveness of early interventions for non-specific low back pain: a randomized controlled study investigating medical yoga, exercise therapy and self-care advice. *J Rehabil Med.* 2015;47(2):167–173.

Ahmadi H, Adib H, Selk-Ghaffari M, *et al.* Comparison of the effects of the Feldenkrais Method versus core stability exercise in the management of chronic low back pain: a randomised control trial. *Clin Rehabil.* 2020;34(12):1449–1457.

Aibar-Almazán A, Hita-Contreras F, Cruz-Díaz D, de la Torre-Cruz M, Jiménez-García JD, Martínez-Amat A. Effects of Pilates training on sleep quality, anxiety, depression and fatigue in postmenopausal women: a randomized controlled trial. *Maturitas.* 2019;124:62–67.

Alexander FM. *Man's Supreme Inheritance.* New York, NY: E. P. Dutton and Co., Inc; 1918.

Alexander FM. *Constructive Conscious Control of the Individual.* New York, NY: E. P. Dutton and Co., Inc; 1923.

Alexander FM. *The Use of the Self.* New York, NY: E. P. Dutton and Co., Inc; 1932.

Alexander FM. *The Universal Constant in Living.* New York, NY: E. P. Dutton and Co., Inc; 1941.

Altug Z. *Integrative Healing: Developing Wellness in the Mind and Body.* Springville, UT: Cedar Fort, Inc; 2018.

American Society for the Alexander Technique; 2023. www.amsatonline.org

Araujo CG, de Souza E Silva CG, Laukkanen JA, *et al.* Successful 10-second one-legged stance performance predicts survival in middle-aged and older individuals. *Br J Sports Med.* 2022;56(17):975–980.

Banth S, Ardebil MD. Effectiveness of mindfulness meditation on pain and quality of life of patients with chronic low back pain. *Int J Yoga.* 2015;8(2):128–133.

Barrows S. *Smartroller Guide to Optimal Movement,* 2nd ed. Minneapolis, MN: Orthopedic Physical Therapy Products; 2018.

Barrows S, Barrows M. Somatic Education: Feldenkrais and Pilates. In: Elgelid S, Kresge C, ed. *The Feldenkrais Method: Learning Through Movement.* Pencaitland, Scotland: Handspring Publishing; 2021.

Bayley PJ, Schulz-Heik RJ, Tang JS, *et al.* Randomised clinical non-inferiority trial of breathing-based meditation and cognitive processing therapy for symptoms of post-traumatic stress disorder in military veterans. *BMJ Open.* 2022;12(8):e056609.

Behman PJ, Rash JA, Bagshawe M, Giesbrecht GF. Short-term autonomic nervous system and experiential responses during a labyrinth walk. *Cogent Psychology.* 2018;5(1).

Berland R, Marques-Sule E, Marín-Mateo JL, Moreno-Segura N, López-Ridaura A, Sentandreu-Mañó T. Effects of the Feldenkrais Method as a physiotherapy tool: a systematic review and meta-analysis of randomized controlled trials. *Int J Environ Res Public Health.* 2022;19(21):13734.

Berman MG, Jonides J, Kaplan S. The cognitive benefits of interacting with nature. *Psychol Sci.* 2008;19(12):1207–1212.

Blödt S, Pach D, Kaster T, *et al.* Qigong versus exercise therapy for chronic low back pain in adults—a randomized controlled non-inferiority trial. *Eur J Pain.* 2015;19(1):123–131.

Cacciatore TW, Gurfinkel VS, Horak FB, Cordo PJ, Ames KE. Increased dynamic regulation of postural tone through Alexander Technique training. *Hum Mov Sci.* 2011;30(1):74–89.

Cai Q, Cai SB, Chen JK, *et al.* Tai chi for anxiety and depression symptoms in cancer, stroke, heart failure, and chronic obstructive pulmonary disease: a systematic review and meta-analysis. *Complement Ther Clin Pract.* 2022;46:101510.

Chen MC, Liu HE, Huang HY, Chiou AF. The effect of a simple traditional exercise programme (Baduanjin exercise) on sleep quality of older adults: a randomized controlled trial. *Int J Nurs Stud.* 2012;49(3):265–273.

Cheung DST, Takemura N, Lam TC, *et al.* Feasibility of aerobic exercise and tai-chi interventions in advanced lung cancer patients: a randomized controlled trial. *Integr Cancer Ther.* 2021;20:15347354211033352.

Chinese Health Qigong Association. *Ba Duan Jin: Eight Section Qigong Exercises.* London, United Kingdom: Singing Dragon; 2008a.

Chinese Health Qigong Association. *Liu Zi Jue: Six Sounds Approach to Qigong Breathing Exercises.* London, United Kingdom: Singing Dragon; 2008b.

Chinese Health Qigong Association. *Wu Qin Xi: Five-Animal Qigong Exercises.* London, United Kingdom: Singing Dragon; 2008c.

Cohen KS. *The Way of Qigong: The Art and Science of Chinese Energy Healing.* New York, NY: Ballantine Books; 1997.

Connors KA, Galea MP, Said CM. Feldenkrais method balance classes improve balance in older adults: a controlled trial. *Evid Based Complement Alternat Med.* 2011:873672.

de Manincor M, Bensoussan A, Smith CA, *et al.* Individualized yoga for reducing depression and anxiety, and improving well-being: a randomized controlled trial. *Depress Anxiety.* 2016;33(9):816–828.

de Medeiros SA, de Almeida Silva HJ, do Nascimento RM, da Silva Maia JB, de Almeida Lins CA, de Souza MC. Mat Pilates is as effective as aquatic aerobic exercise in treating women with fibromyalgia: a clinical, randomized and blind trial. *Adv Rheumatol.* 2020;60(1):21.

Feldenkrais M. *Judo: The Art of Defense and Attack.* New York, NY: Frederick Warne & Co; 1944.

Feldenkrais M. *Body and Mature Behaviour: A Study of Anxiety, Sex, Gravitation & Learning.* New York, NY: International Universities Press; 1949.

Feldenkrais M. *Higher Judo.* New York, NY: Frederick Warne & Co; 1952.

Feldenkrais M. *Awareness Through Movement: Health Exercises for Personal Growth*. New York, NY: Harper & Row; 1972.

Feldenkrais M. *The Case of Nora: Body Awareness as Healing Therapy*. New York, NY: Harper & Row; 1977.

Feldenkrais M. *The Elusive Obvious or Basic Feldenkrais*. Cupertino, CA: Meta Publications; 1981.

Feldenkrais M. *The Master Moves*. Cupertino, CA: Meta Publications; 1984.

Feldenkrais M, Kimmey M, eds. *The Potent Self: A Guide to Spontaneity*. San Francisco, CA: Harper & Row; 1985.

Feng F, Tuchman S, Denninger JW, Fricchione GL, Yeung A. Qigong for the prevention, treatment, and rehabilitation of COVID-19 infection in older adults. *Am J Geriatr Psychiatry*. 2020;28(8):812–819.

Fernández-Rodríguez R, Álvarez-Bueno C, Cavero-Redondo I, *et al.* Best exercise options for reducing pain and disability in adults with chronic low back pain: Pilates, strength, core-based, and mind-body. A network meta-analysis. *J Orthop Sports Phys Ther*. 2022;52(8):505–521.

Goldsby TL, Goldsby ME, McWalters M, Mills PJ. Effects of singing bowl sound meditation on mood, tension, and well-being: an observational study. *J Evid Based Complementary Altern Med*. 2017;22(3):401–406.

Greendale GA, Huang MH, Karlamangla AS, Seeger L, Crawford S. Yoga decreases kyphosis in senior women and men with adult-onset hyperkyphosis: results of a randomized controlled trial. *J Am Geriatr Soc*. 2009;57(9):1569–1579.

Groessl EJ, Liu L, Chang DG, *et al.* Yoga for military veterans with chronic low back pain: a randomized clinical trial. *Am J Prev Med*. 2017;53(5):599–608.

Hao Z, Zhang X, Chen P. Effects of different exercise therapies on balance function and functional walking ability in multiple sclerosis disease patients: a network meta-analysis of randomized controlled trials. *Int J Environ Res Public Health*. 2022;19(12):7175.

Jayawardena R, Ranasinghe P, Chathuranga T, Atapattu PM, Misra A. The benefits of yoga practice compared to physical exercise in the management of Type 2 diabetes mellitus: a systematic review and meta-analysis. *Diabetes Metab Syndr*. 2018;12(5):795–805.

Kabat-Zinn J. An outpatient program in behavioral medicine for chronic pain patients based on the practice of mindfulness meditation: theoretical considerations and preliminary results. *Gen Hosp Psychiatry*. 1982;4(1):33–47.

Kabat-Zinn J, Lipworth L, Burney R, *et al.* Four-year follow-up of a meditation-based program for the self-regulation of chronic pain: treatment outcomes and compliance. *Clin J Pain*. 1986;2(3):159–173.

Kabat-Zinn J, Lipworth L, Burney R. The clinical use of mindfulness meditation for the self-regulation of chronic pain. *J Behav Med*. 1985;8(2):163–190.

Kabat-Zinn J, Massion AO, Kristeller J, *et al.* Effectiveness of a meditation-based stress reduction program in the treatment of anxiety disorders. *Am J Psychiatry*. 1992;149(7):936–943.

Kalron A, Rosenblum U, Frid L, Achiron A. Pilates exercise training vs. physical therapy for improving walking and balance in people with multiple sclerosis: a randomized controlled trial. *Clin Rehabil*. 2017;31(3):319–328.

Klein SD, Bayard C, Wolf U. The Alexander Technique and musicians: a systematic review of controlled trials. *BMC Complement Altern Med*. 2014;14:414.

Kuntz AB, Chopp-Hurley JN, Brenneman EC, *et al.* Efficacy of a biomechanically-based yoga exercise program in knee osteoarthritis: a randomized controlled trial. *PLoS One*. 2018;13(4):e0195653.

Kuo CC, Wang CC, Chang WL, Liao TC, Chen PE, Tung TH. Clinical effects of Baduanjin qigong exercise on cancer patients: a systematic review and meta-analysis on randomized controlled trials. *Evid Based Complement Alternat Med*. 2021:6651238.

Kwok JYY, Kwan JCY, Auyeung M, *et al.* Effects of mindfulness yoga vs stretching and resistance training exercises on anxiety and depression for people with Parkinson Disease: a randomized clinical trial. *JAMA Neurol*. 2019;76(7):755–763.

Lai J, Cai Y, Yang L, Xia M, Cheng X, Chen Y. Effects of Baduanjin exercise on motor function, balance and gait in Parkinson's disease: a systematic review and meta-analysis. *BMJ Open*. 2022;12(11):e067280.

Li F, Harmer P, Fitzgerald K, *et al.* Effectiveness of a therapeutic tai ji quan intervention vs a multimodal exercise intervention to prevent falls among older adults at high risk of falling: a randomized clinical trial. *JAMA Intern Med*. 2018;178(10):1301–1310.

Li H, Ge D, Liu S, *et al.* Baduanjin exercise for low back pain: a systematic review and meta-analysis. *Complement Ther Med*. 2019;43:109–116.

Lin FL, Yeh ML. Walking and mindfulness improve the exercise capacity of patients with chronic obstructive pulmonary disease: a randomised controlled trial. *Clin Rehabil*. 2021;35(8):1117–1125.

Lin H, Ye Y, Wan M, Qiu P, Xia R, Zheng G. Effect of Baduanjin exercise on cerebral blood flow and cognitive frailty in the community older adults with cognitive frailty: a randomized controlled trial. *J Exerc Sci Fit*. 2023;21(1):131–137.

Lin PJ, Kleckner IR, Loh KP, *et al.* Influence of yoga on cancer-related fatigue and on mediational relationships between changes in sleep and cancer-related fatigue: a nationwide, multicenter randomized controlled trial of yoga in cancer survivors. *Integr Cancer Ther.* 2019;18:1534735419855134.

Little P, Lewith G, Webley F, *et al.* Randomised controlled trial of Alexander technique lessons, exercise, and massage (ATEAM) for chronic and recurrent back pain. *Br J Sports Med.* 2008;42(12):965–968.

Liu F, Chen X, Nie P, *et al.* Can tai chi improve cognitive function? A systematic review and meta-analysis of randomized controlled trials. *J Altern Complement Med.* 2021a;27(12):1070–1083.

Liu MH, Perry P. *The Healing Art of Qi Gong.* New York, NY: Warner Books; 1997.

Liu ST, Zhan C, Ma YJ, *et al.* Effect of qigong exercise and acupressure rehabilitation program on pulmonary function and respiratory symptoms in patients hospitalized with severe COVID-19: a randomized controlled trial. *Integr Med Res.* 2021b;10(Suppl):100796.

Liu W, Schaffer L, Herrs N, Chollet C, Taylor S. Improved sleep after Qigong exercise in breast cancer survivors: a pilot study. *Asia Pac J Oncol Nurs.* 2015;2(4):232–239.

Lizier DS, Silva-Filho R, Umada J, Melo R, Neves AC. Effects of reflective labyrinth walking assessed using a questionnaire. *Medicines (Basel).* 2018;5(4):111.

Lundqvist LO, Zetterlund C, Richter HO. Effects of Feldenkrais Method on chronic neck/scapular pain in people with visual impairment: a randomized controlled trial with one-year follow-up. *Arch Phys Med Rehabil.* 2014;95(9):1656–1661.

Ma J, Williams J, Morris PG, Chan PSWY. Effectiveness of mindful walking intervention in nature on sleep quality and mood among university students during Covid-19: a randomised control study [published online ahead of print, 2022 Aug 11]. *Explore (NY).* 2022;S1550-8307(22)00125-2.

MacPherson H, Tilbrook H, Richmond S, *et al.* Alexander Technique lessons or acupuncture sessions for persons with chronic neck pain: a randomized trial [published correction appears in *Ann Intern Med.* 2016 Feb 2;164(3):204]. *Ann Intern Med.* 2015;163(9):653–662.

Natour J, Cazotti Lde A, Ribeiro LH, Baptista AS, Jones A. Pilates improves pain, function and quality of life in patients with chronic low back pain: a randomized controlled trial. *Clin Rehabil.* 2015;29(1):59–68.

Niles BL, Mori DL, Polizzi CP, Pless Kaiser A, Ledoux AM, Wang C. Feasibility, qualitative findings and satisfaction of a brief Tai Chi mind-body programme for veterans with post-traumatic stress symptoms. *BMJ Open.* 2016;6(11):e012464.

Pan Y, Huang Y, Zhang H, Tang Y, Wang C. The effects of Baduanjin and yoga exercise programs on physical and mental health in patients with multiple sclerosis: a randomized controlled trial. *Complement Ther Med.* 2022;70:102862.

Paolucci T, Zangrando F, Iosa M, *et al.* Improved interoceptive awareness in chronic low back pain: a comparison of back school versus Feldenkrais Method. *Disabil Rehabil.* 2017;39(10):994–1001.

Phattharasupharerk S, Purepong N, Eksakulkla S, Siriphorn A. Effects of qigong practice in office workers with chronic non-specific low back pain: a randomized control trial. *J Bodyw Mov Ther.* 2019;23(2):375–381.

Pilates JH. *Your Health: A Corrective System of Exercising that Revolutionizes the Entire Field of Physical Education.* New York, NY: C. J. O'Brien, Inc; 1934.

Pilates JH, Miller WJ. *Return to Life Through Contrology.* New York, NY: J. J. Augustin; 1945.

Porter RS, Kaplan JL, eds. *The Merck Manual of Diagnosis and Therapy*, 20th ed. Kenilworth, NJ: MERCK Sharp & Dohme Corporation; 2018.

Qin J, Chen Y, Guo S, *et al.* Effect of tai chi on quality of life, body mass index, and waist-hip ratio in patients with Type 2 diabetes mellitus: a systematic review and meta-analysis. *Front Endocrinol (Lausanne).* 2021;11:543627.

Qin J, Zhang Y, Wu L, *et al.* Effect of tai chi alone or as additional therapy on low back pain: systematic review and meta-analysis of randomized controlled trials. *Medicine (Baltimore).* 2019;98(37):e17099.

Qingguang Z, Shuaipan Z, Jingxian LI, *et al.* Effectiveness of Liu-zi-jue exercise on coronavirus disease 2019 in the patients: a randomized controlled trial. *J Tradit Chin Med.* 2022;42(6):997–10053.

Reb AM, Saum NS, Murphy DA, Breckenridge-Sproat ST, Su X, Bormann JE. Qigong in injured military service members. *J Holist Nurs.* 2017;35(1):10–24.

Saper RB, Lemaster C, Delitto A, *et al.* Yoga, physical therapy, or education for chronic low back pain: a randomized noninferiority trial. *Annals of Internal Medicine.* 2017;167(2):85–94.

Shelton J. The Alexander Technique of Southern California; n.d. www.julieshelton.com

Singh VP, Khandelwal B. Effect of yoga and exercise on glycemic control and psychosocial parameters in Type 2 diabetes mellitus: a randomized controlled study. *Int J Yoga.* 2020;13(2):144–151.

Solakoglu O, Dogruoz Karatekin B, Yumusakhuylu Y, Mesci E, Icagasioglu A. The effect of yoga asana "Vrksasana (Tree Pose)" on balance in patients with postmenopausal osteoporosis: a randomized controlled trial. *Am J Phys Med Rehabil*. 2022;101(3):255–261.

Song R, Grabowska W, Park M, *et al.* The impact of tai chi and qigong mind-body exercises on motor and non-motor function and quality of life in Parkinson's disease: a systematic review and meta-analysis. *Parkinsonism Relat Disord*. 2017;41:3–13.

Song R, Park M, Jang T, Oh J, Sohn MK. Effects of a tai chi-based stroke rehabilitation program on symptom clusters, physical and cognitive functions, and quality of life: a randomized feasibility study. *Int J Environ Res Public Health*. 2021;18(10):5453.

Sonmezer E, Özköslü MA, Yosmaoğlu HB. The effects of clinical Pilates exercises on functional disability, pain, quality of life and lumbopelvic stabilization in pregnant women with low back pain: a randomized controlled study. *J Back Musculoskelet Rehabil*. 2021;34(1):69–76.

Stallibrass C, Sissons P, Chalmers C. Randomized controlled trial of the Alexander technique for idiopathic Parkinson's disease. *Clin Rehabil*. 2002;16(7):695–708.

Suárez-Iglesias D, Miller KJ, Seijo-Martínez M, Ayán C. Benefits of Pilates in Parkinson's disease: a systematic review and meta-analysis. *Medicina (Kaunas)*. 2019;55(8):476.

Taylor E, Taylor-Piliae RE. The effects of Tai Chi on physical and psychosocial function among persons with multiple sclerosis: a systematic review. *Complement Ther Med*. 2017;31:100–108.

Teixeira-Machado L, Araújo FM, Cunha FA, Menezes M, Menezes T, Melo DeSantana J. Feldenkrais Method-based exercise improves quality of life in individuals with Parkinson's disease: a controlled, randomized clinical trial. *Altern Ther Health Med*. 2015;21(1):8–14.

Teut M, Roesner EJ, Ortiz M, *et al.* Mindful walking in psychologically distressed individuals: a randomized controlled trial. *Evidence-Based Complementary and Alternative Medicine*. 2013;489856.

Vancini RL, Rayes ABR, Lira CAB, Sarro KJ, Andrade MS. Pilates and aerobic training improve levels of depression, anxiety and quality of life in overweight and obese individuals. *Arq Neuro-psiquiatr*. 2017;75(12):850–857.

Venes D, ed. *Taber's Cyclopedic Medical Dictionary*, 24th ed. Philadelphia, PA: FA Davis; 2021.

Voss MW, Prakash RS, Erickson KI, *et al.* Plasticity of brain networks in a randomized intervention trial of exercise training in older adults. *Front Aging Neurosci*. 2010;2:32.

Wan M, Xia R, Lin H, Ye Y, Qiu P, Zheng G. Baduanjin exercise modulates the hippocampal subregion structure in community-dwelling older adults with cognitive frailty. *Front Aging Neurosci*. 2022;14:956273.

Wang C, Schmid CH, Fielding RA, *et al.* Effect of tai chi versus aerobic exercise for fibromyalgia: comparative effectiveness randomized controlled trial. *BMJ*. 2018;360:k851.

Wang C, Schmid CH, Iversen MD, *et al.* Comparative effectiveness of tai chi versus physical therapy for knee osteoarthritis: a randomized trial. *Ann Intern Med*. 2016;165(2):77–86.

Wang X, Wu J, Ye M, Wang L, Zheng G. Effect of Baduanjin exercise on the cognitive function of middle-aged and older adults: a systematic review and meta-analysis. *Complement Ther Med*. 2021;59:102727.

Webster's New World Dictionary, 5th ed. New York, NY: Houghton Mifflin Harcourt Publishing Company; 2016.

Wen J, Lin T, Cai Y, *et al.* Baduanjin exercise for Type 2 diabetes mellitus: a systematic review and meta-analysis of randomized controlled trials. *Evid Based Complement Alternat Med*. 2017:8378219.

Zhang L, Liu X, Xi X, *et al.* Effect of Zhan Zhuang Qigong on upper limb static tremor and aerobic exercise capacity in patients with mild-to-moderate Parkinson's disease: study protocol for a randomised controlled trial. *BMJ Open*. 2022;12(7):e059625.

Additional Reading

Elgelid S, Kresge C. *The Feldenkrais Method: Learning Through Movement*. London, United Kingdom: Handspring; 2021.

Iyengar BKS. *Light on Yoga*. New York, NY: Schocken Books; 1979.

Iyengar BKS. *Light on Life: The Journey to Wholeness, Inner Peace and Ultimate Freedom*. Emmaus, PA: Rodale Books; 2005.

Iyengar BKS. *B.K.S. Iyengar Yoga: The Path to Holistic Health*. New York, NY: DK Publishing; 2014.

Lasater JH. *Relax and Renew: Restful Yoga for Stressful Times*. Boulder, CO: Shambhala Publications, Inc; 2011.

Lasater JH. *Restore and Rebalance: Yoga for Deep Relaxation*. Boulder, CO: Shambhala Publications, Inc; 2017.

Wang MY, Yu SS, Hashish R, *et al.* The biomechanical demands of standing yoga poses in seniors: the Yoga Empowers Seniors Study (YESS). *BMC Complement Altern Med*. 2013;13:8.

CHAPTER 6

Stress Management

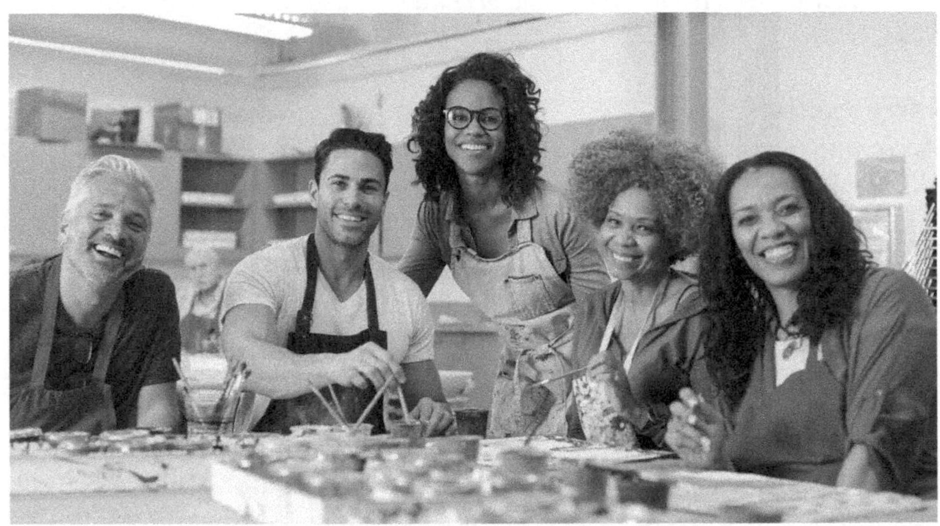

Stress less by trying new hobbies with friends

Learning Objectives

- Understand the basic research for psychological stress management.
- Apply stress management for practical pain management.

Chapter Highlights

- Key Concept: Stress Management Strategies
- Clinical Tip: Shadow Boxing and Non-Contact Boxing
- Clinical Tip: Pet Therapy
- Featured Topic 6.1: Rocking Chair Relaxation
- Featured Topic 6.2: Relaxation Routine
- Featured Topic 6.3: Body Scan Meditation
- Featured Topic 6.4: Mini Meditations

- Self-Care Handout 6.1: Relaxation Breathing-Plus Technique
- Self-Care Handout 6.2: Self-Guided Imagery and Visualization
- Self-Management Activities
- Classroom and Lab Activities
- Useful Clinical Resources
- References
- Additional Reading

Lifestyle Matters: *Free your mind of clutter.*

Introduction

According to one source, stress is a physiological, physical, or psychological force that disrupts equilibrium (Venes 2021). Some factors that increase psychological stress include health crises, conflicts, bankruptcy, marital discord, or self-doubt.

Dr. Hans Selye, MD, Ph.D., an endocrinologist known for his research on the effects of stress, said, "It's not stress that kills us, it is our reaction to it" (George Mason University 2023). The American College of Lifestyle Medicine (2019) states, "Not all stress is bad for us; in fact, some stress can be helpful for completing important projects, studying for an exam, speaking in public, or accomplishing challenging goals." Psychological stress may impact medical conditions such as back pain (Shaw *et al.* 2016), depression (LeMoult *et al.* 2020), diabetes (Ni *et al.* 2021), neck-arm pain (Ortego *et al.* 2016), and Parkinson's (Austin *et al.* 2016). In most cases, uncontrolled mental stress has the potential to exacerbate many conditions. For this reason, providing patients/clients with strategies and options to dial down and reduce stress may help improve their quality of life.

KEY CONCEPT: STRESS MANAGEMENT STRATEGIES

- Smile and laugh more often.
- Train to complain less.
- Use conventional exercises such as walking, running, biking, swimming, or hiking.
- Use mind-body practices such as yoga, tai chi, qigong, or Pilates.
- Engage in music, art, or other hobbies.
- Use essential oils or products (such as soap) for relaxation.
- Get a massage.
- Learn self-massage and self-acupressure techniques.
- Go outside for fresh air, sunshine, and nature-based activities such as gardening, gentle yard work, or a walk in a park with friends.

- Keep a gratitude journal.
- Learn relaxation techniques such as progressive muscle relaxation, body scan meditation, or self-hypnosis.
- Socialize, volunteer, and get involved in community activities.

Stress Management Strategies

The following list offers various integrative and mind-body strategies that may be used for improving sleep quality, relaxation, anxiety, or depression, or reducing pain, along with citations for published research on their use.

- Aromatherapy (Genç *et al.* 2020; Gong *et al.* 2020; Hamzeh *et al.* 2020; Son *et al.* 2019)
- Biofeedback (Bergmann *et al.* 2020; Sielski *et al.* 2017; van der Zwan *et al.* 2015)
- Body scan meditation (Banth and Ardebil 2015; Goodman and Schorling 2012; Pizzoli *et al.* 2020)
- Cognitive behavioral therapy (Carney *et al.* 2017; Cherkin *et al.* 2016; Felder *et al.* 2020)
- Guided imagery (Acar and Aygin 2019; Afshar *et al.* 2018; Beck *et al.* 2015; Manolaki *et al.* 2021)
- Hypnosis (Rizzo *et al.* 2018; Tan *et al.* 2015; Valentine *et al.* 2019)
- Mental imagery (visualization) (Fardo *et al.* 2015; La Touche *et al.* 2020)
- Mindfulness meditation (Luiggi-Hernandez *et al.* 2018; Zgierska *et al.* 2016)
- Prayer (Boelens *et al.* 2009; Hai *et al.* 2021)
- Progressive muscle relaxation (Koukoulithras *et al.* 2021; Mateu *et al.* 2018; Ozgundondu and Gok Metin 2019)
- Self-hypnosis (Bo *et al.* 2018; Grégoire *et al.* 2021; Grégoire *et al.* 2022; McCauley *et al.* 1983)
- Transcendental meditation (Elder *et al.* 2014; Klimes-Dougan *et al.* 2020; Ooi *et al.* 2017)

According to WebMD (WebMD 2023) and StatPearls (Norelli *et al.* 2022), box breathing, also known as square breathing, helps a person slow down their breathing and may be used to reduce anxiety, stress, and tension. An article in *Applied Psychophysiology and Biofeedback* (Röttger *et al.* 2021) indicates that box breathing is also called tactical breathing and is used by military and law enforcement personnel in dangerous situations.

These are the four steps to include in the box breathing technique, and the following figure illustrates the technique:

1. Breathe in slowly through your nose for 2–4 seconds.
2. Pause and hold your breath for 2–4 seconds.
3. Breathe out slowly through your nose or pursed lips for 2–4 seconds.
4. Pause and hold your breath for 2–4 seconds.
5. Repeat steps 1–4 for 1 minute, several minutes, or as long as it takes to regain calmness.

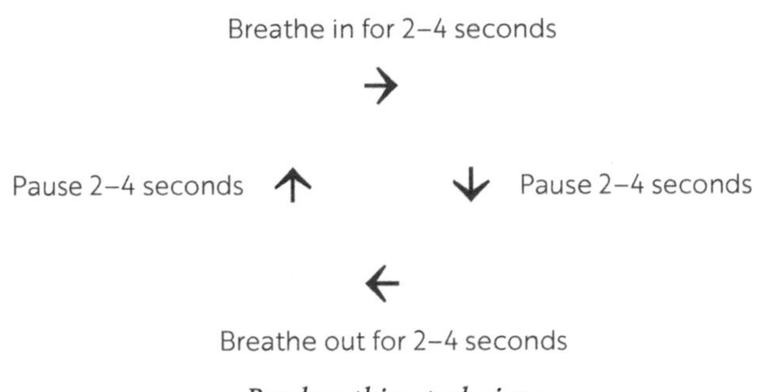

Box breathing technique

CLINICAL TIP: SHADOW BOXING AND NON-CONTACT BOXING

Shadow boxing and non-contact boxing are fun movement patterns for patients/clients looking for a way to be physically active without equipment. Shadow boxing movements may challenge balance, enhance agility, increase mobility, and improve overall well-being (Larson *et al.* 2022; Zheng *et al.* 2015).

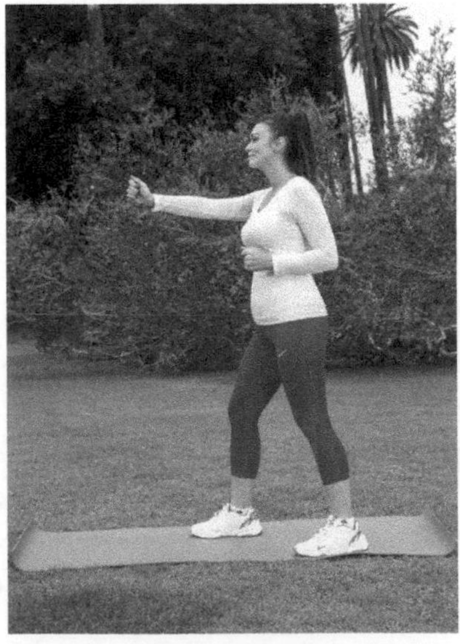

Shadow boxing

CLINICAL TIP: PET THERAPY

Pet therapy is the therapeutic use of animals to help individuals who are socially isolated and also for reducing stress, anxiety, and loneliness.

Featured Topics

Featured Topic 6.1 outlines how a simple rocking chair may be useful for regulating mood, and managing pain and other conditions.

Featured Topic 6.2 outlines a relaxation routine that may be used for reducing tension and helping with sleep.

Featured Topic 6.3 outlines a body scan meditation routine adapted and shortened from a routine developed by Professor Jon Kabat-Zinn, Ph.D. The routine may last from 5 to 30 minutes, depending on the program's goals and the individual's needs. For an expanded version of the body scan technique, refer to Dr. Kabat-Zinn's excellent book *Full Catastrophe Living* (Kabat-Zinn 2013).

An article in *Mindfulness* (Dreeben *et al.* 2013) states that the body scan meditation technique is an attention-focusing practice introduced as part of the mindfulness-based stress reduction program by Dr. Kabat-Zinn. According to Professor Kabat-Zinn, "the idea in scanning your body is to actually *feel* and *inhabit* each region you focus on and linger in it, in the timeless present as best you can" (Kabat-Zinn 2013, p.78).

Mindfulness-based stress reduction programs that may include body scan, seated meditation, walking meditation, and mindful stretching can be helpful for chronic low back pain (Banth and Ardebil 2015; Morone *et al.* 2016), chronic pain (Ussher *et al.* 2014), and other conditions. One study found that a single virtual body scan meditation session may reduce the anxiety of both facilitators and participants (Kogan and Bussolari 2021).

Featured Topic 6.4 outlines mini meditations that can easily fit into daily activities.

■ Featured Topic 6.1: Rocking Chair Relaxation

Janet Travell, MD (1901–1997), White House physician to President John F. Kennedy, recommended a rocking chair as a part of her treatments to manage the president's back pain. In the book *Myofascial Pain and Dysfunction: The Trigger Point Manual* (1992), Janet Travell, MD, and David Simons, MD, state that a rocking chair may be used to:

- help relax trigger points in the gluteus medius muscle
- reduce piriformis muscle trigger points due to postural stress
- decrease gastrocnemius and soleus muscle trigger points.

Furthermore, articles show that a rocking chair may help regulate mood (Cross *et al.* 2018), manage pain (Karper 2013), and potentially reduce the duration of postoperative ileus (Massey 2010). A randomized controlled trial from Finland (Niemelä *et al.* 2011) even showed that community-dwelling women aged 73–87 benefitted from using a rocking chair as a part of an exercise program.

Self-Care Guide: Rocking Chair Mindfulness Meditation

1. Start: Either physically sit in a rocking chair or mentally picture yourself sitting in one.
2. Close your eyes and imagine your favorite view (e.g., lake, mountain, garden, or ocean).
3. Slowly begin to rock in your chair (physically or mentally).
4. Breathe in and out slowly using belly breathing.
5. Think about the positive things you have accomplished.
6. Think about the future dreams you have yet to accomplish.
7. When you are ready to finish, smile and think about the wonderful things in your life.
8. End: Gently open your eyes and enjoy the day, or go to sleep.

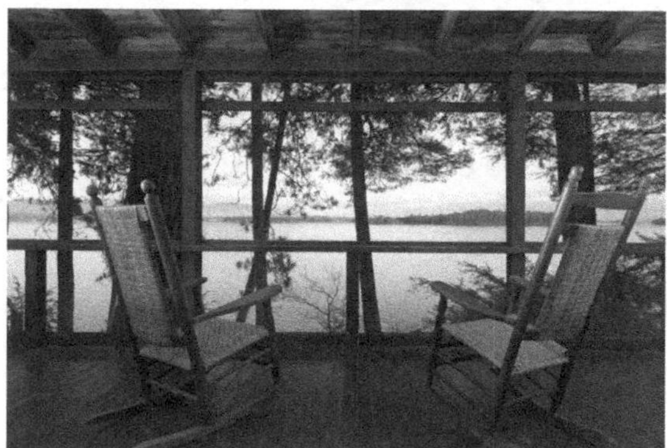

Rocking chair with a view

■ Featured Topic 6.2: Relaxation Routine

The following is an adapted relaxation routine outlined by Bud Winter that may be used for reducing tension and helping with sleep (Sleep Foundation 2023; Winter 2012; Yates 1946):

1. Start: Sit erect in a chair with your feet flat on the floor.
2. Rest your hands on the insides of your thighs.

3. Close your eyes and start to breathe slowly.
4. Take the wrinkles out of your forehead.
5. Relax your scalp.
6. Relax the muscles around your eyes.
7. Relax your jaw (i.e., by letting it sag), tongue, and lips.
8. Let your neck relax and allow your chin to drop toward your chest.
9. Let your shoulders drop and relax.
10. Let your arm and hand muscles relax.
11. Let your leg muscles relax.
12. Say the word "calm" to yourself in this relaxed state.
13. Smile slightly, open your eyes, and resume your normal activities or go to sleep.
14. End.

Adapted from Winter 2012.

Note: Lloyd "Bud" Winter was a track coach at San José State University for 30 years, participated in six Olympic Games, and wrote several books. His techniques are based on training methods used to prepare World War II combat flyers. For more information see: www.budwinter.com.

■ Featured Topic 6.3: Body Scan Meditation

1. Start: Sit or lie down and gently close your eyes.
2. Gently let your attention settle on your abdomen to feel the slow wave-like rise and fall with each belly breath in and breath out. Do this for about a minute.
3. Take a moment to feel your body from head to toe and the sensations of touch in places you are in contact with on the floor, mat, or bed.
4. Now, bring awareness to your left toes. Do you feel warmth, cold, stiffness, tightness, or pain?
5. Note about pain: If you have pain, see if you can direct your breath to this area. If the redirection does not work, then focus directly on the pain. Now breathe in *to* and out *from* the pain itself. Then, imagine the in-breath penetrating the tissue until it is completely absorbed, and the out-breath as a channel to discharge the pain from the body. This strategy can be used for any painful body area.
6. Continue belly breathing as you feel the sensations in your left toes. If you don't feel anything, that's okay too.

7. When you are ready to leave the left toes and move on, continue belly breathing and shift your attention to:
   - → the sole of your left foot, → your left heel, → the top of your left foot, → your left ankle, → your left calf, → your left knee, and finally, → your left hip.
8. Then, systematically move up your right leg as previously outlined, starting at your right toes.
9. Continue with the same approach into:
   - → your pelvis, → your abdomen, → your lower back, → your upper back, → your chest.
10. Continue with the same approach into:
    - → your left fingers, → your left wrist, → your left lateral elbow, → your left medial elbow → your left shoulder.
11. Systematically move up your right arm as previously outlined, starting at your right fingers.
12. Finally, shift your attention to:
    - → the back of your neck, → the front of your neck, → your mouth, → your nose, → your jaws, → your eyes, → your forehead, and finally, → the top of your head.
13. Continue belly breathing for about 1 minute or until you are ready to finish.
14. End: Gently open your eyes and enjoy the day, or go to sleep.

Adapted from Kabat-Zinn 2013.

■ Featured Topic 6.4: Mini Meditations

The following are mini meditations that can easily fit into daily activities:

- Doodle on a sketchpad.
- Gaze at the clouds or night sky.
- Enjoy the comforting rhythmical movements of a rocking chair.
- Listen to a relaxing song.
- Look at a landscape painting.
- Play with pets.
- Read a poem.
- Relax while standing in a long line at the store or bank.
- Take a quick stroll through the garden and smell the flowers.
- Watch and listen to the rain.
- Write an entry in a journal or diary.

Self-Care Education Guides

See **Self-Care Handout 6.1: Relaxation Breathing-Plus Technique** for an adapted relaxation breathing technique that may be used for pain management, relaxation, and stress reduction (Chen *et al.* 2017; Ebrahimi *et al.* 2021; Eron *et al.* 2020; Guétin *et al.* 2005; Hopper *et al.* 2019; Norelli *et al.* 2022; Williams *et al.* 2020).

See **Self-Care Handout 6.2: Self-Guided Imagery and Visualization** for an adapted version of the self-guided imagery and visualization technique the author of this text uses in the clinic setting as a simple pain-management and stress-reduction strategy (Brugnoli *et al.* 2018; Garland *et al.* 2017; Spiegel and Spiegel 2004; Spinhoven and Linssen 1989; Tan *et al.* 2015).

There are many forms of guided imagery, visualization, self-hypnosis, and hypnosis for relaxation and pain management. If a patient or client wants additional training in self-hypnosis and hypnosis, they should see a psychologist or healthcare provider trained in this area for more advanced and personalized techniques.

The American Psychological Association (2023) states that:

> Hypnosis is a set of techniques designed to enhance concentration, minimize one's usual distractions, and heighten responsiveness to suggestions to alter one's thoughts, feelings, behavior, or physiological state. Hypnosis is not a type of psychotherapy. It also is not a treatment in and of itself; rather, it is a procedure that can be used to facilitate other types of therapies and treatments.

It is recommended a person works with a psychologist or specialist trained in hypnosis for safety and effectiveness.

Self-Care Handout 6.1: Relaxation Breathing-Plus Technique

1. Start: Sit or lie down and gently close your eyes.
2. Mentally go to your favorite happy or relaxing place (such as the beach, park, lake, garden, or your "secret" place).
3. Breathe in through your nose as if trying to draw in a pleasant aroma, and breathe out through your mouth as if you want to make the flame of a candle in front of your mouth start to flicker without blowing it out (or pretend to blow on a dandelion and watch the seeds fly away). This is called diaphragmatic breathing or belly breathing.
4. When you are in your favorite or "secret" place, engage all your senses as you continue belly breathing. In your imagination, what do you smell (e.g., flowers, trees, ocean air)? What do you hear (e.g., birds, leaves rustling in the wind, flowing water)? What do you see (e.g., trees, lake, mountain overlook view)? What do you taste (e.g., green tea you drank from your water container)? What do you feel (e.g., the warmth of the sun, wind on your face, weight of a blanket)?
5. For more direct engagement of your senses, try the following:
   - Add taste for relaxation—drink green tea before beginning this technique.
   - Add sound for relaxation—play your favorite soft melody from your smartphone.
   - Add smell for relaxation—use essential oils (such as lavender or chamomile) for relaxing aromatherapy. Place two tiny drops of oil on the pillow you are using if you are lying down. Or use a scented soap next to your pillow.
   - Add the sensation of touch for relaxation—cover yourself with a weighted blanket.
6. You can modify this technique to last anywhere from 5 to 15 minutes. You may do this technique 1–3 times a day or as needed.
7. When you are ready to finish, smile and think about the wonderful things in your life.
8. End: Gently open your eyes and enjoy the day, or go to sleep.

Self-Care Handout 6.2: Self-Guided Imagery and Visualization

1. Start: Sit or lie down and gently close your eyes.
2. Breathe in through your nose as if trying to draw in a pleasant aroma, and breathe out through your mouth as if you want to make the flame of a candle in front of your mouth start to flicker without blowing it out (or pretend to blow on a dandelion and watch the seeds fly away). This is called diaphragmatic breathing or belly breathing.
3. See yourself floating a few inches from where you are sitting or lying down. Continue to belly breathe for 3–10 breaths.
4. Ease yourself into relaxation by counting down from 5 through 1 as you visualize large blue numbers in your mind (or green if it is a more relaxing color for you) as you belly breathe.
   5 4 3 2 1
5. Remember, belly breathing may be breathing in and out through the nose, or breathing in through the nose and out through the mouth.
6. Think of slowly walking down an easy ramp with rails into a shallow warm pool as you belly breathe.
7. Picture yourself stepping into the water, starting at your ankles, then your knees, hips, abdomen, and finally to your shoulders.
8. Then, imagine holding onto the rails as you gently float face-up in the warm pool.
9. Mentally go to your favorite happy or relaxing place (such as the beach, park, lake, garden, or your "secret" place). Continue to belly breathe for 3–10 breaths.
10. Think about something positive you want to change, for example "I feel better," "I feel calm," "I feel relaxed," or "I feel happy." Continue to belly breathe for 3–10 breaths.
11. You can modify this technique to last anywhere from 5 to 15 minutes. You may do this technique 1–3 times a day or as needed.
12. Slowly ease yourself back from your relaxed and floating state into the present moment by counting from 1 through 5 as you visualize small blue numbers in your mind (or green if it is a more relaxing color for you).
    1 2 3 4 5
13. When you are ready to finish, smile and think about the wonderful things in your life.
14. End: Gently open your eyes and enjoy the day, or go to sleep.

Self-Management Activities: Explore Music and Meditation Apps

The following online resources can help patients/clients, healthcare providers, and health/fitness professionals to manage stress and anxiety by exploring music.

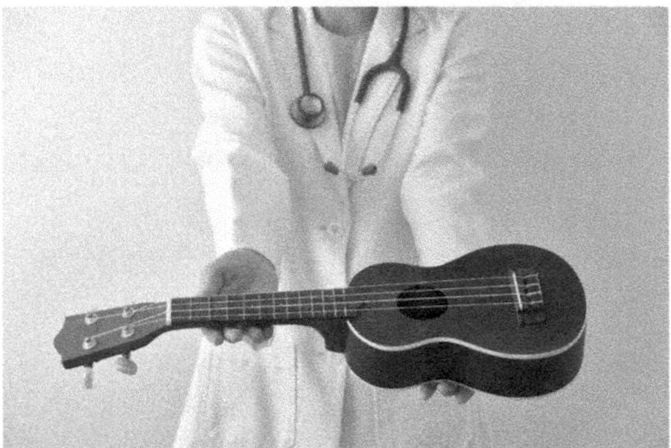

Relax with music

- The BandLab app provides a music creation platform: www.bandlab.com
- The GarageBand app provides a music creation platform: www.apple.com/ios/garageband
- The Soundtrap app provides a music creation platform for students and teachers: www.soundtrap.com
- The Dot Piano site is a visual musical instrument tool to help create music using the computer keyboard: https://dotpiano.com
- The Plink site provides a global and shared music experience using the computer keyboard: https://plink.in
- The NYU Music Experience Design site provides a variety of music creation platforms to create and play music: https://musedlab.org

Classroom and Lab Activities

- Analyze different types of meditation and relaxation techniques. Why do certain techniques work for some individuals?
- Outline meditation and relaxation techniques that may be ideal for home, work, and school use.

Useful Clinical Resources

Organizations

- American College of Lifestyle Medicine, www.lifestylemedicine.org
- American Institute of Stress, www.stress.org
- American Psychological Association, www.apa.org
- Benson-Henry Institute, https://bensonhenryinstitute.org
- Stress Management Society, www.stress.org.uk

Apps

- Breethe, https://breethe.com
- Calm, www.calm.com
- Headspace, www.headspace.com
- InsightTimer, https://insighttimer.com
- One Mind PsyberGuide, https://onemindpsyberguide.org
- The Mindfulness App, https://themindfulnessapp.com
- UCLA Mindful (meditations for well-being), https://apps.apple.com/us/app/ucla-mindful/id1459128935

Practitioner Sites

- Jon Kabat-Zinn, Ph.D., www.mindfulnesscds.com

Podcast

- Military Meditation Coach, https://soundcloud.com/militarymeditationcoach

Outcome Measures

- *Brief Resilience Scale*
  Smith BW, Dalen J, Wiggins K, Tooley E, Christopher P, Bernard J. The brief resilience scale: assessing the ability to bounce back. *Int J Behav Med.* 2008;15(3):194–200.
- *Perceived Stress Scale*
  Cohen S, Kamarck T, Mermelstein R. A global measure of perceived stress. *J Health Soc Behav.* 1983;24(4):385–396.
- *Psychological Stress Measure (PSM-9)*
  Lemyre L, Lalande-Markon MP. Psychological Stress Measure (PSM-9): integration of an evidence-based approach to assessment, monitoring,

and evaluation of stress in physical therapy practice. *Physiother Theory Pract.* 2009;25(5–6):453–462.

- *State-Trait Anxiety Inventory*
  Spielberger CD, Gorsuch RL, Lushene R, Vagg PR, Jacobs GA. *Manual for the State-Trait Anxiety Inventory*. Palo Alto, CA: Consulting Psychologists Press; 1983.

References

Acar K, Aygin D. Efficacy of guided imagery for postoperative symptoms, sleep quality, anxiety, and satisfaction regarding nursing care: a randomized controlled study. *J Perianesth Nurs.* 2019;34(6):1241–1249.

Afshar M, Mohsenzadeh A, Gilasi H, Sadeghi-Gandomani H. The effects of guided imagery on state and trait anxiety and sleep quality among patients receiving hemodialysis: a randomized controlled trial. *Complement Ther Med.* 2018;40:37–41.

American College of Lifestyle Medicine. Handout: Lifestyle stress reduction. American College of Lifestyle Medicine; 2019. www.lifestylemedicine.org

American Psychological Association. Hypnosis for pain relief and control of pain; 2023. www.apa.org/research/action/hypnosis

Austin KW, Ameringer SW, Cloud LJ. An integrated review of psychological stress in Parkinson's disease: biological mechanisms and symptom and health outcomes. *Parkinsons Dis.* 2016:9869712.

Banth S, Ardebil MD. Effectiveness of mindfulness meditation on pain and quality of life of patients with chronic low back pain. *Int J Yoga.* 2015;8(2):128–133.

Beck BD, Hansen ÅM, Gold C. Coping with work-related stress through guided imagery and music (GIM): randomized controlled trial. *J Music Ther.* 2015;52(3):323–352.

Bergmann A, Edelhoff D, Schubert O, Erdelt KJ, Pho Duc JM. Effect of treatment with a full-occlusion biofeedback splint on sleep bruxism and TMD pain: a randomized controlled clinical trial. *Clin Oral Investig.* 2020;24(11):4005–4018.

Bo S, Rahimi F, Goitre I, *et al.* Effects of self-conditioning techniques (self-hypnosis) in promoting weight loss in patients with severe obesity: a randomized controlled trial. *Obesity (Silver Spring).* 2018;26(9):1422–1429.

Boelens PA, Reeves RR, Replogle WH, Koenig HG. A randomized trial of the effect of prayer on depression and anxiety. *Int J Psychiatry Med.* 2009;39(4):377–392.

Brugnoli MP, Pesce G, Pasin E, Basile MF, Tamburin S, Polati E. The role of clinical hypnosis and self-hypnosis to relief pain and anxiety in severe chronic diseases in palliative care: a 2-year long-term follow-up of treatment in a nonrandomized clinical trial. *Ann Palliat Med.* 2018;7(1):17–31.

Carney CE, Edinger JD, Kuchibhatla M, *et al.* Cognitive behavioral insomnia therapy for those with insomnia and depression: a randomized controlled clinical trial. *Sleep.* 2017;40(4):zsx019.

Chen YF, Huang XY, Chien CH, Cheng JF. The effectiveness of diaphragmatic breathing relaxation training for reducing anxiety. *Perspect Psychiatr Care.* 2017;53(4):329–336.

Cherkin DC, Sherman KJ, Balderson BH, *et al.* Effect of mindfulness-based stress reduction vs cognitive behavioral therapy or usual care on back pain and functional limitations in adults with chronic low back pain: a randomized clinical trial. *JAMA.* 2016;315(12):1240–1249.

Cross RL, White J, Engelsher J, O'Connor SS. Implementation of rocking chair therapy for veterans in residential substance use disorder treatment. *J Am Psychiatr Nurses Assoc.* 2018;24(3):190–198.

Dreeben SJ, Mamberg MH, Salmon P. The MBSR body scan in clinical practice. *Mindfulness.* 2013;4:394–401.

Ebrahimi H, Mardani A, Basirinezhad MH, Hamidzadeh A, Eskandari F. The effects of lavender and chamomile essential oil inhalation aromatherapy on depression, anxiety and stress in older community-dwelling people: a randomized controlled trial [published online ahead of print, 2021 Jan 9]. *Explore (NY).* 2021;S1550-8307(21)00001-X.

Elder C, Nidich S, Moriarty F, Nidich R. Effect of transcendental meditation on employee stress, depression, and burnout: a randomized controlled study. *Perm J.* 2014;18(1):19–23.

Eron K, Kohnert L, Watters A, Logan C, Weisner-Rose M, Mehler PS. Weighted blanket use: a systematic review. *Am J Occup Ther.* 2020;74(2):7402205010p1–7402205010p14.

Fardo F, Allen M, Jegindø EM, Angrilli A, Roepstorff A. Neurocognitive evidence for mental imagery-driven hypoalgesic and hyperalgesic pain regulation. *Neuroimage*. 2015;120:350–361.

Felder JN, Epel ES, Neuhaus J, Krystal AD, Prather AA. Efficacy of digital cognitive behavioral therapy for the treatment of insomnia symptoms among pregnant women: a randomized clinical trial [published correction appears in *JAMA Psychiatry*. 2020 Jul 1;77(7):768]. *JAMA Psychiatry*. 2020;77(5):484–492.

Garland EL, Baker AK, Larsen P, *et al.* Randomized controlled trial of brief mindfulness training and hypnotic suggestion for acute pain relief in the hospital setting. *J Gen Intern Med*. 2017;32(10):1106–1113.

Genç F, Karadağ S, Kılıç Akça N, Tan M, Cerit D. The effect of aromatherapy on sleep quality and fatigue level of the elderly: a randomized controlled study. *Holist Nurs Pract*. 2020;34(3):155–162.

George Mason University. Famous quotes on stress and well-being; 2023. https://wellbeing.gmu.edu/famous-quotes-on-stress-and-well-being

Gong M, Dong H, Tang Y, Huang W, Lu F. Effects of aromatherapy on anxiety: a meta-analysis of randomized controlled trials. *J Affect Disord*. 2020;274:1028–1040.

Goodman MJ, Schorling JB. A mindfulness course decreases burnout and improves well-being among healthcare providers. *Int J Psychiatry Med*. 2012;43(2):119–128.

Grégoire C, Faymonville ME, Vanhaudenhuyse A, Jerusalem G, Willems S, Bragard I. Randomized controlled trial of a group intervention combining self-hypnosis and self-care: secondary results on self-esteem, emotional distress and regulation, and mindfulness in post-treatment cancer patients. *Qual Life Res*. 2021;30(2):425–436.

Grégoire C, Faymonville ME, Vanhaudenhuyse A, Jerusalem G, Willems S, Bragard I. Randomized, controlled trial of an intervention combining self-care and self-hypnosis on fatigue, sleep, and emotional distress in posttreatment cancer patients: 1-year follow-up. *Int J Clin Exp Hypn*. 2022;70(2):136–155.

Guétin S, Coudeyre E, Picot MC, *et al.* Intérêt de la musicothérapie dans la prise en charge de la lombalgie chronique en milieu hospitalier (Etude contrôlée, randomisée sur 65 patients) [Effect of music therapy among hospitalized patients with chronic low back pain: a controlled, randomized trial]. *Ann Readapt Med Phys*. 2005;48(5):217–224.

Hai AH, Wigmore B, Franklin C, *et al.* Efficacy of two-way prayer meditation in improving the psychospiritual well-being of people with substance use disorders: a pilot randomized controlled trial. *Subst Abus*. 2021;42(4):832–841.

Hamzeh S, Safari-Faramani R, Khatony A. Effects of aromatherapy with lavender and peppermint essential oils on the sleep quality of cancer patients: a randomized controlled trial. *Evid Based Complement Alternat Med*. 2020:7480204.

Hopper SI, Murray SL, Ferrara LR, Singleton JK. Effectiveness of diaphragmatic breathing for reducing physiological and psychological stress in adults: a quantitative systematic review. *JBI Database System Rev Implement Rep*. 2019;17(9):1855–1876.

Kabat-Zinn J. *Full Catastrophe Living: Using the Wisdom of Your Body and Mind to Face Stress, Pain and Illness*. New York, NY: Bantam Books; 2013.

Karper W. Rocking chair exercise and fibromyalgia syndrome. *Activities, Adaptations & Aging*. 2013;37:141–152.

Klimes-Dougan B, Chong LS, Samikoglu A, *et al.* Transcendental meditation and hypothalamic-pituitary-adrenal axis functioning: a pilot, randomized controlled trial with young adults. *Stress*. 2020;23(1):105–115.

Kogan LR, Bussolari C. Exploring the potential impact of a virtual body scan meditation exercise conducted with pet dogs on recipients and facilitators. *Front Psychol*. 2021;12:698075.

Koukoulithras I Sr, Stamouli A, Kolokotsios S, Plexousakis M Sr, Mavrogiannopoulou C. The effectiveness of non-pharmaceutical interventions upon pregnancy-related low back pain: a systematic review and meta-analysis. *Cureus*. 2021;13(1):e13011.

La Touche R, Fernández Pérez JJ, Martínez García S, Cuenca-Martínez F, López-de-Uralde-Villanueva I, Suso-Martí L. Hypoalgesic effects of aerobic and isometric motor imagery and action observation exercises on asymptomatic participants: a randomized controlled pilot trial. *Pain Med*. 2020;21(10):2186–2199.

Larson D, Yeh C, Rafferty M, Bega D. High satisfaction and improved quality of life with Rock Steady Boxing in Parkinson's disease: results of a large-scale survey. *Disabil Rehabil*. 2022;44(20):6034–6041.

LeMoult J, Humphreys KL, Tracy A, Hoffmeister JA, Ip E, Gotlib IH. Meta-analysis: exposure to early life stress and risk for depression in childhood and adolescence. *J Am Acad Child Adolesc Psychiatry*. 2020;59(7):842–855.

Luiggi-Hernandez JG, Woo J, Hamm M, Greco CM, Weiner DK, Morone NE. Mindfulness for chronic low back pain: a qualitative analysis. *Pain Med*. 2018;19(11):2138–2145.

Manolaki S, Gkiatas I, Sioutis S, *et al.* Relaxation techniques in low back pain patients: a randomized controlled trial. *J Long Term Eff Med Implants*. 2021;31(2):39–44.

Massey RL. A randomized trial of rocking-chair motion on the effect of postoperative ileus duration in patients with cancer recovering from abdominal surgery. *Appl Nurs Res.* 2010;23(2):59–64.

Mateu M, Alda O, Inda MD, *et al.* Randomized, controlled, crossover study of self-administered Jacobson relaxation in chronic, nonspecific, low-back pain. *Altern Ther Health Med.* 2018;24(6):22–30.

McCauley JD, Thelen MH, Frank RG, Willard RR, Callen KE. Hypnosis compared to relaxation in the outpatient management of chronic low back pain. *Arch Phys Med Rehabil.* 1983;64(11):548–552.

Morone NE, Greco CM, Moore CG, *et al.* A mind-body program for older adults with chronic low back pain: a randomized clinical trial. *JAMA Intern Med.* 2016;176(3):329–337.

Ni YX, Ma L, Li JP. Effects of mindfulness-based intervention on glycemic control and psychological outcomes in people with diabetes: a systematic review and meta-analysis. *J Diabetes Investig.* 2021;12(6):1092–1103.

Niemelä K, Väänänen I, Leinonen R, Laukkanen P. Benefits of home-based rocking-chair exercise for physical performance in community-dwelling elderly women: a randomized controlled trial. *Aging Clin Exp Res.* 2011;23(4):279–287.

Norelli SK, Long A, Krepps JM. Relaxation Techniques. In: StatPearls [Internet]. Treasure Island (FL): StatPearls Publishing; 2022. www.ncbi.nlm.nih.gov/books/NBK513238

Ooi SL, Giovino M, Pak SC. Transcendental meditation for lowering blood pressure: an overview of systematic reviews and meta-analyses. *Complement Ther Med.* 2017;34:26–34.

Ortego G, Villafañe JH, Doménech-García V, Berjano P, Bertozzi L, Herrero P. Is there a relationship between psychological stress or anxiety and chronic nonspecific neck-arm pain in adults? A systematic review and meta-analysis [published correction appears in *J Psychosom Res.* 2017 May;96:107]. *J Psychosom Res.* 2016;90:70–81.

Ozgundondu B, Gok Metin Z. Effects of progressive muscle relaxation combined with music on stress, fatigue, and coping styles among intensive care nurses. *Intensive Crit Care Nurs.* 2019;54:54–63.

Pizzoli SFM, Marzorati C, Mazzoni D, Pravettoni G. Web-based relaxation intervention for stress during social isolation: randomized controlled trial. *JMIR Ment Health.* 2020;7(12):e22757.

Rizzo RRN, Medeiros FC, Pires LG, *et al.* Hypnosis enhances the effects of pain education in patients with chronic nonspecific low back pain: a randomized controlled trial. *J Pain.* 2018;19(10):1103.e1–1103.e9.

Röttger S, Theobald DA, Abendroth J, Jacobsen T. The effectiveness of combat tactical breathing as compared with prolonged exhalation. *Appl Psychophysiol Biofeedback.* 2021;46(1):19–28.

Shaw WS, Hartvigsen J, Woiszwillo MJ, Linton SJ, Reme SE. Psychological distress in acute low back pain: a review of measurement scales and levels of distress reported in the first 2 months after pain onset. *Arch Phys Med Rehabil.* 2016;97(9):1573–1587.

Sielski R, Rief W, Glombiewski JA. Efficacy of biofeedback in chronic back pain: a meta-analysis. *Int J Behav Med.* 2017;24(1):25–41.

Sleep Foundation. Sleep in the military; 2023. www.sleepfoundation.org/sleep-in-the-military

Son HK, So WY, Kim M. Effects of aromatherapy combined with music therapy on anxiety, stress, and fundamental nursing skills in nursing students: a randomized controlled trial. *Int J Environ Res Public Health.* 2019;16(21):4185.

Spiegel H, Spiegel D. *Trance & Treatment: Clinical Uses of Hypnosis.* Washington, DC: American Psychiatric Publishing, Inc; 2004.

Spinhoven P, Linssen AC. Education and self-hypnosis in the management of low back pain: a component analysis. *Br J Clin Psychol.* 1989;28(2):145–153.

Tan G, Rintala DH, Jensen MP, Fukui T, Smith D, Williams W. A randomized controlled trial of hypnosis compared with biofeedback for adults with chronic low back pain. *Eur J Pain.* 2015;19(2):271–280.

Travell JG, Simons DG. *Myofascial Pain and Dysfunction: The Trigger Point Manual: The Lower Extremities—Volume 2.* Baltimore, MD: Williams & Wilkins; 1992.

Ussher M, Spatz A, Copland C, *et al.* Immediate effects of a brief mindfulness-based body scan on patients with chronic pain. *J Behav Med.* 2014;37(1):127–134.

Valentine KE, Milling LS, Clark LJ, Moriarty CL. The efficacy of hypnosis as a treatment for anxiety: a meta-analysis. *Int J Clin Exp Hypn.* 2019;67(3):336–363.

van der Zwan JE, de Vente W, Huizink AC, Bögels SM, de Bruin EI. Physical activity, mindfulness meditation, or heart rate variability biofeedback for stress reduction: a randomized controlled trial. *Appl Psychophysiol Biofeedback.* 2015;40(4):257–268.

Venes D, ed. *Taber's Cyclopedic Medical Dictionary,* 24th ed. Philadelphia, PA: FA Davis; 2021.

WebMD. What is box breathing? 2023. WebMD. www.webmd.com/balance/what-is-box-breathing

Williams JL, Everett JM, D'Cunha NM, *et al.* The effects of green tea amino acid L-Theanine consumption on the ability to manage stress and anxiety levels: a systematic review. *Plant Foods Hum Nutr.* 2020;75(1):12–23.

Winter B. *Relax and Win: Championship Performance in Whatever You Do* (updated edition). Bud Winter Enterprises; 2012.

Yates DH. Relaxation in psychotherapy. *J Gen Psychol.* 1946;34:213–238.

Zgierska AE, Burzinski CA, Cox J, *et al.* Mindfulness meditation-based intervention is feasible, acceptable, and safe for chronic low back pain requiring long-term daily opioid therapy. *J Altern Complement Med.* 2016;22(8):610–620.

Zheng Y, Zhou Y, Lai Q. Effects of twenty-four move shadow boxing combined with psychosomatic relaxation on depression and anxiety in patients with type-2 diabetes. *Psychiatr Danub.* 2015;27(2):174–179.

Additional Reading

Ein N, Li L, Vickers K. The effect of pet therapy on the physiological and subjective stress response: a meta-analysis. *Stress Health.* 2018;34(4):477–489.

Kabat-Zinn J. *Coming to Our Senses: Healing Ourselves and the World Through Mindfulness.* New York, NY: Hyperion; 2005.

Kabat-Zinn J. *Wherever You Go, There You Are: Mindfulness Meditation in Everyday Life,* 10th ed. New York, NY: Hyperion; 2005.

Kabat-Zinn J. *Arriving at Your Own Door: 108 Lessons in Mindfulness.* New York, NY: Hyperion; 2007.

Kornspan AS. *Fundamentals of Sport and Exercise Psychology.* Champaign, IL: Human Kinetics; 2009.

Lee LO, James P, Zevon ES, *et al.* Optimism is associated with exceptional longevity in 2 epidemiologic cohorts of men and women. *Proc Natl Acad Sci U S A.* 2019;116(37):18357–18362.

Philips KH, Brintz CE, Moss K, Gaylord SA. Didgeridoo sound meditation for stress reduction and mood enhancement in undergraduates: a randomized controlled trial. *Glob Adv Health Med.* 2019;8:2164956119879367.

CHAPTER 7

Restorative Sleep

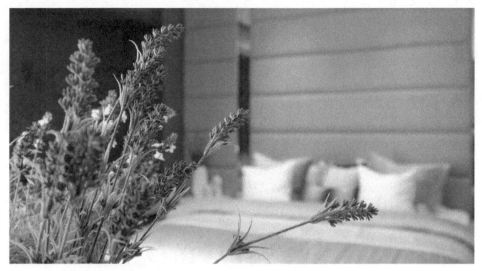

A comfortable and cozy bedroom means a good night's sleep

Learning Objectives

- Understand the basic research for sleep hygiene.
- Apply sleep hygiene for practical pain management.

Chapter Highlights

- Key Concept: Sleep is Medicine
- Clinical Tip: Horticultural Therapy and Sleep
- Featured Topic 7.1: Pre-Sleep Routine
- Featured Topic 7.2: Weighted Blanket
- Self-Care Handout 7.1: Sleep Hygiene Guidelines
- Self-Care Handout 7.2: Progressive Muscle Relaxation Routine
- Self-Management Activities

- Classroom and Lab Activities
- Useful Clinical Resources
- References
- Additional Reading

Lifestyle Matters: *Live slow, live healthy.*

Introduction

Venes (2021, p.2203) defines sleep as "a periodic state of rest accompanied by varying degrees of unconsciousness and relative inactivity." Loss of sleep may be caused by lifestyle habits such as alcohol, smoking, and caffeine, medical conditions such as sleep apnea, medications, poor sleep hygiene habits, recent surgery, sleep disorders, stress, work and family obligations, anxiety, frequent travel, and work schedule. Studies show that sleep deficiency may, for example, impact dementia (Robbins *et al.* 2021) and obesity (Bacaro *et al.* 2020).

Simply issuing self-care and sleep hygiene guidelines will not work unless a provider addresses the root cause of an individual's sleep disturbance. For example, is the person's disturbed sleep due to pain, stress, poor sleep hygiene, frequent travel across time zones, insomnia, obstructive sleep apnea, circadian phase disorders, partial arousal parasomnias, narcolepsy disorder, behaviorally induced insufficient sleep syndrome, restless legs syndrome, or periodic limb movement disorder? For this reason, providers need to assess the person, if within their scope of practice, with various tools such as a sleep diary, sleep assessments, and questionnaires (such as the Single-Item Sleep Quality Scale, Global Sleep Assessment Questionnaire, Epworth Sleepiness Scale, Pittsburgh Sleep Quality Index, STOP-BANG Questionnaire, Adolescent Sleep Hygiene Scale, Women's Health Initiative Insomnia Rating Scale, or Composite Scale for Morningness Questionnaire), or utilize more advanced strategies such as a polysomnography study or actigraphy. Once the appropriate assessment is completed, the provider may decide if strategies such as sleep hygiene guidelines, behavioral therapies, sleep restriction therapy, or relaxation training are indicated (Clayton and Bonnet 2023).

KEY CONCEPT: SLEEP IS MEDICINE

Sleep is good medicine since it helps a person reduce health problems such as heart disease and Type 2 diabetes, and also increases productivity, boosts mood, and helps maintain a healthy weight. The American Academy of Sleep Medicine provides resources for the community on its Sleep is Good Medicine website: https://sleepisgoodmedicine.com. The organization covers topics such as why sleep is essential and how to get healthy sleep. It also discusses finding a sleep center (if needed) and provides a calculator to determine optimal sleep duration.

Why Sleep is Necessary

The Joint Consensus Statement of the American Academy of Sleep Medicine and Sleep Research Society (Consensus Conference Panel *et al.* 2015) indicates that sleep is vital for health and brain functions such as cognitive performance, memory consolidation, mood regulation, and clearance of brain metabolites. The authors say that sleep is involved in metabolism, appetite regulation, immune and hormone function, and the cardiovascular system. Finally, the statement indicates that sleep duration is linked to cancer, cardiovascular disease, depression, diabetes, and obesity.

A part of the Consensus Statement of the American Academy of Sleep Medicine and Sleep Research Society (Watson *et al.* 2015, p.843) states, "Adults should sleep 7 or more hours per night on a regular basis to promote optimal health."

The following list presents some conditions associated with sleep problems:

- Anxiety
- Decreased job performance
- Depression
- Diabetes
- Fatigue
- Heart attack
- High blood pressure
- Impaired cognitive function
- Increased incidence of colds and viruses
- Increased pain perception
- Increased risk of falls
- Irritability
- Obesity
- Overeating
- Pain (such as general pain, neck and back pain)
- Reduced quality of life
- Risk of sports injuries in adolescents
- Slowed reaction times
- Stroke

- Systemic low-grade inflammation

From Besedovsky et al. 2019; Bonanno et al. 2019; Cohen et al. 2009; Gao et al. 2019; Schrimpf et al. 2015; Skarpsno et al. 2020.

Sleep Management Strategies

The following list outlines various conventional, integrative, and mind-body strategies that may improve sleep quality in selected cases along with citations for published research on their use:

- Acupressure (Dincer *et al.* 2022; Lai *et al.* 2017)
- Aromatherapy (Hwang and Shin 2015; Genç *et al.* 2020)
- Body scan meditation (Hubbling *et al.* 2014)
- Cognitive behavioral therapy (Carney *et al.* 2017; Felder *et al.* 2020)
- Exercise (Jurado-Fasoli *et al.* 2020; Kovacevic *et al.* 2018)
- Guided imagery (Afshar *et al.* 2018; Ramezani Kermani *et al.* 2020)
- Hypnosis (Elkins *et al.* 2021)
- Mindfulness meditation (Black *et al.* 2015; Rusch *et al.* 2019; Zhang *et al.* 2015)
- Music therapy (Lund *et al.* 2022; Wang *et al.* 2014)
- Outdoor activity (Luo *et al.* 2020)
- Progressive muscle relaxation (Kılıç and Parlar Kılıç 2021; Özlü *et al.* 2021)
- Qigong (Baduanjin) (Carcelén-Fraile *et al.* 2022)
- Self-hypnosis (Grégoire *et al.* 2022; Otte *et al.* 2020)
- Tai chi (Irwin *et al.* 2014; Li *et al.* 2020; Si *et al.* 2020; Siu *et al.* 2021)
- Therapeutic touch (Çalışkan and Cerit 2021)
- Yoga (Lin *et al.* 2019; Mustian *et al.* 2013; Roseen *et al.* 2020; Shree Ganesh *et al.* 2021; Susanti *et al.* 2022; Wang *et al.* 2020)

CLINICAL TIP: HORTICULTURAL THERAPY AND SLEEP

Horticultural therapy (such as planting vegetables, making a rosemary wreath, designing a healing garden, arranging a rose basket, and enjoying a garden party) may improve happiness, well-being, and sleep quality of elderly individuals (Shen *et al.* 2022).

Featured Topics

Featured Topic 7.1 outlines a sample pre-sleep routine.

Featured Topic 7.2 outlines the benefits of using a weighted blanket.

Please note that the following featured topics provide tools that may help some individuals relax before sleep. However, simple self-care strategies do not address the root cause of various sleep-related disturbances, as mentioned in the introduction.

■ Featured Topic 7.1: Pre-Sleep Routine

The following is an adapted pre-sleep routine outlined by Bud Winter (Winter 2012):

1. Start: Lie face up in your bed. (This technique may also be performed sitting in a chair to fall asleep on a bus, train, or plane.)
2. Relax the muscles in your forehead, jaw, and around your eyes.
3. Drop your shoulders.
4. Take three deep breaths.
5. Select one of these three techniques based on what works for you:
   - Imagine lying on your back in the bottom of a canoe on a peaceful lake during a warm day. Stare at the blue sky with some floating clouds. There should be no motion or movement in this mental image. Stay focused on this image and enjoy it for 10 seconds.
   - Imagine lying in a black velvet hammock in a pitch-black room. Stay focused on this motionless image for 10 seconds.
   - Say the words "don't think" or "I'm calm" slowly for 10 seconds.
6. Once you find the image that resonates with you the most, keep going with it for around 2 minutes or until you fall asleep.
7. End.

Adapted from Winter 2012.

Note: Lloyd "Bud" Winter was a track coach at San José State University for 30 years, participated in six Olympic Games, and wrote several books. His techniques are based on training methods used to prepare World War II combat flyers. For more information see: www.budwinter.com.

■ Featured Topic 7.2: Weighted Blanket

It is proposed that a weighted blanket provides widespread pressure on the body that results in relaxation, decreased anxiety, and reduced pain. Weighted blankets can weigh from 3 to 20 pounds. They may be an effective adjunct intervention option for conditions such as attention deficit hyperactivity disorder (ADHD) and/or autism spectrum disorder (ASD), anxiety, chronic pain, and insomnia (Baumgartner *et al.* 2022; Becklund *et al.* 2021; Bernstein 2023; Bolic Baric *et al.* 2021; Ekholm *et al.* 2020; Eron *et al.* 2020; Meth *et al.* 2022; Noyed 2023).

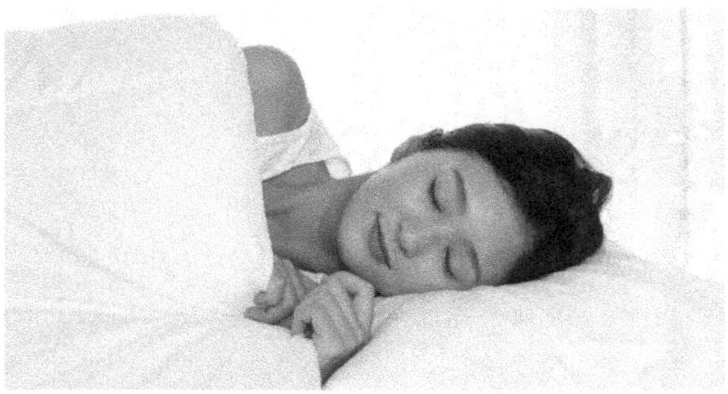

Weighted blanket for comfort

Self-Care Education Guides

See **Self-Care Handout 7.1: Sleep Hygiene Guidelines** for a practical sleep hygiene guideline checklist that may be issued to patients/clients (Altug 2018; American College of Lifestyle Medicine 2019; Kryger *et al.* 2022; Matsuo *et al.* 2019; Vitale *et al.* 2019; Wittmann *et al.* 2006).

See **Self-Care Handout 7.2: Progressive Muscle Relaxation Routine** for a relaxation strategy using the progressive muscle relaxation routine created by psychiatrist Edmund Jacobson, MD, Ph.D. (1888–1983), who wrote five books (Jacobson 1962; 1964a; 1964b; 1967; 1976). The progressive muscle relaxation routine may help a person fall asleep and promote overall relaxation (Akmeşe and Oran 2014; Bernstein and Borkovec 1973; Mateu *et al.* 2018).

Self-Care Handout 7.1: Sleep Hygiene Guidelines

- Establish regular bedtime and waking hours.
- Avoid or minimize "social jet lag" that may be due to work, school, or personal schedules.
- Create a comfortable bedroom that is cool, dark, and quiet.
- Sleep in a comfortable bed and make sure it's not too old.
- Use a supportive and comfortable pillow, and make sure it's not too old.
- Maintain a healthy body mass index (BMI).
- Turn off the radio and television before going to sleep.
- Minimize bright light near bedtime, but do increase daytime exposure to sunlight.
- Try a weighted blanket during sleep.
- Minimize wearing tight or restrictive clothing during sleep, unless it's for medical purposes.
- Learn strategies to reduce daily stress so it does not result in poor quality sleep.
- Minimize tense or stressful living since this may carry over into sleep.
- Finish dinner a couple of hours before bedtime.
- Engage in regular physical activity during the day to help improve sleep quality.
- Avoid near bedtime:
  - caffeine (for at least several hours before bedtime, but it may need to be longer)
  - alcohol (for at least several hours before bedtime)
  - smoking or using nicotine (for at least several hours before bedtime); ideally, don't smoke
  - after-dinner and late-night snacking
  - intense exercise (for at least several hours before bedtime).
- To minimize trips to the bathroom, near bedtime reduce intake of:
  - fluids, but do maintain adequate hydration during the day
  - sugar and salt.
- Gradually wind down the evening:
  - Minimize intense television shows or news programs near bedtime.
  - Minimize intense activities such as personal finances or business meetings near bedtime.
  - Limit or avoid computer and smartphone use near bedtime.

  - Read a book, listen to relaxing music, watch a fun television show, or engage in a fun hobby near bedtime.
- Embrace mindfulness before bedtime:
  - Consider meditating close to bedtime or using a body scan or progressive muscle relaxation technique.
  - Consider gentle tai chi, qigong, or yoga later in the day.
- Establish a bedtime ritual such as the following:
  - One hour before going to sleep, shut down all phone and computer devices. Then you can either read a book or watch a funny television show (drama may be too stimulating).
  - Five minutes before you go to sleep wash your hands and face with lavender soap and, finally, shut off all the lights before you slip into your cozy bed with gratitude and pleasant thoughts.

Self-Care Handout 7.2: Progressive Muscle Relaxation Routine

1. Start: Sit or lie down and gently close your eyes.
2. Breathe in through your nose as if trying to draw in a pleasant aroma, and breathe out through your mouth as if you want to make the flame of a candle in front of your mouth start to flicker without blowing it out (or pretend to blow on a dandelion and watch the seeds fly away). This is called diaphragmatic breathing or belly breathing.
3. Wrinkle your forehead for 5 seconds, and relax with 2 belly breaths.
4. Frown for 5 seconds, and relax with 2 belly breaths.
5. Press your lips together for 5 seconds, and relax with 2 belly breaths.
6. Shrug your shoulders for 5 seconds, and relax with 2 belly breaths.
7. Tighten your arm muscles for 5 seconds, and relax with 2 belly breaths.
8. Tighten your fists for 5 seconds, and relax with 2 belly breaths.
9. Tighten your abdominal muscles for 5 seconds, and relax with 2 belly breaths.
10. Tighten your hip muscles for 5 seconds, and relax with 2 belly breaths.
11. Tighten your thigh muscles for 5 seconds, and relax with 2 belly breaths.
12. Point your toes away from you for 5 seconds, and relax with 2 belly breaths.
13. Scrunch your toes for 5 seconds, and relax with 2 belly breaths.
14. When you are ready to finish, smile and think about the wonderful things in your life.
15. End: Gently open your eyes and enjoy the day, or go to sleep.

Self-Management Activities: Explore Art

The following online resources can help patients/clients, healthcare providers, and health/fitness professionals to manage stress and anxiety by exploring art. Search for famous artists such as Claude Monet, Pierre-Auguste Renoir, Vincent Van Gogh, Rembrandt van Rijn, or Berthe Morisot to learn about the artists and relax by looking at their paintings.

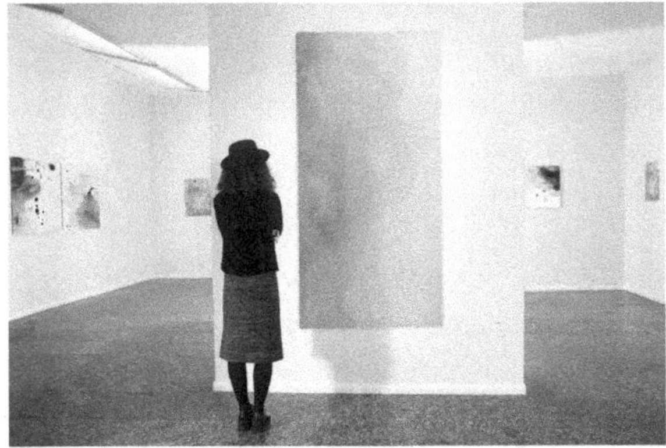

Art for relaxation

- The Louvre Museum, www.louvre.fr/en
- The Museum of Modern Art, www.moma.org
- The National Gallery, www.nationalgallery.org.uk
- The National Gallery of Art, www.nga.gov

Classroom and Lab Activities

- Determine which yoga poses might help promote sleep.
- Create a pre-sleep yoga routine.

Useful Clinical Resources

Organizations

- American Academy of Sleep Medicine, https://aasm.org
- Better Sleep Council, https://bettersleep.org
- National Heart, Lung, and Blood Institute (sleep deprivation and deficiency), www.nhlbi.nih.gov/health-topics/sleep-deprivation-and-deficiency
- National Sleep Foundation, www.thensf.org

- Sleep Education (American Academy of Sleep Medicine), https://sleepeducation.org
- Sleep Foundation, www.sleepfoundation.org
- Sleep is Good Medicine (American Academy of Sleep Medicine), https://sleepisgoodmedicine.com

Outcome Measures

- *Adolescent Sleep Hygiene Scale*
  Storfer-Isser A, Lebourgeois MK, Harsh J, Tompsett CJ, Redline S. Psychometric properties of the Adolescent Sleep Hygiene Scale. *J Sleep Res.* 2013;22(6):707–716.
- *Athlete Sleep Behavior Questionnaire*
  Driller MW, Mah CD, Halson SL. Development of the athlete sleep behavior questionnaire: a tool for identifying maladaptive sleep practices in elite athletes. *Sleep Sci.* 2018;11(1):37–44.
- *Composite Scale for Morningness Questionnaire*
  Smith CS, Reilly C, Midkiff K. Evaluation of three circadian rhythm questionnaires with suggestions for an improved measure of morningness. *J Appl Psychol.* 1989;74(5):728–738.
- *Epworth Sleepiness Scale*
  Johns MW. A new method for measuring daytime sleepiness: the Epworth Sleepiness Scale. *Sleep.* 1991;14:540–545.
- *Global Sleep Assessment Questionnaire*
  Roth T, Zammit G, Kushida C, et al. A new questionnaire to detect sleep disorders. *Sleep Med.* 2002;3(2):99–108.
- *Pittsburgh Sleep Quality Index*
  Mollayeva T, Thurairajah P, Burton K, Mollayeva S, Shapiro CM, Colantonio A. The Pittsburgh sleep quality index as a screening tool for sleep dysfunction in clinical and non-clinical samples: a systematic review and meta-analysis. *Sleep Med Rev.* 2016;25:52–73.
- *Restorative Sleep Questionnaire*
  Robbins R, Quan SF, Buysse D, *et al.* A nationally representative survey assessing restorative sleep in US adults. *Front Sleep.* 2022;1:935228.
- *Single-Item Sleep Quality Scale*
  Snyder E, Cai B, DeMuro C, Morrison MF, Ball W. A New Single-Item Sleep Quality Scale: Results of Psychometric Evaluation in Patients With Chronic Primary Insomnia and Depression. *J Clin Sleep Med.* 2018;14(11):1849–1857.

- *Sleep Hygiene Index*
  Mastin DF, Bryson J, Corwyn R. Assessment of sleep hygiene using the Sleep Hygiene Index. *J Behav Med*. 2006;29(3):223–227.
- *STOP-BANG Questionnaire*
  Chung F, Abdullah HR, Liao P. STOP-Bang Questionnaire: a practical approach to screen for obstructive sleep apnea. *Chest*. 2016;149(3):631–638.
- *Women's Health Initiative Insomnia Rating Scale*
  Levine DW, Kripke DF, Kaplan RM, et al. Reliability and validity of the Women's Health Initiative Insomnia Rating Scale. *Psychol Assess*. 2003;15(2):137–148.

References

Afshar M, Mohsenzadeh A, Gilasi H, Sadeghi-Gandomani H. The effects of guided imagery on state and trait anxiety and sleep quality among patients receiving hemodialysis: a randomized controlled trial. *Complement Ther Med*. 2018;40:37–41.

Akmeşe ZB, Oran NT. Effects of progressive muscle relaxation exercises accompanied by music on low back pain and quality of life during pregnancy. *J Midwifery Women's Health*. 2014;59(5):503–509.

Altug Z. *Integrative Healing: Developing Wellness in the Mind and Body*. Springville, UT: Cedar Fort; 2018.

American College of Lifestyle Medicine. Handout: Lifestyle sleep health. American College of Lifestyle Medicine; 2019. www.lifestylemedicine.org

Bacaro V, Ballesio A, Cerolini S, *et al.* Sleep duration and obesity in adulthood: an updated systematic review and meta-analysis. *Obes Res Clin Pract*. 2020;14(4):301–309.

Baumgartner JN, Quintana D, Leija L, *et al.* Widespread pressure delivered by a weighted blanket reduces chronic pain: a randomized controlled trial. *J Pain*. 2022;23(1):156–174.

Becklund AL, Rapp-McCall L, Nudo J. Using weighted blankets in an inpatient mental health hospital to decrease anxiety. *J Integr Med*. 2021;19(2):129–134.

Bernstein DA, Borkovec TD. *Progressive Relaxation Training: A Manual for the Helping Professions*. Champaign, IL: Research Press; 1973.

Bernstein S. Weighted blankets: What you need to know; 2023. WebMD. www.webmd.com/sleep-disorders/weighted-blankets

Besedovsky L, Lange T, Haack M. The sleep-immune crosstalk in health and disease. *Physiol Rev*. 2019;99(3):1325–1380.

Black DS, O'Reilly GA, Olmstead R, Breen EC, Irwin MR. Mindfulness meditation and improvement in sleep quality and daytime impairment among older adults with sleep disturbances: a randomized clinical trial. *JAMA Intern Med*. 2015;175(4):494–501.

Bolic Baric V, Skuthälla S, Pettersson M, Gustafsson PA, Kjellberg A. The effectiveness of weighted blankets on sleep and everyday activities: a retrospective follow-up study of children and adults with attention deficit hyperactivity disorder and/or autism spectrum disorder [published online ahead of print, 2021 Jun 29]. *Scand J Occup Ther*. 2021;1–11.

Bonanno L, Metro D, Papa M, *et al.* Assessment of sleep and obesity in adults and children: observational study. *Medicine (Baltimore)*. 2019;98(46):e17642.

Çalışkan MA, Cerit B. Effect of therapeutic touch on sleep quality and anxiety in individuals with chronic obstructive pulmonary disease: a randomized controlled trial. *Complement Ther Clin Pract*. 2021;45:101481.

Carcelén-Fraile MDC, Aibar-Almazán A, Martínez-Amat A, *et al.* Qigong for mental health and sleep quality in postmenopausal women: a randomized controlled trial. *Medicine (Baltimore)*. 2022;101(39):e30897.

Carney CE, Edinger JD, Kuchibhatla M, *et al.* Cognitive behavioral insomnia therapy for those with insomnia and depression: a randomized controlled clinical trial. *Sleep*. 2017;40(4):zsx019.

Clayton JS, Bonnet J. *Foundations of Lifestyle Medicine: Board Review Manual*, 4th ed. Chesterfield, MO: American College of Lifestyle Medicine; 2023.

Cohen S, Doyle WJ, Alper CM, Janicki-Deverts D, Turner RB. Sleep habits and susceptibility to the common cold. *Arch Intern Med*. 2009;169(1):62–67.

Consensus Conference Panel; Watson NF, Badr MS, *et al.* Joint Consensus Statement of the American

Academy of Sleep Medicine and Sleep Research Society on the Recommended Amount of Sleep for a Healthy Adult: methodology and discussion. *Sleep*. 2015;38(8):1161–1183.

Dincer B, İnangil D, İnangil G, *et al.* The effect of acupressure on sleep quality of older people: a systematic review and meta-analysis of randomized controlled trials. *Explore (NY)*. 2022;18(6):635–645.

Ekholm B, Spulber S, Adler M. A randomized controlled study of weighted chain blankets for insomnia in psychiatric disorders. *J Clin Sleep Med*. 2020;16(9):1567–1577.

Elkins G, Otte J, Carpenter JS, *et al.* Hypnosis intervention for sleep disturbance: determination of optimal dose and method of delivery for postmenopausal women. *Int J Clin Exp Hypn*. 2021;69(3):323–345.

Eron K, Kohnert L, Watters A, Logan C, Weisner-Rose M, Mehler PS. Weighted blanket use: a systematic review. *Am J Occup Ther*. 2020;74(2):7402205010p1–7402205010p14.

Felder JN, Epel ES, Neuhaus J, Krystal AD, Prather AA. Efficacy of digital cognitive behavioral therapy for the treatment of insomnia symptoms among pregnant women: a randomized clinical trial [published correction appears in *JAMA Psychiatry*. 2020 Jul 1;77(7):768]. *JAMA Psychiatry*. 2020;77(5):484–492.

Gao B, Dwivedi S, Milewski MD, Cruz AI Jr. Lack of sleep and sports injuries in adolescents: a systematic review and meta-analysis. *J Pediatr Orthop*. 2019;39(5):e324–e333.

Genç F, Karadağ S, Kılıç Akça N, Tan M, Cerit D. The effect of aromatherapy on sleep quality and fatigue level of the elderly: a randomized controlled study. *Holist Nurs Pract*. 2020;34(3):155–162.

Grégoire C, Faymonville ME, Vanhaudenhuyse A, Jerusalem G, Willems S, Bragard I. Randomized, controlled trial of an intervention combining self-care and self-hypnosis on fatigue, sleep, and emotional distress in posttreatment cancer patients: 1-year follow-up. *Int J Clin Exp Hypn*. 2022;70(2):136–155.

Hubbling A, Reilly-Spong M, Kreitzer MJ, Gross CR. How mindfulness changed my sleep: focus groups with chronic insomnia patients. *BMC Complement Altern Med*. 2014;14:50.

Hwang E, Shin S. The effects of aromatherapy on sleep improvement: a systematic literature review and meta-analysis. *J Altern Complement Med*. 2015;21(2):61–68.

Irwin MR, Olmstead R, Carrillo C, *et al.* Cognitive behavioral therapy vs. tai chi for late life insomnia and inflammatory risk: a randomized controlled comparative efficacy trial. *Sleep*. 2014;37(9):1543–1552.

Jacobson E. *Progressive Relaxation*, 4th ed. Chicago, IL: University of Chicago Press; 1962.

Jacobson E. *Anxiety and Tension Control*. Philadelphia, PA: JB Lippincott; 1964a.

Jacobson E. *Self-Operations Control Manual*. Chicago, IL: National Foundation for Progressive Relaxation; 1964b.

Jacobson E. *Tension in Medicine*. Springfield, IL: Charles C Thomas; 1967.

Jacobson E. *You Must Relax*, 5th ed. New York, NY: McGraw-Hill Book Company, Inc; 1976.

Jurado-Fasoli L, De-la-O A, Molina-Hidalgo C, Migueles JH, Castillo MJ, Amaro-Gahete FJ. Exercise training improves sleep quality: a randomized controlled trial. *Eur J Clin Invest*. 2020;50(3):e13202.

Kılıç N, Parlar Kılıç S. The effect of progressive muscle relaxation on sleep quality and fatigue in patients with rheumatoid arthritis: a randomized controlled trial [published online ahead of print, 2021 Sep 26]. *Int J Nurs Pract*. 2021;e13015.

Kovacevic A, Mavros Y, Heisz JJ, Fiatarone Singh MA. The effect of resistance exercise on sleep: a systematic review of randomized controlled trials. *Sleep Med Rev*. 2018;39:52–68.

Kryger M, Roth T, Goldstein CA, Dement WC. *Principles and Practice of Sleep Medicine*, 7th ed. Philadelphia, PA: Elsevier; 2022.

Lai FC, Chen IH, Chen PJ, Chen IJ, Chien HW, Yuan CF. Acupressure, sleep, and quality of life in institutionalized older adults: a randomized controlled trial. *J Am Geriatr Soc*. 2017;65(5):e103–e108.

Li H, Chen J, Xu G, *et al.* The effect of tai chi for improving sleep quality: a systematic review and meta-analysis. *J Affect Disord*. 2020;274:1102–1112.

Lin PJ, Kleckner IR, Loh KP, *et al.* Influence of yoga on cancer-related fatigue and on mediational relationships between changes in sleep and cancer-related fatigue: a nationwide, multicenter randomized controlled trial of yoga in cancer survivors. *Integr Cancer Ther*. 2019;18:1534735419855134.

Lund HN, Pedersen IN, Heymann-Szlachcinska AM, *et al.* Music to improve sleep quality in adults with depression-related insomnia (MUSTAFI): randomized controlled trial [published online ahead of print, 2022 Jun 13]. *Nord J Psychiatry*. 2022;1–10.

Luo J, Cao M, Sun F, Shi B, Wang X, Jing J. Association between outdoor activity and insufficient sleep in Chinese school-aged children. *Med Sci Monit*. 2020;26:e921617.

Mateu M, Alda O, Inda MD, *et al.* Randomized, controlled, crossover study of self-administered Jacobson relaxation in chronic, nonspecific, low-back pain. *Altern Ther Health Med*. 2018;24(6):22–30.

Matsuo T, Miyata Y, Sakai H. Effect of salt intake reduction on nocturia in patients with excessive salt intake. *Neurourol Urodyn*. 2019;38(3):927–933.

Meth EMS, Brandão LEM, van Egmond LT, *et al.* A weighted blanket increases pre-sleep salivary concentrations of melatonin in young, healthy adults [published online ahead of print, 2022 Oct 3]. *J Sleep Res*. 2022;e13743.

Mustian KM, Sprod LK, Janelsins M, *et al.* Multicenter, randomized controlled trial of yoga for sleep quality among cancer survivors. *J Clin Oncol*. 2013;31(26):3233–3241.

Noyed D. How heavy should a weighted blanket be? Sleep Foundation; 2023. www.sleepfoundation.org/bedding-information/weighted-blanket-weight-chart

Otte JL, Carpenter JS, Roberts L, Elkins GR. Self-hypnosis for sleep disturbances in menopausal women. *J Womens Health (Larchmt)*. 2020;29(3):461–463.

Özlü İ, Öztürk Z, Karaman Özlü Z, Tekin E, Gür A. The effects of progressive muscle relaxation exercises on the anxiety and sleep quality of patients with COVID-19: a randomized controlled study. *Perspect Psychiatr Care*. 2021;57(4):1791–1797.

Ramezani Kermani A, Aghebati N, Mohajer S, Ghavami V. Effect of guided imagery along with breathing relaxation on sleep quality of the elderly patients under abdominal surgery: a randomized clinical trial. *Holist Nurs Pract*. 2020;34(6):334–344.

Robbins R, Quan SF, Weaver MD, Bormes G, Barger LK, Czeisler CA. Examining sleep deficiency and disturbance and their risk for incident dementia and all-cause mortality in older adults across 5 years in the United States. *Aging (Albany NY)*. 2021;13(3):3254–3268.

Roseen EJ, Gerlovin H, Femia A, *et al.* Yoga, physical therapy, and back pain education for sleep quality in low-income racially diverse adults with chronic low back pain: a secondary analysis of a randomized controlled trial. *J Gen Intern Med*. 2020;35(1):167–176.

Rusch HL, Rosario M, Levison LM, *et al.* The effect of mindfulness meditation on sleep quality: a systematic review and meta-analysis of randomized controlled trials. *Ann N Y Acad Sci*. 2019;1445(1):5–16.

Schrimpf M, Liegl G, Boeckle M, Leitner A, Geisler P, Pieh C. The effect of sleep deprivation on pain perception in healthy subjects: a meta-analysis. *Sleep Med*. 2015;16(11):1313–1320.

Shen JL, Hung BL, Fang SH. Horticulture therapy affected the mental status, sleep quality, and salivary markers of mucosal immunity in an elderly population. *Sci Rep*. 2022;12(1):10246.

Shree Ganesh HR, Subramanya P, Rao MR, Udupa V. Role of yoga therapy in improving digestive health and quality of sleep in an elderly population: a randomized controlled trial. *J Bodyw Mov Ther*. 2021;27:692–697.

Si Y, Wang C, Yin H, *et al.* Tai chi chuan for subjective sleep quality: a systematic review and meta-analysis of randomized controlled trials. *Evid Based Complement Alternat Med*. 2020:4710527.

Siu PM, Yu AP, Tam BT, *et al.* Effects of tai chi or exercise on sleep in older adults with insomnia: a randomized clinical trial. *JAMA Netw Open*. 2021;4(2):e2037199.

Skarpsno ES, Mork PJ, Nilsen TIL, Nordstoga AL. Influence of sleep problems and co-occurring musculoskeletal pain on long-term prognosis of chronic low back pain: the HUNT Study. *J Epidemiol Community Health*. 2020;74(3):283–289.

Susanti HD, Sonko I, Chang PC, Chuang YH, Chung MH. Effects of yoga on menopausal symptoms and sleep quality across menopause statuses: a randomized controlled trial. *Nurs Health Sci*. 2022;24(2):368–379.

Venes D, ed. *Taber's Cyclopedic Medical Dictionary*, 24th ed. Philadelphia, PA: FA Davis; 2021.

Vitale KC, Owens R, Hopkins SR, Malhotra A. Sleep hygiene for optimizing recovery in athletes: review and recommendations. *Int J Sports Med*. 2019;40(8):535–543.

Wang CF, Sun YL, Zang HX. Music therapy improves sleep quality in acute and chronic sleep disorders: a meta-analysis of 10 randomized studies. *Int J Nurs Stud*. 2014;51(1):51–62.

Wang WL, Chen KH, Pan YC, Yang SN, Chan YY. The effect of yoga on sleep quality and insomnia in women with sleep problems: a systematic review and meta-analysis. *BMC Psychiatry*. 2020;20(1):195.

Watson NF, Badr MS, Belenky G, *et al.* Recommended amount of sleep for a healthy adult: A Joint Consensus Statement of the American Academy of Sleep Medicine and Sleep Research Society. *Sleep*. 2015;38(6):843–844.

Winter B. *Relax and Win: Championship Performance in Whatever You Do* (updated edition). Bud Winter Enterprises; 2012.

Wittmann M, Dinich J, Merrow M, Roenneberg T. Social jetlag: misalignment of biological and social time. *Chronobiol Int*. 2006;23(1–2):497–509.

Zhang JX, Liu XH, Xie XH, *et al.* Mindfulness-based stress reduction for chronic insomnia in adults older than 75 years: a randomized, controlled, single-blind clinical trial. *Explore (NY)*. 2015;11(3):180–185.

Additional Reading

Al-Sharman A, Siengsukon CF. Performance on a functional motor task is enhanced by sleep in middle-aged and older adults. *J Neurol Phys Ther.* 2014;38(3):161–169.

Ancoli-Israel S. *All I Want Is a Good Night's Sleep.* St. Louis, MO: Mosby-Yearbook; 1996.

Bonnar D, Bartel K, Kakoschke N, Lang C. Sleep interventions designed to improve athletic performance and recovery: a systematic review of current approaches. *Sports Med.* 2018;48(3):683–703.

Chakradeo PS, Keshavarzian A, Singh S, *et al.* Chronotype, social jet lag, sleep debt and food timing in inflammatory bowel disease. *Sleep Med.* 2018;52:188–195.

Cho S, Kim GS, Lee JH. Psychometric evaluation of the sleep hygiene index: a sample of patients with chronic pain. *Health Qual Life Outcomes.* 2013;11:213.

Edinger JD, Arnedt JT, Bertisch SM, *et al.* Behavioral and psychological treatments for chronic insomnia disorder in adults: an American Academy of Sleep Medicine clinical practice guideline. *J Clin Sleep Med.* 2021;17(2):255–262.

Friedrich A, Schlarb AA. Let's talk about sleep: a systematic review of psychological interventions to improve sleep in college students. *J Sleep Res.* 2018;27(1):4–22.

Guthrie KA, Larson JC, Ensrud KE, *et al.* Effects of pharmacologic and nonpharmacologic interventions on insomnia symptoms and self-reported sleep quality in women with hot flashes: a pooled analysis of individual participant data from four MsFLASH Trials. *Sleep.* 2018;41(1):zsx190.

Irish LA, Kline CE, Gunn HE, Buysse DJ, Hall MH. The role of sleep hygiene in promoting public health: a review of empirical evidence. *Sleep Med Rev.* 2015;22:23–36.

Nijs J, Mairesse O, Neu D, *et al.* Sleep disturbances in chronic pain: neurobiology, assessment, and treatment in physical therapist practice. *Phys Ther.* 2018;98(5):325–335.

Rosekind MR, Pelayo R, Babcock DA. Good sleep, better life-enhancing health and safety with optimal sleep. *JAMA Intern Med.* 2022;182(4):374–375.

Siengsukon CF, Al-Dughmi M, Stevens S. Sleep health promotion: practical information for physical therapists. *Phys Ther.* 2017;97(8):826–836.

Siengsukon CF, Boyd LA. Does sleep promote motor learning? Implications for physical rehabilitation. *Phys Ther.* 2009;89(4):370–383.

CHAPTER 8

Social Connectedness

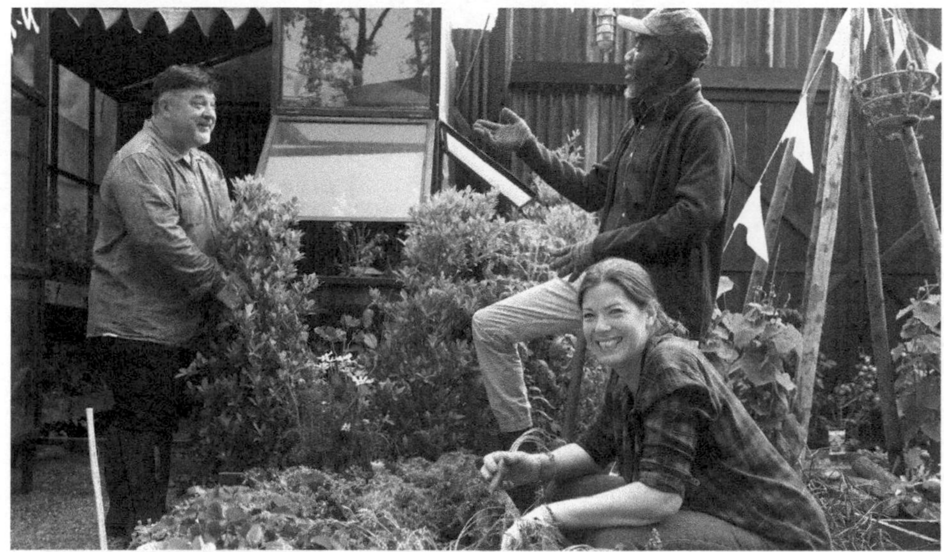

Stay socially connected through community gardening

Learning Objectives

- Understand the basic research for social connectedness.
- Apply social connectedness for practical pain management.

Chapter Highlights

- Key Concept: Identifying Social Risk Factors
- Clinical Tip: Walk with a Doc
- Clinical Tip: Telehealth, Telerehab, and Telewellness Visits
- Featured Topic 8.1: Benefits of Smiling and Laughing
- Self-Care Handout 8.1: How to Stay Socially Connected
- Self-Care Handout 8.2: Strategies to Improve Well-Being and Happiness

- Self-Management Activities
- Classroom and Lab Activities
- Useful Clinical Resources
- References
- Additional Reading

Lifestyle Matters*: Make a difference by getting involved.*

Introduction

Social connections with family, friends, co-workers, and individuals in the community can help people live happier and more fulfilling lives. Research shows that social isolation can affect overall health, happiness, and quality of life.

According to an article in *BMC Geriatrics* (O'Rourke *et al.* 2018, p.2), "Social connectedness is a positive subjective evaluation of the extent to which one has meaningful, close, and constructive relationships with other individuals, groups, or society..." The authors of the article indicate that a lack of social connections may lead to depression, poor life satisfaction, low self-esteem, poor health and well-being, negative affect, and impaired function in activities of daily living. Furthermore, a longitudinal study in the *Annals of Behavioral Medicine* (Karayannis *et al.* 2019) found that social interactions may play a role in a person's pain perception.

An article in the *New England Journal of Medicine* (Roland *et al.* 2020, p.98) states, "The concept of social prescribing entails educating physicians about social interventions, providing guidance on local resources, and permitting them to 'prescribe' social interventions for patients."

KEY CONCEPT: IDENTIFYING SOCIAL RISK FACTORS

Healthcare and wellness/fitness professionals need to screen for food insecurity, housing instability, and transportation difficulties during consultations to help identify necessary interventions (Eder *et al.* 2021).

Social Connection Strategies

One strategy to improve social connectedness is to encourage patients/clients to take up hobbies to stay engaged in life and manage stress and anxiety. Engagement in hobbies may, for example, help an individual lower the risk of cardiovascular diseases (Wang *et al.* 2021) and possibly prevent a decline in activities of daily living in community-dwelling older adults (Tomioka *et al.* 2016).

The following are hobbies and interests a person may pursue:

- Club connections—astronomy, birdwatching, books, bridge, cards, chess, drama, poetry
- Coaching youth sports
- Collecting group—art, books, coins, stamps
- Community gardening
- Cooking
- Dancing
- Fishing
- Golf
- Group travel and active outdoor vacations—active outdoor vacations
- League sports—bowling, softball
- Model building—cars, trains
- Outdoor activities—backpacking, camping, kayaking, rock climbing
- Painting
- Photography—travel, wildlife
- Playing a musical instrument
- Sculpting
- Singing
- Volunteering—community center, hospital, school, homeless shelter, place of worship
- Water sports—sailing, scuba diving
- Woodworking—building tree houses, birdhouses, toys

CLINICAL TIP: WALK WITH A DOC

Go for a walk with a doctor in your community. Walk with a Doc is an organization that inspires communities to engage in movement and conversation with a physician-led walking group (Sabgir and Dorn 2020). To learn more and find a location near you, visit: www.walkwithadoc.org.

Another approach is to encourage patients/clients to engage in purposeful activities. A systematic review in the *Gerontologist* (Owen *et al.* 2022) indicates that retired individuals and older adults may enhance their well-being by participating in purposeful activity. Examples of purposeful activity may include:

- serving as a committee member
- serving as a board member
- serving as a consultant
- mentoring and coaching students
- teaching community classes and offering continuing education classes
- organizing and leading community events

- creating and teaching online courses
- working part-time
- becoming a tour guide
- starting and running a charitable organization
- getting involved in helping to run a small business
- building a small business with family and friends
- creating and running an e-commerce store
- writing a book
- writing an educational blog.

Finally, another example of improving social connections may be for healthcare providers to utilize nature-based social-prescribing referral options. This approach may include providing food vouchers for individuals to attend farmers' markets, community arts activities, walking and cycling clubs, and communal gardening to promote mental well-being and physical health (Leavell *et al.* 2019).

CLINICAL TIP: TELEHEALTH, TELEREHAB, AND TELEWELLNESS VISITS

Providing tele-delivered medical, wellness, and fitness services may be a way to improve social connections for older adults (Choi *et al.* 2020). A virtual service may be a good option for individuals with transportation difficulties, with a busy schedule, who need a quick consultation, or who live in a remote location.

Featured Topic

Featured Topic 8.1 outlines the benefits of smiling and laughing.

■ Featured Topic 8.1: Benefits of Smiling and Laughing

Smiling and laughter are often contagious. Try it. Walk into a room smiling or laughing with friends and see what happens.

Thich Nhat Hanh (1926–2022), a Buddhist monk, peace activist, prolific author, poet, and teacher, once said, "Because of your smile, you make life more beautiful." A review article in the *Postgraduate Medical Journal* (Beamish *et al.* 2019, p.91) states that a smile is "A sign of compassion, empathy and friendliness, smiling can benefit healthcare professionals and their patients, helping to build a relationship of trust."

What about laughing? Milton Berle, an American comedian and actor, once said, "Laughter is an instant vacation." A review article in the *American*

Journal of Lifestyle Medicine (Louie *et al.* 2016) found that laughter has been linked with improved mood, reduced anxiety and stress, and increased pain tolerance.

What makes you smile or laugh? How about giving the following a try:

- Be around genuinely happy people.
- Listen to a standup comedian.
- Read humorous cartoons.
- Try dancing.
- Use more happy and cheerful emojis in messages.
- Practice yoga with laughter (or laughter yoga).
- Watch children playing.
- Watch comedy movies.
- Watch comedy sitcoms.
- Watch pets playing.
- Watch funny YouTube, Instagram, or TikTok videos.

Self-Care Education Guides

Self-Care Handout 8.1: How to Stay Socially Connected outlines tips and strategies to help patients/clients become more socially connected in the community (Leavell *et al.* 2019; National Institutes of Health 2023; Roland *et al.* 2020).

Self-Care Handout 8.2: Strategies to Improve Well-Being and Happiness outlines adapted positive psychology strategies that may help patients/clients improve overall well-being and happiness (Bolier *et al.* 2013; Boselie *et al.* 2018; Braunwalder *et al.* 2021; Lianov *et al.* 2019; Müller *et al.* 2020; Peters *et al.* 2017). To learn more about happiness, see the World Happiness Report from the United Nations (United Nations 2023).

Self-Care Handout 8.1: How to Stay Socially Connected

- Attend local sporting events, music performances, or art and museum exhibits.
- Connect with family and friends locally or on Zoom.
- Connect with your physician, therapist, wellness, or fitness professional via tele-delivered services.
- Create or join a community garden club.
- Create or join a lunchtime walking, yoga, or tai chi club.
- Engage in conventional group exercises such as softball, volleyball, basketball, pickleball, paddle tennis, or tennis.
- Engage in mind-body exercises such as yoga, tai chi, or Pilates.
- Engage in work-related community activities and fitness programs.
- Engage in small conversations with cashiers and employees at various stores you visit.
- Engage with members at your community place of worship.
- Enroll in art-based community activities, such as art, dance, drama, music, poetry, pottery, or expressive writing classes.
- Enroll in a local university or community college class, such as cooking, history, or astronomy.
- Get a library card and participate in book club events.
- Get involved in nature-based activities, such as birdwatching, botanical garden and park visits, farmers' market shopping, forest bathing or hiking, gardening, and walks at a lake, river, or beach.
- Join a group such as a local bicycling club, chess club, table tennis club, or an activity focused on your favorite hobby.
- Join a gym or fitness center.
- Join self-help groups.
- Join social media platforms like Facebook, Twitter (X), Instagram, or TikTok.
- Play with your pets.
- Volunteer at a community center, hospital, school, or library.
- Volunteer to coach sports or mentor students.
- Walk with a mall club or create one in your neighborhood.

Self-Care Handout 8.2: Strategies to Improve Well-Being and Happiness

Plant the seeds of positive thinking and watch them grow.

- Attend a retreat program.
- Attend employer wellness programs.
- Become involved in activities that give you purpose, such as volunteering or mentoring.
- Consider keeping a gratitude journal.
- Consider including flexible thinking.
- Emphasize gratitude and positive events for each day.
- Engage in hobbies you enjoy.
- Engage in exercise and physical activities you enjoy.
- Find activities that make you smile and laugh more often, such as watching comedy television shows or reading comic strips.
- Get help when you feel overwhelmed at your workplace or personal life.
- Get annual medical checkups.
- Include art-based activities, such as art, dance, music, poetry, or writing, in your weekly routine.
- Include nature-based activities in your weekly routine, such as gardening, outdoor biking, hiking, or outdoor walking.
- Learn to cook in order to prepare healthful foods.
- Learn to let go of anger and resentment.
- Learn to meditate. Use either stationary strategies, such as a body scan meditation or progressive muscle relaxation, or dynamic strategies, such as yoga, tai chi, or qigong.
- Minimize overtime work.
- Stay socially connected.
- Take brief mindfulness/meditation breaks at work.
- Take time to enjoy successes and special event celebrations.
- Take regular vacations.
- Use employer fitness facilities to save money and travel time to fitness centers.
- Use self-care and self-management strategies such as self-massage and self-acupressure.
- Utilize the "buddy" system for support when adopting and changing health behaviors, such as increasing exercise or stopping soft drink consumption.
- Visualize a positive future.

Self-Management Activities: Explore Game Apps

Games can offer a form of social connectedness. In fact, online games are the only form of social connection some younger and older individuals have. The following online resources can help patients/clients, healthcare providers, and health/fitness professionals to manage stress and anxiety by exploring games.

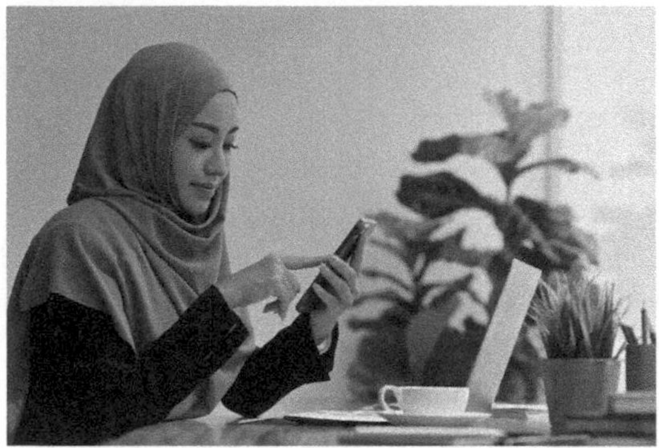

Take fun breaks during the day

- The Crazy Games site provides a fun way to relax using simple gaming skills on your computer. For example, try playing Space Invaders or Tetris: www.crazygames.com
- The Pac-Man game site provides a fun way to relax using simple gaming skills on your computer: https://freepacman.org
- The Pong Game site provides a fun way to relax using simple gaming skills on your computer: www.ponggame.org

Classroom and Lab Activities

- Determine which social media platforms and groups may be beneficial for older adults.
- Create a list of mentorship and volunteer organizations to help individuals stay connected.

Useful Clinical Resources

Organizations

- American Academy of Psychotherapists, www.aapweb.com
- American Psychological Association, www.apa.org
- Association for Applied and Therapeutic Humor, www.aath.org

- Facebook (Meta) Social Connectedness Index, https://dataforgood.fb.com/tools/social-connectedness-index
- Institute on Character, www.viacharacter.org
- National Association of Social Workers, www.socialworkers.org
- Positive Psychology, https://positivepsychology.com
- Positive Psychology Institute, https://positivepsychologyinstitute.com.au
- Pursuit of Happiness, www.pursuit-of-happiness.org
- Social Interventions Research & Evaluation Network, https://sirenetwork.ucsf.edu

Outcome Measures

- *Duke Social Support Index*
  Wardian J, Robbins D, Wolfersteig W. Validation of the DSSI-10 to measure social support in a general population. *Res Soc Work Pract*. 2013;23:100–106.
- *Patient-Reported Outcomes Measurement Information System Social Isolation*
  Hahn EA, DeWalt DA, Bode RK, *et al.* New English and Spanish social health measures will facilitate evaluating health determinants. *Health Psychol*. 2014;33(5):490–499.
- *Social Connectedness Index*
  Bailey M, Cao R, Kuchler T, Stroebel J, Wong A. Social connectedness: measurement, determinants, and effects. *J Econ Perspect*. 2018;32(3):259–280.
- *Social Inclusion Measure (25 Measures)*
  Cordier R, Milbourn B, Martin R, Buchanan A, Chung D, Speyer R. A systematic review evaluating the psychometric properties of measures of social inclusion. *PLoS One*. 2017;12(6):e0179109.
- *Social Needs Screening Tool*
  American Academy of Family Physicians. Social Needs Screening Tool. www.aafp.org/dam/AAFP/documents/patient_care/everyone_project/hops19-physician-form-sdoh.pdf
- *The Social Connectedness Scale*
  Lee RM, Robbins SB. Measuring belongingness: the Social Connectedness and the Social Assurance scales. *J Couns Psychol.* 1995;42:232–241.
- *UCLA Loneliness Scale*
  Russell D, Peplau LA, Cutrona CE. The revised UCLA Loneliness Scale: concurrent and discriminant validity evidence. *J Pers Soc Psychol*. 1980;39(3):472–480.

References

Beamish AJ, Foster JJ, Edwards H, Olbers T. What's in a smile? A review of the benefits of the clinician's smile. *Postgrad Med J*. 2019;95(1120):91–95.

Bolier L, Haverman M, Westerhof GJ, Riper H, Smit F, Bohlmeijer E. Positive psychology interventions: a meta-analysis of randomized controlled studies. *BMC Public Health*. 2013;13:119.

Boselie JJLM, Vancleef LMG, Peters ML. Filling the glass: effects of a positive psychology intervention on executive task performance in chronic pain patients. *Eur J Pain*. 2018;22(7):1268–1280.

Braunwalder C, Müller R, Glisic M, Fekete C. Are positive psychology interventions efficacious in chronic pain treatment? A systematic review and meta-analysis of randomized controlled trials [published online ahead of print, 2021 Aug 4]. *Pain Med*. 2021;pnab247.

Choi NG, Pepin R, Marti CN, Stevens CJ, Bruce ML. Improving social connectedness for homebound older adults: randomized controlled trial of tele-delivered behavioral activation versus tele-delivered friendly visits. *Am J Geriatr Psychiatry*. 2020;28(7):698–708.

Eder M, Henninger M, Durbin S, *et al.* Screening and interventions for social risk factors: technical brief to support the US Preventive Services Task Force. *JAMA*. 2021;326(14):1416–1428.

Karayannis NV, Baumann I, Sturgeon JA, Melloh M, Mackey SC. The impact of social isolation on pain interference: a longitudinal study. *Ann Behav Med*. 2019;53(1):65–74.

Leavell MA, Leiferman JA, Gascon M, Braddick F, Gonzalez JC, Litt JS. Nature-based social prescribing in urban settings to improve social connectedness and mental well-being: a review. *Curr Environ Health Rep*. 2019;6(4):297–308.

Lianov LS, Fredrickson BL, Barron C, Krishnaswami J, Wallace A. Positive psychology in lifestyle medicine and health care: strategies for implementation. *Am J Lifestyle Med*. 2019;13(5):480–486.

Louie D, Brook K, Frates E. The laughter prescription: a tool for lifestyle medicine. *Am J Lifestyle Med*. 2016;10(4):262–267.

Müller R, Segerer W, Ronca E, *et al.* Inducing positive emotions to reduce chronic pain: a randomized controlled trial of positive psychology exercises [published online ahead of print, 2020 Dec 2]. *Disabil Rehabil*. 2020;1–14.

National Institutes of Health, Social Wellness Toolkit; 2023. www.nih.gov/health-information/social-wellness-toolkit

O'Rourke HM, Collins L, Sidani S. Interventions to address social connectedness and loneliness for older adults: a scoping review. *BMC Geriatr*. 2018;18(1):214.

Owen R, Berry K, Brown LJE. Enhancing older adults' well-being and quality of life through purposeful activity: a systematic review of intervention studies. *Gerontologist*. 2022;62(6):e317–e327.

Peters ML, Smeets E, Feijge M, *et al.* Happy despite pain: a randomized controlled trial of an 8-week internet-delivered positive psychology intervention for enhancing well-being in patients with chronic pain. *Clin J Pain*. 2017;33(11):962–975.

Roland M, Everington S, Marshall M. Social prescribing: transforming the relationship between physicians and their patients. *N Engl J Med*. 2020;383(2):97–99.

Sabgir D, Dorn J. Walk with a Doc: a call to action for physician-led walking programs. *Curr Cardiol Rep*. 2020;22(7):44.

Tomioka K, Kurumatani N, Hosoi H. Relationship of having hobbies and a purpose in life with mortality, activities of daily living, and instrumental activities of daily living among community-dwelling elderly adults. *J Epidemiol*. 2016;26(7):361–370.

United Nations. World Happiness Report; 2023. https://worldhappiness.report

Wang X, Dong JY, Shirai K, *et al.* Having hobbies and the risk of cardiovascular disease incidence: a Japan public health center-based study. *Atherosclerosis*. 2021;335:1–7.

Additional Reading

Davidson KW, Krist AH, Tseng CW, *et al.* Incorporation of social risk in US Preventive Services Task Force recommendations and identification of key challenges for primary care. *JAMA*. 2021;326(14):1410–1415.

Johansson G, Engström Å, Juuso P. Experiences of a nature-based intervention program in a northern natural setting: a longitudinal case study of two women with stress-related illness. *Int J Qual Stud Health Well-being*. 2023;18(1):2146857.

Johansson G, Juuso P, Engström Å. Nature-based interventions to promote health for people with stress-related illness: an integrative review. *Scand J Caring Sci*. 2022;36(4):910–925.

Rozanski A, Bavishi C, Kubzansky LD, Cohen R. Association of optimism with cardiovascular events and all-cause mortality: a systematic review and meta-analysis. *JAMA Netw Open*. 2019;2(9):e1912200.

Steinman L, Parrish A, Mayotte C, *et al.* Increasing social connectedness for underserved older adults living with depression: a pre-post evaluation of PEARLS. *Am J Geriatr Psychiatry*. 2021;29(8):828–842.

CHAPTER 9

Avoidance of Risky Substances

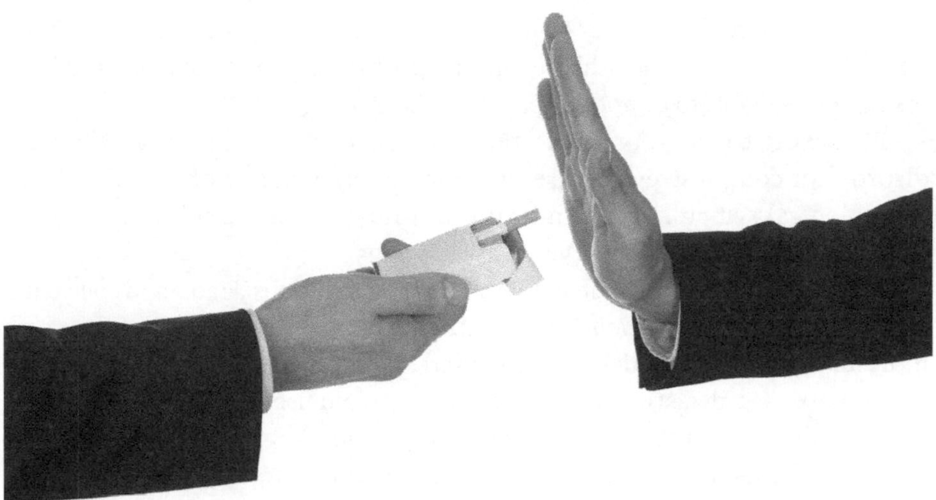

Going smoke-free adds quality years to a person's life

Learning Objectives

- Understand the basic research for risky substance use.
- Recognize resources for managing risky substance use for practical pain management.

Chapter Highlights

- Key Concept: Alcohol and Smoking Related Deaths
- Clinical Tip: Smartphone App for Smoking Cessation
- Featured Topic 9.1: Guidelines for Building Mental Resilience
- Self-Care Handout 9.1: Changing a Bad Habit
- Self-Management Activities
- Classroom and Lab Activities

- Useful Clinical Resources
- References
- Additional Reading

Lifestyle Matters: *Don't wait for a crisis before you make changes in your life.*

Introduction

Risky substances such as smoking, excess alcohol, and other illicit drugs affect a person's health and quality of life, relationships, and performance at work. For this reason, every healthcare and health/fitness professional should have resources available to offer their patients/clients.

According to one source, substance dependence disorder is "an addictive disorder of compulsive drug use. It is marked by a cluster of behavioral and physiological symptoms that indicate continual use of the substance despite significant related problems" (Venes 2021, p.2295).

Substance use disorders affect many medical conditions. Frates and colleagues in the *Lifestyle Medicine Handbook* (Frates *et al.* 2021) state that the most common substance use disorders in the United States include tobacco use disorder, alcohol use disorder, stimulant use disorder, opioid use disorder, and cannabis use disorder. Substance use disorder (alcohol, smoking) may affect back pain (Bryan *et al.* 2015; Ferreira *et al.* 2013; Schmelzer *et al.* 2016; Shiri *et al.* 2010; Yang and Haldeman 2018), bone healing (Xu *et al.* 2021), diabetic foot healing (Fu *et al.* 2018), spine surgery outcomes (Jackson and Devine 2016), stroke risk (Harshfield *et al.* 2021; Larsson *et al.* 2016), total hip or knee arthroplasty (Yue *et al.* 2022), and other conditions.

KEY CONCEPT: ALCOHOL AND SMOKING RELATED DEATHS

Prevention and intervention strategies are key to prevention of alcohol and smoking related deaths:

- "Worldwide, 3 million deaths every year result from harmful use of alcohol. This represents 5.3% of all deaths." (World Health Organization. Alcohol 2022)
- Tobacco-related diseases cause more than 7 million deaths per year across the world. (World Health Organization 2017)

Treatment Approaches

The National Center for Complementary and Integrative Health (NCCIH) (2021) outlines various mind and body practices for smoking cessation, such as acupuncture, hypnotherapy, and yoga. The NCCIH (2018) also discusses mind-body approaches for substance disorders, including acupuncture, hypnotherapy, mindfulness meditation, music therapy, and yoga. Furthermore, research indicates that exercise may be an adjunct intervention in alcohol use disorder (Lardier *et al.* 2021) and that yoga may increase the odds of smoking abstinence (Bock *et al.* 2019). Finally, a review in *JAMA* (Rigotti *et al.* 2022) provides an overview of tobacco-smoking treatments, including pharmacotherapy and behavioral support.

The following are general strategies a practitioner may use to help patients/clients make changes from addictive behaviors:

- Refer patients/clients for individual or group counseling.
- Review and go over the patient's prescription and nonprescription medication use.
- Provide organization contacts and resources to patients/clients.
- Use the Transtheoretical Model of Change approach to determine a person's readiness for change (Prochaska *et al.* 1992; Prochaska *et al.* 1994; Prochaska 1994; Prochaska and Velicer 1997).
- Use motivational interviewing as a part of patient-centered counseling and treatments (D'Amico *et al.* 2018; Lindson-Hawley *et al.* 2015).

The following are specific signposts to sources a practitioner may use to help patients/clients with smoking cessation, risky alcohol use, and/or opioid misuse:

Smoking Cessation

- Use the guidelines from the *American Family Physician* (Gaddey *et al.* 2022) article covering interventions for smoking cessation.
- Consult the American Academy of Family Physicians' *Ask and Act Tobacco Cessation* resources guide (2023) and its *Treating Tobacco Dependence Practice Manual* (2017).

Alcohol Misuse

- Consult the American Academy of Family Physicians' *Incorporating Alcohol Screening and Brief Intervention into Practice* guide (2020) and the Centers for Disease Control and Prevention's *Planning and Implementing Screening and Brief Intervention for Risky Alcohol Use: A Step-by-Step Guide for Primary Care Practices* (Centers for Disease Control and Prevention 2014).

Opioid Misuse

- Consult the randomized clinical trial in *JAMA Internal Medicine* (Garland *et al.* 2022, p.407) where the authors concluded that "the MORE [Mindfulness-Oriented Recovery Enhancement] intervention led to sustained improvements in opioid misuse and chronic pain symptoms and reductions in opioid dosing, emotional distress, and opioid craving compared with supportive group psychotherapy." The MORE intervention consisted of mindfulness (meditation, breathing, body sensations), reappraisal (reframing maladaptive thoughts), and savoring skills (focusing awareness on pleasurable events).

CLINICAL TIP: SMARTPHONE APP FOR SMOKING CESSATION
An acceptance and commitment therapy (ACT) based smartphone application (iCanQuit) may be an effective strategy to help individuals quit cigarette smoking (Bricker *et al.* 2020).

Featured Topic

Featured Topic 9.1 outlines practical guidelines for building mental resilience.

Featured Topic 9.1: Guidelines for Building Mental Resilience

According to Venes (2021), resilience is an ability of a person to withstand physical or mental stress.

Strategies to build mental resilience include (Bartley *et al.* 2019; Coronado *et al.* 2021; Joyce *et al.* 2018; Tse *et al.* 2010; Venes 2021):

- maintaining good overall health (e.g., nutrition, exercise, sleep hygiene, stress management, avoidance of risky substances)
- having strong social connections (e.g., family, friends, work, community center)
- having a good support system (e.g., primary care physician, support group)
- reframing negative thoughts and feelings into positive ones
- learning coping strategies for pain, anxiety, and depression (e.g., cognitive behavioral therapy)
- engaging in enjoyable activities (e.g., gardening, sports, movie club)
- engaging in meaningful activities (e.g., volunteering, mentoring)

- engaging in art-based activities (e.g., music, painting, dancing, pottery, drama clubs)
- participating in mindfulness-based meditation activities (e.g., yoga, mindful walking)
- creating a "happiness file" that makes a person happy, laugh, or smile (e.g., engaging with uplifting people, watching humorous movies or television shows, or reading a joke book, web-based cartoon strips, or app-based jokes)
- for chronic pain, being aware of nonpharmacological pain-management self-care strategies (e.g., heat, cold, massage, meditation, aromatherapy, transcutaneous nerve stimulation, guided imagery).

Self-Care Education Guide

Are you looking to help one of your patients/clients change a bad habit? According to an article in *BMC Public Health* (Allom *et al.* 2018), a habit is an overlearned process that is reinforced by repetition.

See **Self-Care Handout 9.1: Changing a Bad Habit** for a sample strategy that may be useful for helping patients/clients change bad habits (Clear 2018; Gardner *et al.* 2021; Hagger *et al.* 2020; Michie *et al.* 2013; Taibbi 2017). Please note that this handout is only a simplified approach intended to motivate patients/clients. For optimal results, patients/clients may need the guidance of a practitioner. Please see the Useful Clinical Resources section for additional information.

Self-Care Handout 9.1: Changing a Bad Habit

Cue	Task	Action
Identify	Identify the bad habit	Stop smoking
Remove	Remove as many negative triggers as possible	Avoid coffee if it is a trigger and switch to tea
Substitute	Find a substitute for the habit	Try eating carrot or celery sticks
Plan	Pre-plan the alternative	Prepare carrot or celery sticks in the morning
Collaborate	Join forces with a friend	Remind each other to stay on course
Track	Find a way to track your success	Use a habit tracker app
Reward	Create a reward for yourself	Purchase a small gift for yourself and use it at the end of the month for every month you accomplish your goal

Self-Management Activities: Explore Pottery

The following online resource can help patients/clients, healthcare providers, and health/fitness professionals to manage stress and anxiety by exploring pottery.

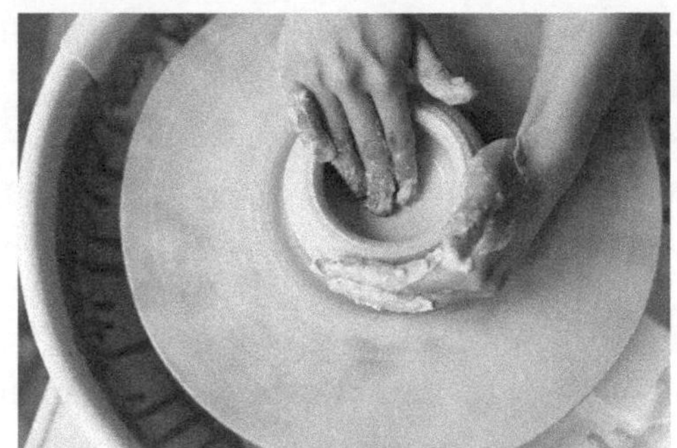

Relax with pottery

- The Let's Create! Pottery 2 app provides a fun way to relax by creating virtual pottery: www.idreams.pl/en

The following resource can help patients/clients, healthcare providers, and health/fitness professionals to manage stress and anxiety by obtaining a pottery kit and exploring pottery.

- The Sculpd site provides a fun way to relax through pottery: https://sculpd.com

Classroom and Lab Activities

- Examine and try various dance styles (e.g., folk dance, modern dance, salsa, square dancing, tango, waltz). How can dance be modified for individuals-with back pain? Why may dance provide pain relief for some individuals?
- How can dance be used for managing depression?

Useful Clinical Resources

Organizations

- Alcoholics Anonymous, www.aa.org
- American Academy of Addiction Psychiatry, www.aaap.org
- American Addiction Centers, Nature-Based Rehab, www.projectknow.com/rehab/nature-based

- American Psychological Association, www.apa.org
- American Society of Addiction Medicine, www.asam.org
- HABITS Lab at University of Maryland, Baltimore County, https://habitslab.umbc.edu
- National Center for Complementary and Integrative Health, www.nccih.nih (search for smoking cessation)
- National Institute on Alcohol Abuse and Alcoholism, www.niaaa.nih.gov
- National Institute on Drug Abuse, www.drugabuse.gov
- ProChange Behavior Solutions (Transtheoretical Model and the Stages of Change), www.prochange.com
- Smokefree, https://smokefree.gov
- Substance Abuse and Mental Health Services Administration, www.samhsa.gov

Patient Information

- Smoking cessation app: SmokeFree, www.healthline.com/health/quit-smoking/top-iphone-android-apps#smoke-free
- Smoking cessation app: QuitGuide, https://smokefree.gov/tools-tips/apps/quitguide
- Smoking cessation app: Quit2Heal, https://quit2heal.org
- Quitline for smoking cessation from www.CDC.gov/quit, 1-800-QUIT-NOW
- QuitNow (smoking cessation app), https://quitnow.app/en

Outcome Measures

- *Commitment to Quitting Smoking Scale*
  Kahler CW, Lachance HR, Strong DR, Ramsey SE, Monti PM, Brown RA. The commitment to quitting smoking scale: initial validation in a smoking cessation trial for heavy social drinkers. *Addict Behav.* 2007;32(10):2420–2424.
- *Fagerström Test for Nicotine Dependence*
  Heatherton TF, Kozlowski LT, Frecker RC, Fagerström KO. The Fagerström Test for Nicotine Dependence: a revision of the Fagerström Tolerance Questionnaire. *Br J Addict.* 1991;86(9):1119–1127.
- *Heaviness of Smoking Index*
  Heatherton TF, Kozlowski LT, Frecker RC, Rickert W, Robinson J. Measuring the heaviness of smoking: using self-reported time to the first cigarette of the day and number of cigarettes smoked per day. *Br J Addict.* 1989;84(7):791–799.

- *Minnesota Tobacco Withdrawal Scale*
  Hughes JR, Hatsukami D. Signs and symptoms of tobacco withdrawal. *Arch Gen Psychiatry*. 1986;43(3):289–294.
- *Process of Change Questionnaire*
  University of Maryland, Baltimore County. https://habitslab.umbc.edu/processes-of-change-questionnaire
- *Readiness Ruler*
  Indiana University. Readiness Ruler. https://iprc.iu.edu/sbirtapp/mi/ruler.php
- *The Stages of Change Readiness and Treatment Eagerness Scale*
  Miller WR, Tonigan JS. Assessing drinkers' motivation for change: The Stages of Change Readiness and Treatment Eagerness Scale (SOCRATES). *Psychology of Addictive Behaviors*. 1996;10(2):81–89.
- *Screening and Assessment Tools Chart*
  National Institute on Drug Abuse. Screening and Assessment Tools Chart. 2023. https://nida.nih.gov/nidamed-medical-health-professionals/screening-tools-resources/chart-screening-tools

References

Allom V, Mullan B, Smith E, Hay P, Raman J. Breaking bad habits by improving executive function in individuals with obesity. *BMC Public Health*. 2018;18(1):505.

American Academy of Family Physicians. *Treating Tobacco Dependence Practice Manual. A Systems-Change Approach.* Ask and Act Tobacco Cessation Program; 2017. www.aafp.org/dam/AAFP/documents/patient_care/tobacco/practice-manual.pdf

American Academy of Family Physicians. *Incorporating Alcohol Screening and Brief Intervention into Practice*; 2020. www.aafp.org/dam/brand/aafp/pubs/fpm/issues/2020/1100/p41.pdf

American Academy of Family Physicians. Ask and Act Tobacco Cessation Program resources; 2023. www.aafp.org/family-physician/patient-care/care-resources/tobacco-and-nicotine/ask-act.html

Bartley EJ, Palit S, Fillingim RB, Robinson ME. Multisystem resiliency as a predictor of physical and psychological functioning in older adults with chronic low back pain [published correction appears in *Front Psychol*. 2020 Oct 12;11:595827]. *Front Psychol*. 2019;10:1932.

Bock BC, Dunsiger SI, Rosen RK, *et al.* Yoga as a complementary therapy for smoking cessation: results from BreathEasy, a randomized clinical trial. *Nicotine Tob Res*. 2019;21(11):1517–1523.

Bricker JB, Watson NL, Mull KE, Sullivan BM, Heffner JL. Efficacy of smartphone applications for smoking cessation: a randomized clinical trial. *JAMA Intern Med*. 2020;180(11):1472–1480.

Bryan CJ, Wolfe AL, Morrow CE, Stephenson JA, Haskell J, Bryan AO. Associations among back and extremity pain with alcohol, tobacco, and caffeine use among US Air Force Pararescuemen. *J Spec Oper Med*. 2015;15(3):66–71.

Centers for Disease Control and Prevention. *Planning and Implementing Screening and Brief Intervention for Risky Alcohol Use: A Step-by-Step Guide for Primary Care Practices*. Atlanta, GA: Centers for Disease Control and Prevention, National Center on Birth Defects and Developmental Disabilities, 2014. www.cdc.gov/ncbddd/fasd/documents/alcoholsbiimplementationguide.pdf

Clear J. *Atomic Habits: An Easy & Proven Way to Build Good Habits and Break Bad Ones.* New York, NY: Avery; 2018.

Coronado RA, Robinette PE, Henry AL, *et al.* Bouncing back after lumbar spine surgery: early postoperative resilience is associated with 12-month physical function, pain interference, social participation, and disability. *Spine J*. 2021;21(1):55–63.

D'Amico EJ, Parast L, Shadel WG, Meredith LS, Seelam R, Stein BD. Brief motivational interviewing intervention to reduce alcohol and marijuana use for at-risk adolescents in primary care. *J Consult Clin Psychol.* 2018;86(9):775–786.

Ferreira PH, Pinheiro MB, Machado GC, Ferreira ML. Is alcohol intake associated with low back pain? A systematic review of observational studies. *Man Ther.* 2013;18(3):183–190.

Frates B, Bonnet JP, Joseph R, Peterson JA. *Lifestyle Medicine Handbook: An Introduction to the Power of Healthy Habits*, 2nd ed. Monterey, CA: Healthy Learning; 2021.

Fu XL, Ding H, Miao WW, Chen HL. Association between cigarette smoking and diabetic foot healing: a systematic review and meta-analysis [published online ahead of print, 2018 Nov 21]. *Int J Low Extrem Wounds.* 2018:1534734618809583.

Gaddey HL, Dakkak M, Jackson NM. Smoking cessation interventions. *Am Fam Physician.* 2022;106(5):513–522.

Gardner B, Richards R, Lally P, Rebar A, Thwaite T, Beeken RJ. Breaking habits or breaking habitual behaviours? Old habits as a neglected factor in weight loss maintenance. *Appetite.* 2021;162:105183.

Garland EL, Hanley AW, Nakamura Y, *et al.* Mindfulness-oriented recovery enhancement vs supportive group therapy for co-occurring opioid misuse and chronic pain in primary care: a randomized clinical trial. *JAMA Intern Med.* 2022;182(4):407–417.

Hagger MS, Cameron LD, Hamilton K, Hankonen N, Lintunen T, eds. *The Handbook of Behavior Change*. Cambridge, United Kingdom: Cambridge University Press; 2020.

Harshfield EL, Georgakis MK, Malik R, Dichgans M, Markus HS. Modifiable lifestyle factors and risk of stroke: a Mendelian randomization analysis. *Stroke.* 2021;52(3):931–936.

Jackson KL 2nd, Devine JG. The effects of smoking and smoking cessation on spine surgery: a systematic review of the literature. *Global Spine J.* 2016;6(7):695–701.

Joyce S, Shand F, Tighe J, Laurent SJ, Bryant RA, Harvey SB. Road to resilience: a systematic review and meta-analysis of resilience training programmes and interventions. *BMJ Open.* 2018;8(6):e017858.

Lardier DT, Coakley KE, Holladay KR, Amorim FT, Zuhl MN. Exercise as a useful intervention to reduce alcohol consumption and improve physical fitness in individuals with alcohol use disorder: a systematic review and meta-analysis. *Front Psychol.* 2021;12:675285.

Larsson SC, Wallin A, Wolk A, Markus HS. Differing association of alcohol consumption with different stroke types: a systematic review and meta-analysis. *BMC Med.* 2016;14(1):178.

Lindson-Hawley N, Thompson TP, Begh R. Motivational interviewing for smoking cessation. *Cochrane Database Syst Rev.* 2015;(3):CD006936.

Michie S, Richardson M, Johnston M, *et al.* The behavior change technique taxonomy (v1) of 93 hierarchically clustered techniques: building an international consensus for the reporting of behavior change interventions. *Ann Behav Med.* 2013;46(1):81–95.

National Center for Complementary and Integrative Health. Mind and body approaches for substance use disorders: what the science says; 2018. www.nccih.nih.gov/health/providers/digest/mind-and-body-approaches-for-substance-use-disorders-science

National Center for Complementary and Integrative Health. Complementary health approaches for smoking cessation: what the science says; 2021. www.nccih.nih.gov/health/providers/digest/complementary-health-approaches-for-smoking-cessation-science?nav=govdcd

Prochaska JO. Strong and weak principles for progressing from precontemplation to action on the basis of twelve problem behaviors. *Health Psychol.* 1994;13(1):47–51.

Prochaska JO, DiClemente CC, Norcross JC. In search of how people change. Applications to addictive behaviors. *Am Psychol.* 1992;47(9):1102–1114.

Prochaska JO, Velicer WF. The transtheoretical model of health behavior change. *Am J Health Promot.* 1997;12(1):38–48.

Prochaska JO, Velicer WF, Rossi JS, *et al.* Stages of change and decisional balance for 12 problem behaviors. *Health Psychol.* 1994;13(1):39–46.

Rigotti NA, Kruse GR, Livingstone-Banks J, Hartmann-Boyce J. Treatment of tobacco smoking: a review. *JAMA.* 2022;327(6):566–577.

Schmelzer AC, Salt E, Wiggins A, Crofford LJ, Bush H, Mannino DM. Role of stress and smoking as modifiable risk factors for nonpersistent and persistent back pain in women. *Clin J Pain.* 2016;32(3):232–237.

Shiri R, Karppinen J, Leino-Arjas P, Solovieva S, Viikari-Juntura E. The association between smoking and low back pain: a meta-analysis. *Am J Med.* 2010;123(1):87.e7–35.

Taibbi B. How to break bad habits. *Psychology Today.* December 15, 2017. www.psychologytoday.com/us/blog/fixing-families/201712/how-break-bad-habits

Tse MM, Lo AP, Cheng TL, Chan EK, Chan AH, Chung HS. Humor therapy: relieving chronic pain and enhancing happiness for older adults. *J Aging Res.* 2010:343574.

Venes D. ed. *Taber's Cyclopedic Medical Dictionary*, 24th ed. Philadelphia, PA: FA Davis; 2021.

World Health Organization. WHO report on the global tobacco epidemic, 2017: Monitoring tobacco use and prevention policies; 2017. https://apps.who.int/iris/handle/10665/255874

World Health Organization. Alcohol; 2022. www.who.int/news-room/fact-sheets/detail/alcohol

Xu B, Anderson DB, Park ES, Chen L, Lee JH. The influence of smoking and alcohol on bone healing: systematic review and meta-analysis of non-pathological fractures. *EClinicalMedicine*. 2021;42:101179.

Yang H, Haldeman S. Behavior-related factors associated with low back pain in the US adult population. *Spine (Phila Pa 1976)*. 2018;43(1):28–34.

Yue C, Cui G, Ma M, *et al.* Associations between smoking and clinical outcomes after total hip and knee arthroplasty: a systematic review and meta-analysis. *Front Surg*. 2022;9:970537.

Additional Reading

Esser MB, Leung G, Sherk A, *et al.* Estimated deaths attributable to excessive alcohol use among US adults aged 20 to 64 years, 2015 to 2019. *JAMA Netw Open*. 2022;5(11):e2239485.

Garland EL. *Mindfulness-Oriented Recovery Enhancement for Addiction, Stress, and Pain*. Washington, DC: NASW Press; 2013.

McClure JB, Bricker J, Mull K, Heffner JL. Comparative effectiveness of group-delivered acceptance and commitment therapy versus cognitive behavioral therapy for smoking cessation: a randomized controlled trial. *Nicotine Tob Res*. 2020;22(3):354–362.

Miller WR, Rollnick S. *Motivational Interviewing: Helping People Change*, 3rd ed. New York, NY: Guilford Press; 2013.

Osaji J, Ojimba C, Ahmed S. The use of acceptance and commitment therapy in substance use disorders: a review of literature. *J Clin Med Res*. 2020;12(10):629–633.

CHAPTER 10

Nature-Based Therapies

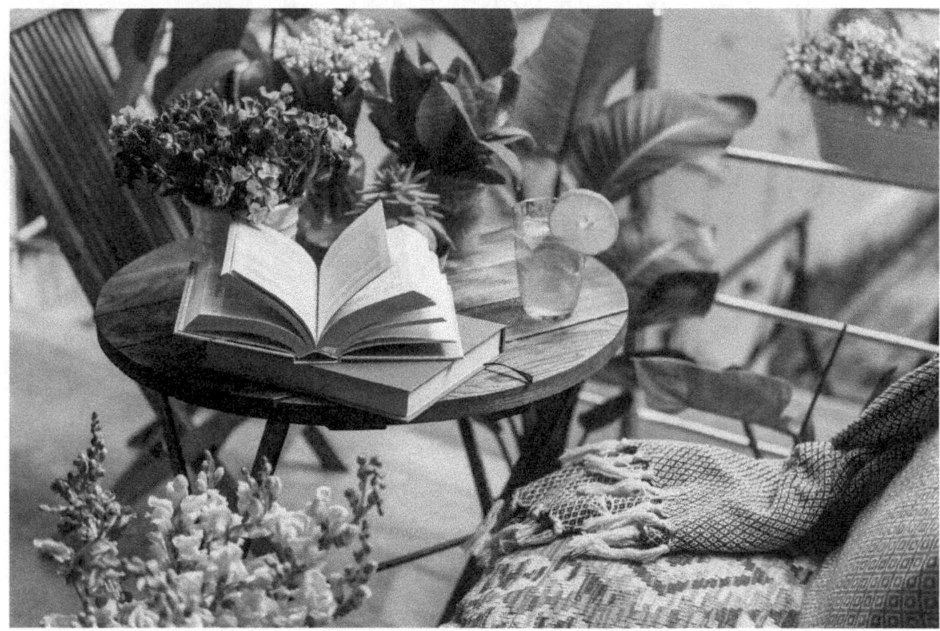

A balcony garden for fresh air, sunshine, and bright light to improve mood

Learning Objectives

- Understand the basic research for outdoor and green exercise.
- Recognize resources for outdoor and green activity for practical pain management.

Chapter Highlights

- Key Concept: Ecotherapy for Well-Being
- Clinical Tip: Trekking Poles

- Clinical Tip: Air Pollution and Physical Activity
- Clinical Tip: Retreat Vacations
- Featured Topic 10.1: Healing Places and Healing Spaces
- Featured Topic 10.2: Gardening for Health
- Featured Topic 10.3: Park Prescriptions
- Featured Topic 10.4: Nature as Medicine
- Featured Topic 10.5: Biophilic Design
- Featured Topic 10.6: Soothing Sounds
- Featured Topic 10.7: Case Vignette—Tai Chi in the Park
- Self-Care Handout 10.1: Your Nature Prescription
- Self-Care Handout 10.2: Nature Prescription
- Self-Care Handout 10.3: Natural Light Exposure at Home
- Self-Care Handout 10.4: Natural Light Exposure at Work
- Self-Care Handout 10.5: Natural Light Exposure at School
- Self-Care Handout 10.6: Nature Trail Circuit
- Self-Care Handout 10.7: Garden Meditation
- Self-Care Handout 10.8: Nature at Work
- Self-Management Activities
- Classroom and Lab Activities
- Useful Clinical Resources
- References
- Additional Reading

Lifestyle Matters: *For something to be sustainable, it needs some level of adaptability.*

Introduction

Nature may be the bond that holds together the six pillars of the American College of Lifestyle Medicine (see the figure in 'Introduction' in Chapter 1). Sundermann, Chielli, and Spell (2023) state, "There are 6 Official Pillars of Lifestyle Medicine, and now mounting evidence supports daily exposure to nature and fresh air as vital to optimizing overall physical and mental health."

In around 1980, Bill Gates, the co-founder of Microsoft, said "a computer on every desk and in every home." Why not create another ambitious goal? How about "a sustainable park, garden, or outdoor physical activity area in every neighborhood across the globe"?

Professor Sir Partha Dasgupta, the Frank Ramsey Emeritus Professor of Economics at Cambridge and Fellow of St John's College, says that, "If we care about our common future and the common future of our descendants, we should all in part be naturalists" (Dasgupta 2021, p.6). Dasgupta published his 610-page report

The Economics of Biodiversity: The Dasgupta Review in 2021 (Dasgupta 2021). He makes the point that humans need to find sustainable ways to live with nature and not just exploit it for economic growth.

This chapter will explore practical strategies to add nature to our everyday life. The key is to find nature-based outdoor activities for every season. This way, a person gets fresh air, sensible sunshine, natural bright light exposure, and all the benefits of being outdoors. Nature-based interventions may include parks, nature reserves, gardens, outdoor sports fields, mountain trails, rivers, lakes, and oceans. Intervention in a natural outdoor environment may help improve mental health, reduce anxiety and depressive mood, and enhance social connections (Coventry *et al.* 2021). An article by Vibholm and colleagues (2023) found that occupational therapists and physiotherapists considered nature-based rehabilitation an extended location for activity and training.

Outdoor environments have a positive influence on mental and physical health. For example, a study in the *International Journal of Environmental Research and Public Health* (Cerwén *et al.* 2016) indicates that patients suffering from mental stress-related disorders found natural sounds (e.g., birds, running water, wind) pleasant, while they found technological sounds (e.g., road traffic, computers, fans) disturbing. What sounds do you enjoy and what sounds do you dislike? Instead of using a leaf blower around a small home, why not use a standard rake and broom, which is quiet and uses calming rhythmical patterns? It's also a nice way to work on core stabilization.

A study in the *Frontiers in Psychology* journal (Pálsdóttir *et al.* 2021) found that smells from plants (especially citrus-scented pelargonium) may help reduce stress as a part of a nature-based intervention. Finally, a study in the *American Journal of Lifestyle Medicine* (Bauer and White 2023) found that time in nature has a positive influence on blood pressure.

The following list outlines some potential benefits of nature prescriptions, outdoor activity, and green exercise. It may help to:

- improve exercise adherence
- improve mental health in general and improve mental health and executive function in individuals with schizophrenia
- increase exercise intensity in adolescent and young adult cancer survivors
- increase the enjoyment of being active
- lower blood pressure
- manage anxiety and depression
- manage chronic pain
- manage and prevent the development of myopia in children
- provide a beneficial effect on chronic pain

- serve as a multisurface terrain training intervention for fall prevention in older adults.

From Baruki et al. 2022; Coventry et al. 2021; de Keijzer et al. 2018; He et al. 2015; Huber et al. 2019; Ideno et al. 2017; Klompmaker et al. 2022; Lacharité-Lemieux et al. 2015; Lahart et al. 2019; Li et al. 2021; Miller et al. 2021; Nguyen et al. 2023; Ryu et al. 2020; Selby et al. 2019; Thompson Coon et al. 2011; Turunen et al. 2023; Wu et al. 2018; Zhou et al. 2020.

KEY CONCEPT: ECOTHERAPY FOR WELL-BEING

Ecotherapy is an approach that includes the following activities for conditions such as stress reduction, depression, obesity, hypertension, ADHD (attention deficit hyperkinetic disorder), and PTSD (post-traumatic stress disorder) (Chaudhury and Banerjee 2020):

- green exercises, such as walking in parks or the countryside
- nature arts, such as photography, painting, or writing in parks or the countryside
- care farming, such as the use of agricultural landscapes to grow crops and look after animals
- social and therapeutic horticulture, such as gardening
- animal-assisted interventions, such as the use of pets and horses as a therapeutic intervention
- wilderness therapy, such as individual or group interactions with nature.

Can Light Therapy Affect Health?

An article in the *British Journal of Ophthalmology* (Turner and Mainster 2008, p.1442) indicates that the eyes play a vital role in good health. The authors state, "Bright light (≥2500 lux) particularly from bluer sources such as outdoor daylight can reduce or eliminate insomnia and depression; immediately increase brain serotonin, mood, alertness, and cognitive function..." Furthermore, Figueiro and colleagues in the *Lighting and Research Technology* journal (Figueiro *et al.* 2018, p.38) state, "Light can also elicit an acute alerting effect on people, similar to a 'cup of coffee.'" One consideration is to skip the coffee and add outdoor natural light in the morning.

A simple and cost-effective way to obtain natural light is to exercise or engage in outdoor activities in your neighborhood (see the following image). A simple option is to go for a morning walk (see image below) or perform light gardening before work. The key is that adequate light exposure is most important during the earlier part of the day. Another option to increase outdoor light is to have breakfast near a window (see image below), on the patio, balcony, porch, or backyard. Finally, some individuals may need to use a special light box strategy to get adequate light exposure during the winter months (see image below).

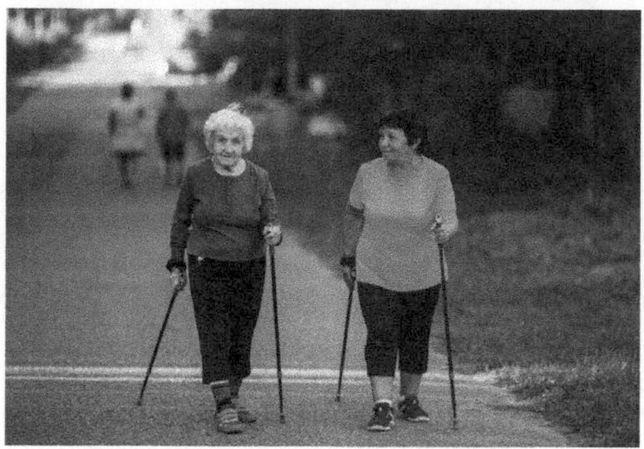

Walking with trekking poles

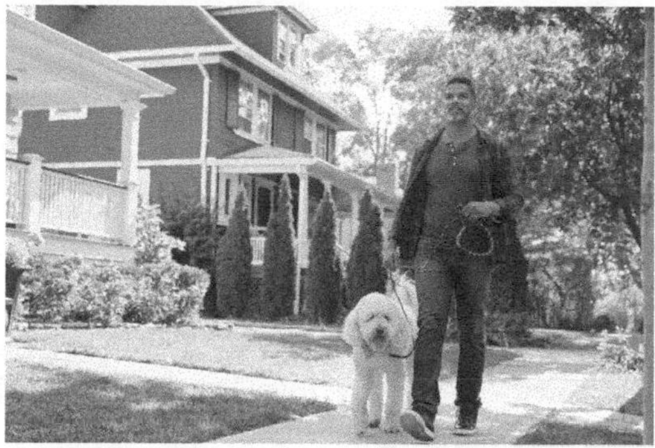

Early morning walk in the neighborhood

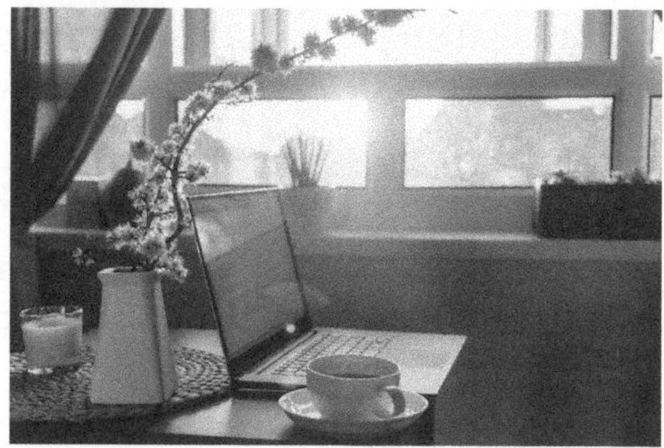

Breakfast near a window for increased natural light exposure

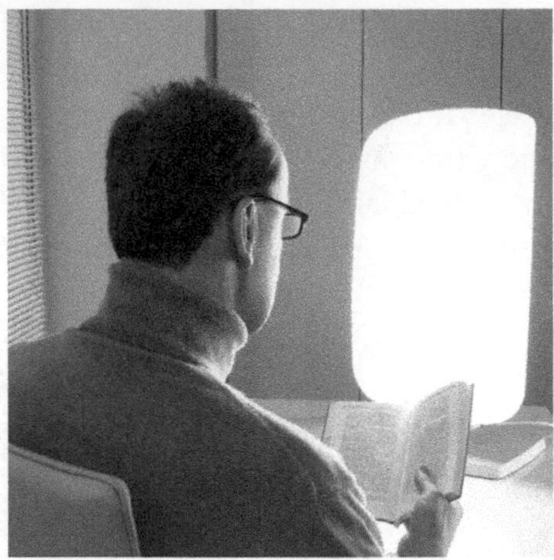

Light therapy while reading for increased light during the winter months

CLINICAL TIP: TREKKING POLES

Trekking poles may enhance stability and balance, improve posture, and provide exercise for the upper body. Some individuals may benefit from using trekking poles (or Nordic walking) during hikes and walks in nature (Bullo *et al.* 2018; Cohen *et al.* 2021).

Bright light therapy has been used for alertness (Figueiro *et al.* 2018; Lehrl *et al.* 2007), Alzheimer's (Figueiro *et al.* 2014; van Maanen *et al.* 2016), cancer-related fatigue (Johnson *et al.* 2018), chronic nonspecific back pain (Leichtfried *et al.* 2014), circadian rhythm disorders (Burns *et al.* 2021; Lam and Chung 2021; Pun *et al.* 2022), dementia (Figueiro *et al.* 2020), mood disorders (such as depression or bipolar disorder) (Espiritu *et al.* 1994; Even *et al.* 2008; Penders *et al.* 2016; Sit *et al.* 2018; Terman and Terman 1998; Terman and Terman 2005), neurological disorders (such as multiple sclerosis or Parkinson's) (Mateen *et al.* 2020; Videnovic *et al.* 2017), pain sensitivity in women with fibromyalgia (Burgess *et al.* 2017), seasonal affective disorder (SAD) (Pjrek *et al.* 2020), and weight control (Danilenko *et al.* 2013). Furthermore, studies on daytime light exposure can help sleep quality and improve mood (Baloch *et al.* 2020; Boubekri *et al.* 2014; Boubekri *et al.* 2020; Figueiro and Rea 2010; Figueiro *et al.* 2017; Hahn *et al.* 2011; Youngstedt *et al.* 2004).

The following tables outline light levels in outdoor and indoor environments, and sample outdoor activities that may be prescribed to improve natural bright light exposure.

Light levels in outdoor and indoor environments

Light Source: Outdoor	Light Level
Bright sunlight, noon	100,000 lux
Cloudy bright day	25,000 lux
Overcast day	10,000 lux
Very overcast day	2,000 lux
Sun rising over the horizon	800 lux
Light Source: Indoor	
Candle	1 lux
Offices, kitchens	200–500 lux
Living room	50–200 lux
Average nursing home	50 lux
Typical SAD treatment	2,500 lux (2 hours per day) or 5,000 lux (1 hour) or 10,000 lux (30 minutes per day)

Note: Lux is a unit of light intensity equivalent to 1 lumen/m^2.

Adapted from Choukroun and Geoffroy 2019; Turner and Mainster 2008; Venes 2021.

Sample outdoor activities

Locations for Activities	Outdoor Activities
• Home balcony • Home patio • Home backyard • Home gazebo • Park • Trail • Community fitness courts and trails (e.g., pull-up bars, rope, parallel bars, rings)	• Biking • Hiking • Outdoor calisthenics • Outdoor Pilates • Outdoor tai chi • Outdoor yoga • Swimming • Trekking • Walking
Outdoor Sports	**Winter Activities**
• Badminton • Basketball • Football (soccer) • Pickleball • Softball • Table tennis • Tennis • Volleyball	• Cross-country skiing • Ice skating • Outdoor trail biking • Outdoor walking • Skiing • Sled riding • Snowboarding • Snowshoe walking

The images below show examples of light exposure at work, school, and home.

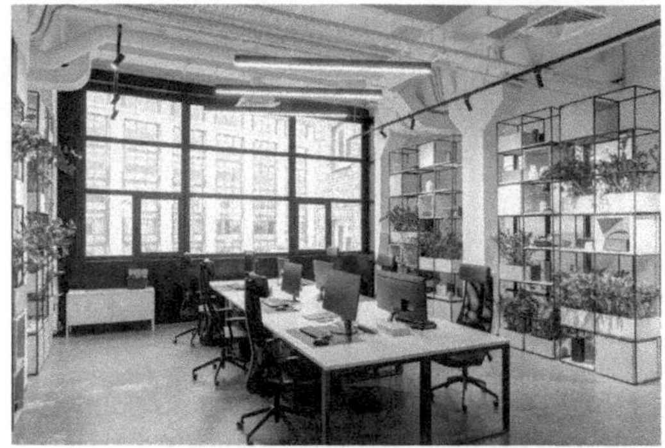

Large open workspace with natural light for good health and productivity

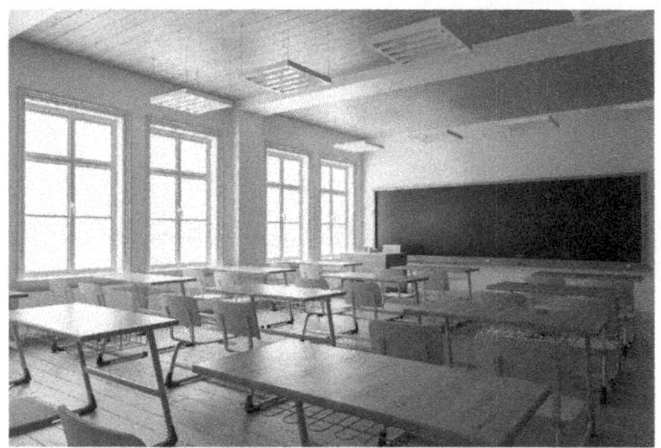

Classroom with natural light for good health and optimal learning

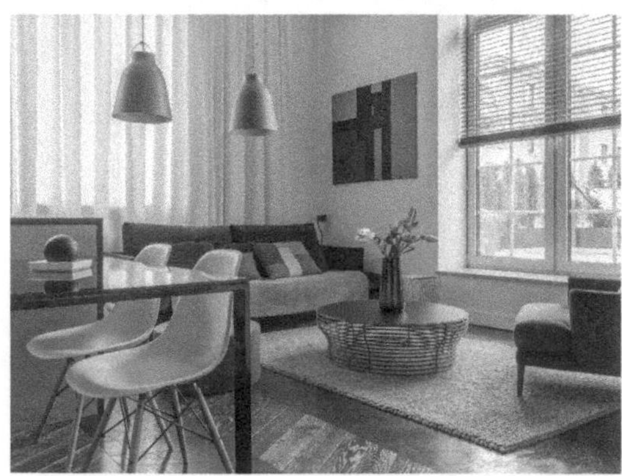

Bright living room with large windows for health and happiness

Examples of light exposure at work, school, and home

Can Sunshine Affect Health?

According to Venes (2021), heliotherapy is "exposure to sunlight" (p.1106), while phototherapy is "exposure to sunlight or to ultraviolet light" (p.1852) for therapeutic purposes. An article in *JAMA Dermatology* (Aldahan *et al.* 2016) indicates that sun worship has been a part of many cultures. For instance, the Chinese integrated the morning sun into tai chi practice and yoga includes the Sun Salutation.

Sensible sunshine and sunlight exposure may improve health, enhance mood, control infections, improve life expectancy, reduce cognitive impairment, enhance immune system function, and serve as a source of vitamin D (Amichai *et al.* 2014; An *et al.* 2016; Baggerly *et al.* 2015; Fahimipour *et al.* 2018; Hobday and Cason 2009; Hobday and Dancer 2013; Holick 2004; Holick 2016; Kent *et al.* 2009; Lindqvist *et al.* 2016; McCullough and Lehrer 2018; Schuit *et al.* 2020; Tang *et al.* 2021; Wacker and Holick 2013).

However, it should be noted that not everyone can be in the sun due to a medical condition, medications, or sensitivity. Professor Michael Holick, Ph.D., MD, recommends limited and sensible sunshine exposure (Holick 2010). After sensible sun exposure, the key is to cover up with sun protective clothing that may include a wide-brimmed hat, long-sleeve shirt and pants, and sunscreen. See the products section at the end of this chapter for sun-protective clothing websites.

CLINICAL TIP: AIR POLLUTION AND PHYSICAL ACTIVITY

To minimize exposure to air pollution during physical activity, consider the following strategies (Giorgini *et al.* 2016; Tainio *et al.* 2021):

- Walk, run, or bike away from roads with heavy traffic.
- Exercise or train during times of reduced traffic volume.
- Exercise in your backyard or patio.
- If weather permits, open windows when exercising in your home to provide adequate ventilation.
- Engage in physical activities at a local park, trail, lake, or ocean.
- Get involved in local legislation to reduce community air pollution.

Practical Home Wellness Spaces

A unique approach to wellness may be to help a patient/client create healing and restorative spaces in and around their home for their fitness and self-care routines (Engineer *et al.* 2020; Sternberg 2009). The wellness space(s) could incorporate outdoor natural light, sensible sunshine exposure, fresh air, connection to nature, plants, decorative art items, music, aromatherapy, and personalized, simple exercise equipment. This section illustrates four options to consider.

Fitness and Wellness Around the Home

Consider fitness strategies around the home that may include exercise or physical activity in the living room, balcony, patio, or garage gym.

Fitness in the living room

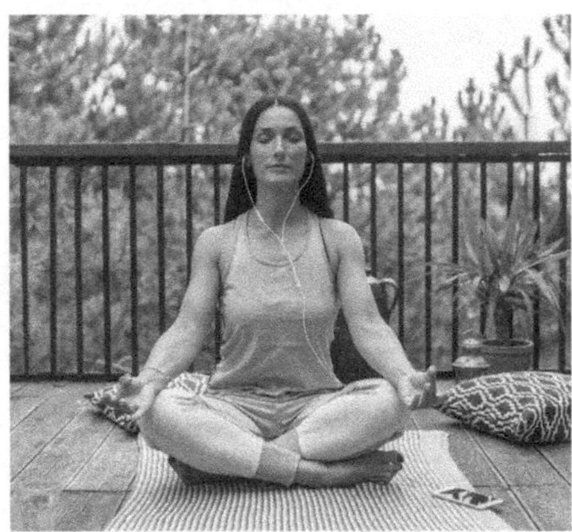

Fitness on the balcony

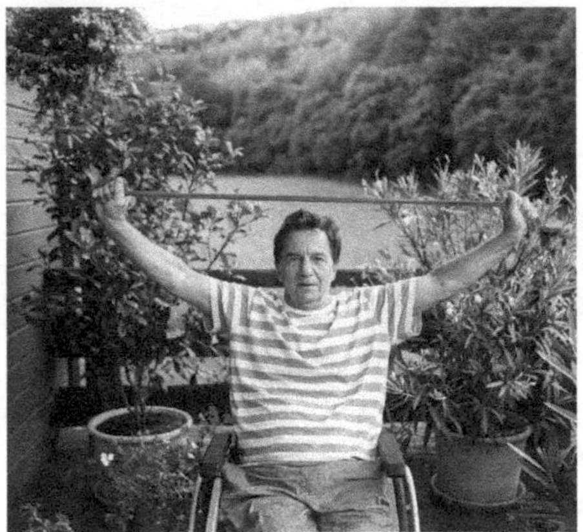

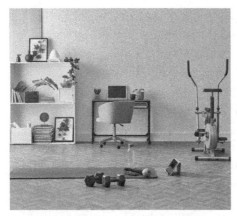

Fitness on the patio

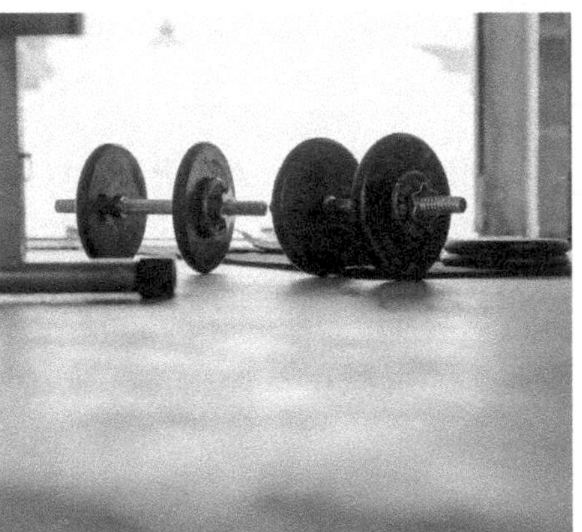

Fitness in a home garage

Fitness strategies around the home

Fitness and Wellness Outside the Home

Consider fitness strategies outside the home that may include exercise or physical activity in the backyard or garden.

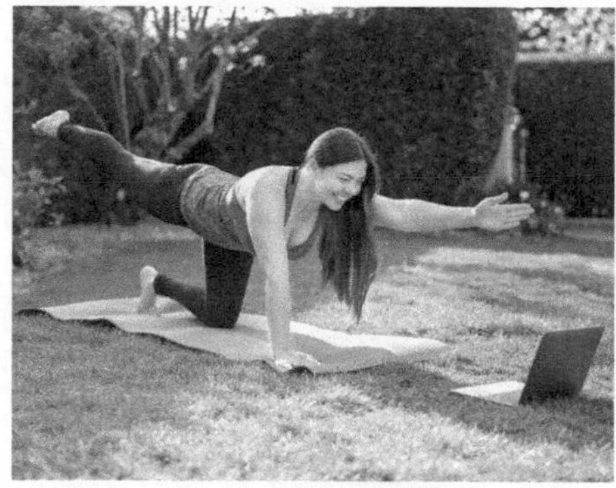

Backyard fitness

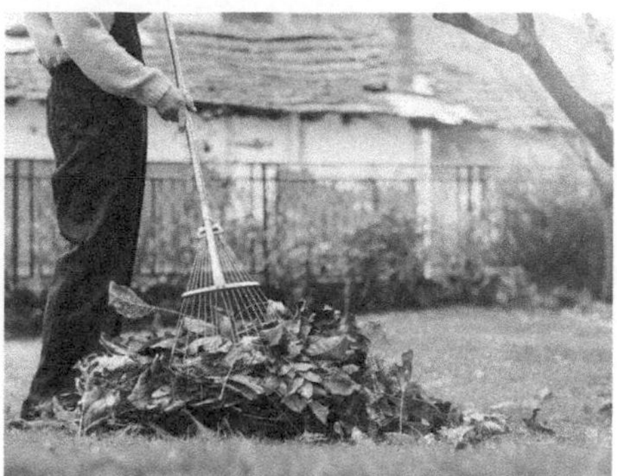

Raking leaves for functional fitness

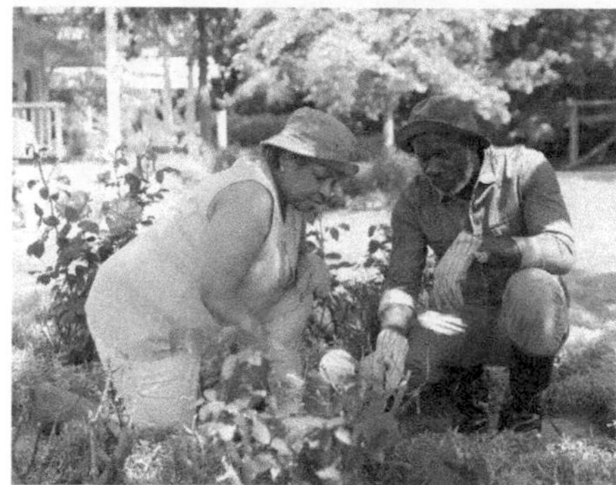

Gardening for leisure fitness

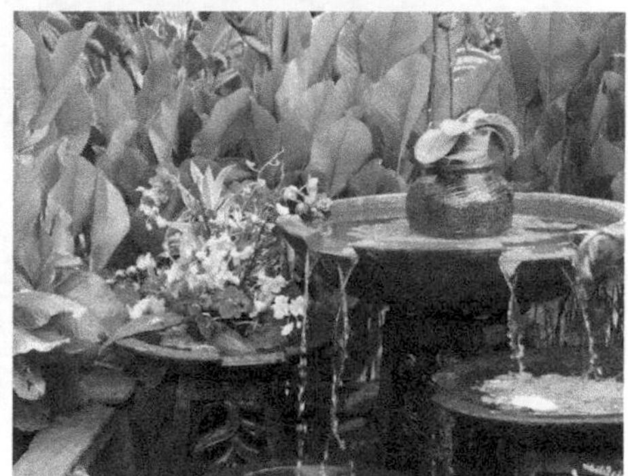

Garden meditation

Fitness strategies outside the home

Home Leisure Activities

Consider home leisure activities that may include backyard or driveway badminton, table tennis, volleyball, or basketball.

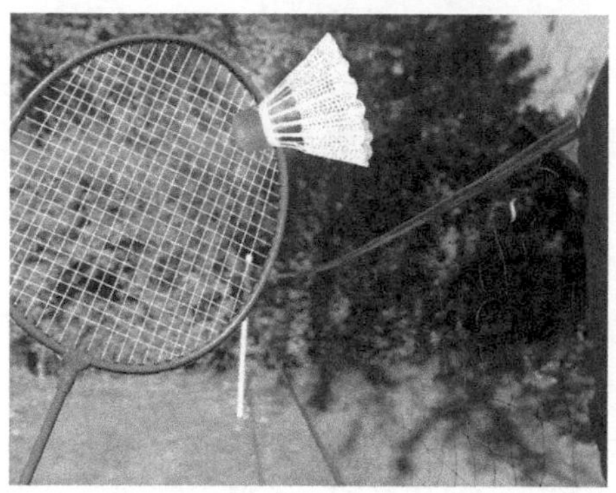

Home badminton for fitness

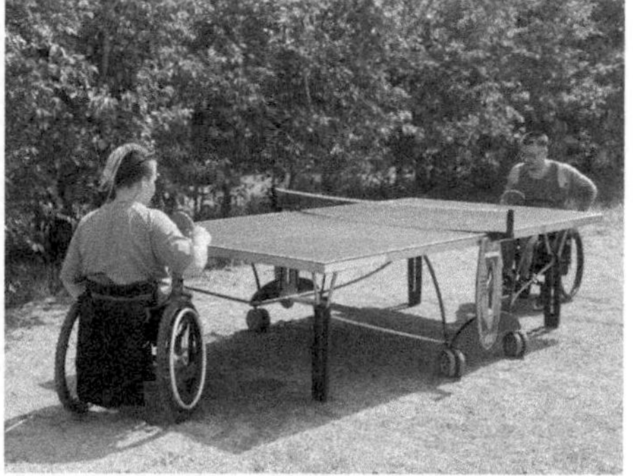

Home table tennis for fitness

Fitness strategies outside the home

Home Therapy Activities

Consider home therapy activities that may include art therapy, music therapy, poetry therapy, expressive writing, gardening, or meditation. For example, viewing a potted bonsai tree may be relaxing for older individuals (Song *et al.* 2018), or utilizing bonsai art by cultivation of a miniature tree may be helpful for health promotion (Hermann 2021; Hermann and Edwards 2021). The following images show some examples.

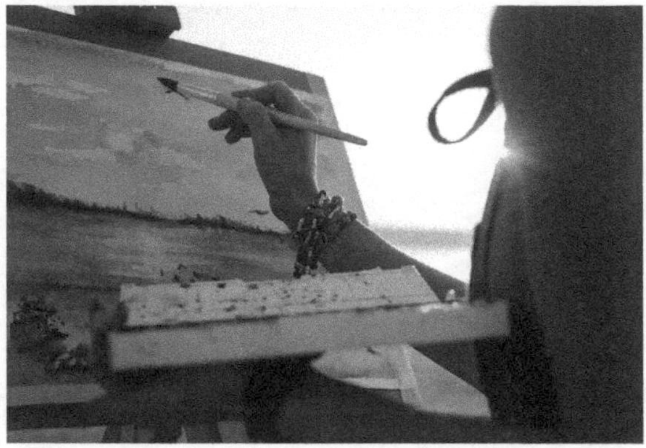

Painting outdoors

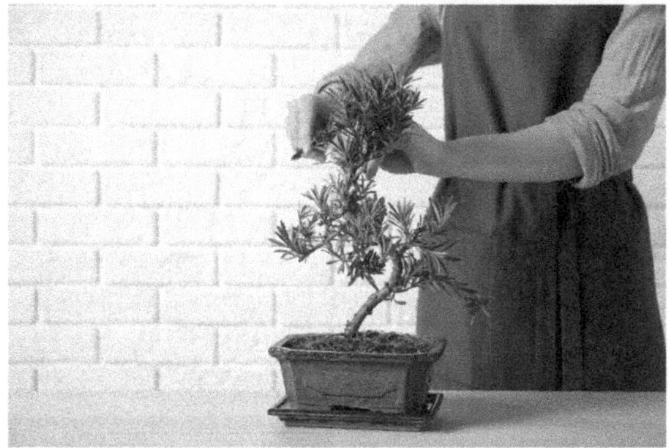

Trimming a Japanese bonsai tree for relaxation and mental health

Practical Outdoor Wellness

Outdoor fitness equipment installed in parks or green spaces may serve as a free-access option to increase physical activity in a community. Outdoor gyms may improve overall health and social connectedness (Grigoletto *et al.* 2021; Lee *et al.* 2018). There are a number of outdoor activities that a person may consider to be physically active. For example, a person can exercise at a variety of fitness courts. The following images show some examples.

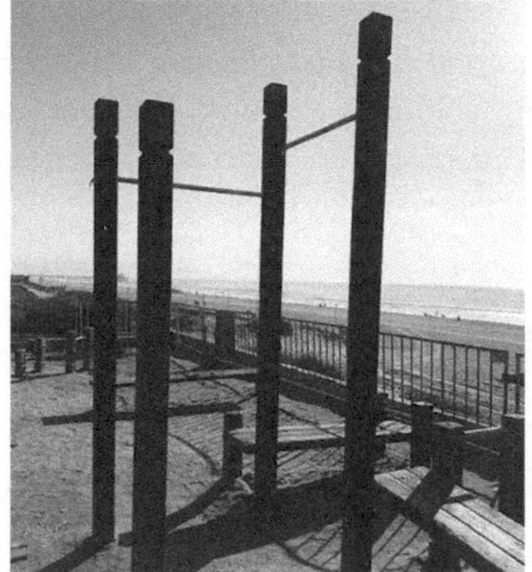
Small beach path fitness court

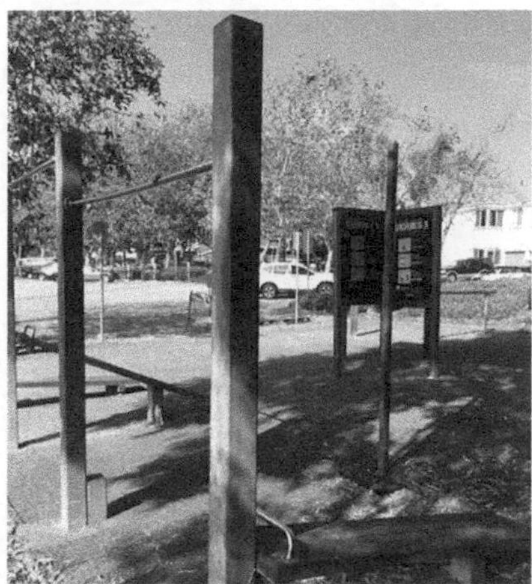
Small community fitness court

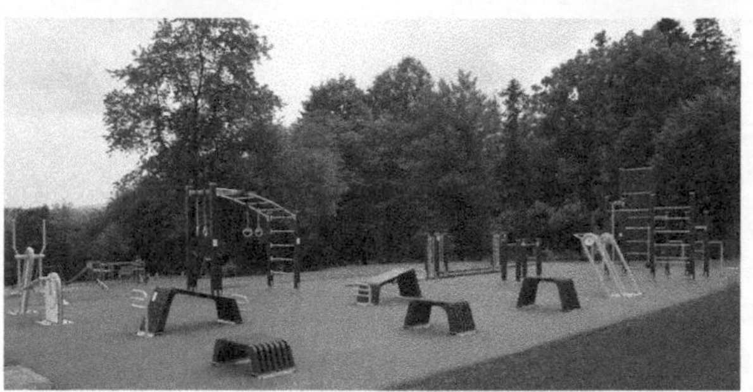
Large community fitness court

Fitness court exercises

The images below show other exercise programs that are easy to perform in any location such as yoga, tai chi, or calisthenics on a mat. Also, see Self-Care Handout 5.1: Mindful Walking Routine for a nature-based mindfulness walking program.

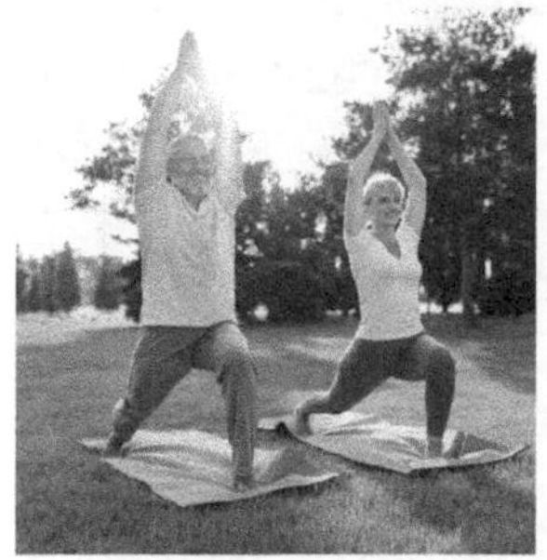
Yoga at a park

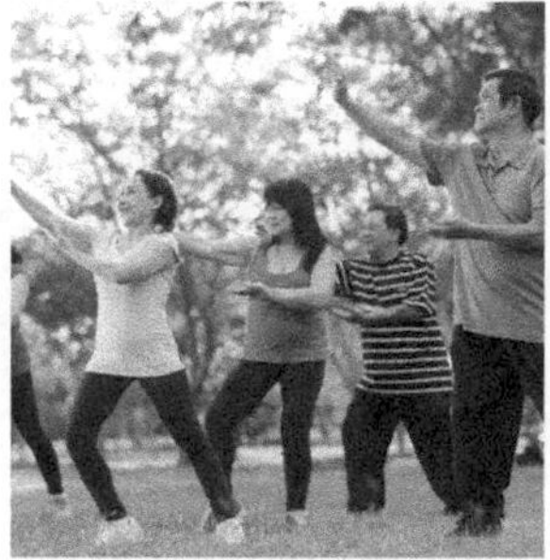
Tai chi at a park

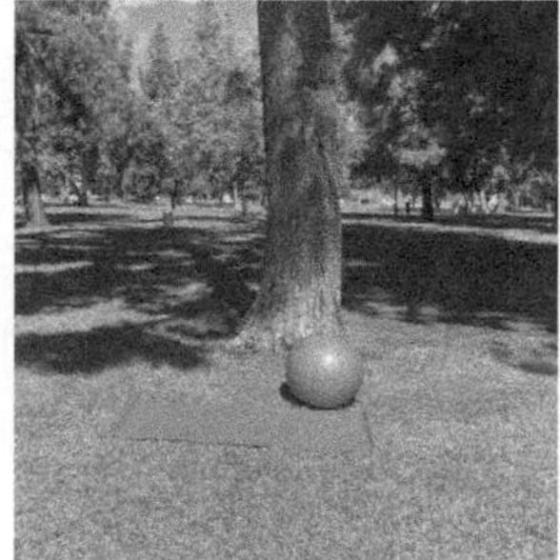
Calisthenics at a park

It can be easy to transport exercise to any outdoor location

CLINICAL TIP: RETREAT VACATIONS

Consider a retreat vacation to reduce stress and anxiety, meet new friends, and learn new skills such as meditation, cooking, yoga, and/or tai chi (Blasche *et al.* 2021; Haber *et al.* 2020; Khoury *et al.* 2017). For example, a person can relax, learn, and renew at locations such as the following:

- Armathwaite Hall Hotel and Spa, www.armathwaite-hall.com
- Canyon Ranch, www.canyonranch.com
- Chenot Palace, www.chenotpalaceweggis.com
- Esalen, www.esalen.org
- Euphoria Retreat, www.euphoriaretreat.com
- Kripalu, https://kripalu.org
- Kuru Private Resort, https://kururesort.com
- Six Senses Hotels and Resorts, www.sixsenses.com/en

Featured Topics

Featured Topic 10.1 outlines healing places and healing spaces that healthcare providers may help patients/clients create in their homes.

Featured Topic 10.2 outlines the benefits of gardening for health.

Featured Topic 10.3 outlines the benefits of being in parks and green spaces.

Featured Topic 10.4 outlines the emerging nature-as-medicine movement in healthcare.

Featured Topic 10.5 outlines basic concepts of biophilic design.

Featured Topic 10.6 outlines some soothing sounds for relaxation and stress reduction.

Featured Topic 10.7 outlines a case vignette of an older couple benefitting from tai chi at a local park.

■ Featured Topic 10.1: Healing Places and Healing Spaces

A healing place or space needs to be personalized for each person. Some individuals may need a place to relax, meditate, unwind, exercise, or engage in hobbies. For example, a person may create a healing space in a part of a room, on the front porch, on the patio or balcony, or in their backyard.

In this section, the focus will be on creating a personalized healing place and space by using a wellness gazebo or a shed. The gazebo may be an excellent way to include nature in daily life. On the other hand, the shed approach could be better suited for colder climates or where there is more rain.

In their personal healing wellness gazebo or shed, a person may:

- perform yoga, tai chi, qigong, calisthenics, bodyweight exercises, and/or weight training with dumbbells or kettlebells
- engage in mindfulness meditation (e.g., progressive muscle relaxation, body scan technique)
- engage in purposeful hobbies (e.g., art and crafts, painting, writing, reading)
- entertain or relax with friends and family
- plant a herb and vegetable garden for plant-based organic foods and aromatic flowers (e.g., lavender for relaxing aromatherapy) in the perimeter
- enjoy the sounds of birds by including bird feeders around the gazebo or shed
- allow children to perform homework in a calming nature-based environment.

Give it a try and build your own unique healing space.

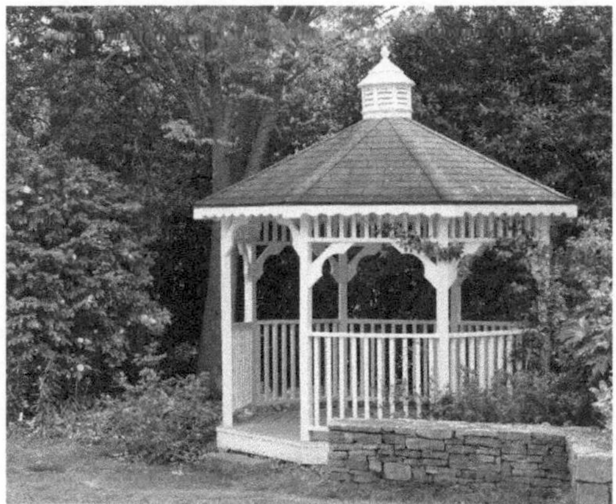

Home gazebo for wellness and fitness

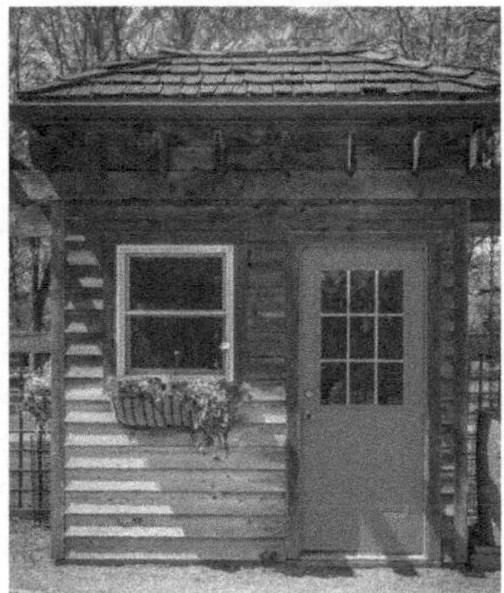

Home shed for wellness and fitness

■ Featured Topic 10.2: Gardening for Health

Gardening can help improve overall health and well-being, reduce stress, benefit nutritional behaviors (consumption of fruits and vegetables), increase functional physical activity (such as bending, squatting, reaching, lifting, and carrying), promote subjective happiness, and enhance social connections (Gatto *et al.* 2017; Howarth *et al.* 2020; Savoie-Roskos *et al.* 2017). Also, a study found that virtual therapy using a therapeutic garden may help lower depressive symptoms and anxiety levels in older women (Szczepańska-Gieracha *et al.* 2021).

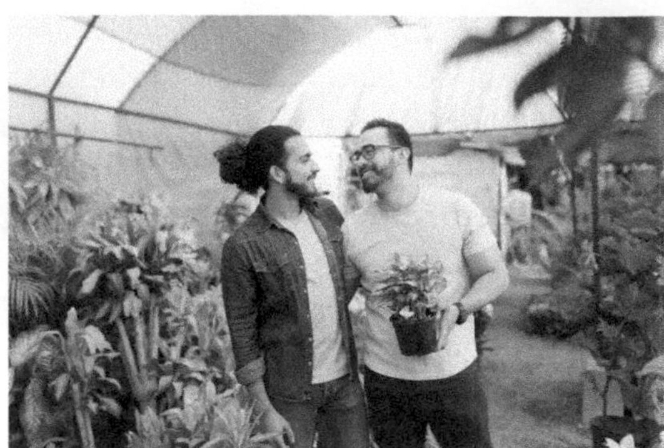

Gardening for health

■ Featured Topic 10.3: Park Prescriptions

Being near parks and green spaces is associated with increased childhood physical activity, lower incidence of being overweight, improved behavioral health and resilience, fewer ADHD symptoms in children, and less anxiety and depression in adults (Reuben *et al.* 2020).

■ Featured Topic 10.4: Nature as Medicine

"Nature as medicine" is taking on strong roots in the medical community. Nature is a form of medicine since it has many therapeutic effects on physical and mental well-being. Nature medicine uses fresh air, sunshine, landscape, soundscape, and smellscape. To obtain the benefits of nature, a person may perform outdoor activities such as gardening, walking, hiking, biking, camping, or various sporting and recreational activities.

An article by Victorson *et al.* (2020, p.659) states that, "Throughout millennia, ancient societies left signs and cultural artifacts that highlighted the vast interconnectedness and interdependence they had with nature for health, healing, sustainability, survival, and spiritual affiliation." Studies outlined in this chapter show that nature-based therapies may help individuals with anxiety, stress management, depression, and attention-related disorders.

■ Featured Topic 10.5: Biophilic Design

According to the *Frontiers in Psychology* journal (Barbiero and Berto 2021, p.7), "the goal of biophilic design is to create artificial environments as similar as possible to natural ones, to ensure the positive effect that Nature has on people's health and wellbeing."

Zhao and colleagues (2022, p.1) indicate that, "By restoring the interaction between buildings and nature, biophilic design improves the quality of environments and the health of users." For example, a biophilic design may be used in residential indoor spaces to help individuals living with chronic pain, depression, and migraines (Huntsman and Bulaj 2022).

Benefits of biophilic design include reduced anxiety, reduced pain, reduced stress, improved mood, improved sleep, and improved cognitive performance. The following are some ways to improve the connection to nature in interior spaces:

- Natural light—large windows, skylights
- Natural sounds—sounds of birds and leaves rustling in the wind through open windows
- Nature landscapes—windowsill garden
- Natural materials in the home—wood, stone, marble, wool, cotton, silk
- Natural shapes—curves and nature-based shapes
- Natural colors—blue, green, yellow, brown
- Natural elements—ventilation through open windows and doors for fresh air, indoor plants, fountains, fish tank, aromatherapy through flowers
- Pets—cats, dogs, fish tank, bird feeders on a balcony or porch
- Nature-based art—painting, sculptures

For more information about biophilic design, see: Gray and Birrell 2014; Kellert 2018; Kellert *et al.* 2008; Tekin *et al.* 2023.

Featured Topic 10.6: Soothing Sounds

In general, natural soundscapes or soothing sounds may be useful for relaxation and reducing stress and anxiety. Consider the following sounds:

- Birds
- Flowing water in a stream
- Laughter
- Leaves rustling
- Rain
- Singing
- Waves at the ocean
- Whistling
- Wind chimes

■ Featured Topic 10.7: Case Vignette—Tai Chi in the Park

Joe, a 70-year-old retired engineer, noticed that he and his wife of 40 years no longer had energy when they went shopping. Also, their balance was getting worse with activities such as stair climbing. Joe and his wife, a retired teacher, did yard work and periodically went to a community center for various events, but mainly stayed home watching television. They both felt somewhat isolated, even though they talked to their adult children who lived in Europe. Upon the suggestion of their family physician, they looked for a tai chi class and found one at a nearby park. On the first day of class, they were pleased to see about 15 individuals from their community. They performed tai chi twice weekly for 12 weeks and gradually noticed they had more endurance and improved balance. The tai chi group not only improved their physical fitness, but they also enjoyed being in natural surroundings with their neighbors. The park experience led Joe and his wife to increase their community involvement by mentoring high school students and creating an outdoor walking and networking club.

Adapted from Altug 2020.

Self-Care Education Guides

See **Self-Care Handout 10.1: Your Nature Prescription** for practical strategies for patients/clients to engage in nature (Ambrosi *et al.* 2019; Britton *et al.* 2020; Chan *et al.* 2021; de Boer *et al.* 2017; Ellingsen-Dalskau *et al.* 2021; Feng *et al.* 2021; Grigoletto *et al.* 2021; Johnson *et al.* 2020; Juster-Horsfield and Bell 2022; Lee *et al.* 2017; Li *et al.* 2018; Lu *et al.* 2020; Twohig-Bennett and Jones 2018; Zhang *et al.* 2021).

See **Self-Care Handout 10.2: Nature Prescription** for practical strategies for patients/clients to engage in nature.

See **Self-Care Handout 10.3: Natural Light Exposure at Home** for practical strategies for patients/clients to improve light exposure at home (Rosenthal 2013; Terman and McMahan 2012; Wirz-Justice *et al.* 2013). For optimal benefits, homeowners may need to consider remodeling their homes to allow more interaction with the outdoor environment. Consult with a sleep medicine or lighting specialist for additional guidance in helping patients/clients obtain the ideal amount of light for their needs.

See **Self-Care Handout 10.4: Natural Light Exposure at Work** for practical strategies for patients/clients to improve light exposure at work (Rosenthal 2013; Terman and McMahan 2012; Wirz-Justice *et al.* 2013). For optimal benefits, companies may need to consider remodeling their buildings to allow more interaction with the outdoor environment. If a person's job involves hospital work, additional strategies to help patients recover may include increasing natural light in a hospital room. For example, the healthcare professional could try to ensure the hospital room has a direct window view, open the curtains and blinds to let natural light and sunshine into the room, and provide opportunities for patients to sit outside in a courtyard if possible (Joschko *et al.* 2023; Malenbaum *et al.* 2008; Walch *et al.* 2005).

See **Self-Care Handout 10.5: Natural Light Exposure at School** for practical strategies for patients/clients to improve light exposure at school (Birnbaum 1984; Birnbaum 1985; Rosenthal 2013). For optimal benefits, schools may need to consider remodeling their buildings to allow more interaction with the outdoor environment.

See **Self-Care Handout 10.6: Nature Trail Circuit** for an outdoor fitness routine that may be performed on a trail or at a local park (Altug 2018).

See **Self-Care Handout 10.7: Garden Meditation** for a simple relaxation strategy.

See **Self-Care Handout 10.8: Nature at Work** for strategies to include nature in your workplace.

Self-Care Handout 10.1: Your Nature Prescription

Nature has been shown to reduce stress and anxiety, improve sleep, and enhance overall well-being. Try any of the following to get the benefits of nature medicine, nature-based therapy, green exercise, or ecotherapy:

Activities	Examples
Adventure therapy and activities	Hiking, rafting, nature photography, rock climbing, camping, skiing
Animal-assisted therapy	Caring for animals, walking the dog
Arts therapies in the outdoors	Drum circles, painting
Blue care	Water-based activities at rivers, lakes, ponds, oceans
Conventional outdoor exercise	Walking, hiking, biking
Farm-related therapy	Working with crops at a local farm
Fitness courts in the outdoors	Pull-ups, push-ups, planks
Forest therapy (or bathing)	Hiking, meditation
Gardening	Home or community garden
Home healing spaces	Garage gym, patio, or backyard fitness
Horticultural therapy	Use of plants for promoting well-being
Mind-body outdoor exercise	Yoga, tai chi, qigong, labyrinth walking
Nature games	Fort building, hide and seek, capture the flag
Nature meditation	Meditation at a park, beach, forest, stream
Night meditation	Stargazing, astronomy club
Park activities	Identifying plants and animals
Sports in the outdoors	Basketball, golf, triathlons, volleyball
Volunteering	Local park projects, coaching football (soccer) or softball
Wilderness therapy	Camping, campfire stories, hiking

Self-Care Handout 10.2: Nature Prescription

Patient/client name: ....

Date: ....

Place

- ☐ Forest hiking
- ☐ Gardening
- ☐ Outdoor hobbies
- ☐ Park activities
- ☐ ....
- ☐ ....

How Often

- ☐ 1–2 times per week
- ☐ 2–3 times per week
- ☐ 3–4 times per week
- ☐ 4–5 times per week
- ☐ ....
- ☐ ....

How Long

- ☐ 15 minutes
- ☐ 30 minutes
- ☐ 45 minutes
- ☐ 60 minutes
- ☐ ....
- ☐ ....

Key Concepts

- ☐ Be active
- ☐ Meditate
- ☐ Relax
- ☐ Socialize
- ☐ ....
- ☐ ....

Challenges

- ☐ Challenge yourself
- ☐ Learn a new activity
- ☐ Learn a new hobby
- ☐ Meet new friends
- ☐ ....
- ☐ ....

Goals

- ☐ Reduce hypertension
- ☐ Reduce weight
- ☐ Reduce stress
- ☐ Stop smoking
- ☐ ....
- ☐ ....

Comments: ....

Signature: ....

Self-Care Handout 10.3: Natural Light Exposure at Home

- Get enough natural outdoor light during the day, especially in the morning.
- Have your breakfast near a window, on a balcony, porch, or patio, or in your backyard gazebo.
- Open the curtains to let in as much outdoor light as possible, especially in the morning.
- Consider remodeling the home to add more windows or skylights or enlarge existing windows.
- Consider adding a sundeck or a gazebo to the backyard for exercise, meditation, relaxation, or reading.
- Consider painting walls with light shades or tones (e.g., white) and purchasing light-colored furniture.
- Create a reading, relaxation, or healing space in the home with sunlight streaming in. For reading, it's best if the sunlight is behind the person.
- Place the home computer or workstation to face out of a large window where a person can periodically gaze off into the distance. However, the person should avoid facing direct sunlight.
- Wash home windows and trim the bushes and trees near the windows to allow more light to enter the home.
- Sit on a balcony, patio, porch, or backyard and do some birdwatching or gaze at the horizon or trees in the distance for light and relaxation.
- To prevent sleep problems, turn off cellphones and computers several hours before bedtime.

Self-Care Handout 10.4: Natural Light Exposure at Work

- If a person has windows in their office, position the desk to face out of the window. Looking away from a computer monitor and into the distance may help reduce eye strain. However, the person should avoid facing direct sunlight.
- Arrange all workstations at the perimeter of the office to face out of windows.
- Place vending machines, water dispensers, and photocopiers near windows.
- Create well-lit waiting room areas in hospitals and clinics.
- Have meetings in well-lit rooms with large windows and natural outdoor light.
- Consider holding small group meetings while walking outside on a sunny day.
- Consider adding skylights to areas with many workstations.
- Open window blinds and trim back bushes and trees covering office windows.
- Eat lunch outdoors (at a picnic table or sitting on a portable chair), even if sitting under a tree or in the shade. If a person can't go outside due to heat, cold, allergies, or pollution, they could sit near a window in the cafeteria and do some birdwatching or gaze at the horizon or trees in the distance for light, relaxation, and stress reduction. Excess close work may increase mental and visual stress.
- After eating lunch, take 10–15-minute walks.
- Exercise outdoors in short bouts before work, during lunch, or after work. Short-bout exercise has been shown to improve health and enhance exercise adherence in overweight and obese adults.
- Go outdoors during work breaks. Even on an overcast day, an outdoor environment provides more light than the typical indoor office lighting.

Self-Care Handout 10.5: Natural Light Exposure at School

- Open the blinds and curtains to allow natural outdoor light to enter the classroom.
- Have children sit near the windows.
- Take recess outdoors when possible.
- Include more outdoor recess breaks and outdoor physical education classes.
- Include or create activities that involve outdoor projects (such as painting, singing, writing).
- Encourage children to eat outdoors, even if it's under a tree or in the shade.
- To minimize or avoid near-point visual stress, have children gaze off into the distance (such as out of the window) periodically.
- If the children can't go outside due to heat, cold, allergies, or pollution, have them sit near a window in the cafeteria and do some birdwatching or cloud watching. Or make a game out of looking outdoors by having children gaze at the horizon or trees in the distance and seeing who can identify the most distant object.

Self-Care Handout 10.6: Nature Trail Circuit

1. Start: Warm up for 5 minutes with gentle calisthenics and mobility exercises.
2. Walk on the chosen trail for 5–10 minutes observing the plants and trees.
3. Stop and perform overhead pressing movements 15 times using a stick you find on the path or your trekking poles.
4. Walk on the trail for 5–10 minutes listening for the sounds of birds and wildlife.
5. Stop and perform step-ups from a 6–12-inch flat rock that is stable for 15 repetitions.
6. Walk on the trail for 5–10 minutes noticing the smells of the various plants and trees along your path. Consider this your halfway point. Either turn round on the trail to head back or look to finish the loop.
7. Stop and pick a rock weighing about 5–10 pounds. Perform the squatting movement with the rock for 5–10 repetitions.
8. Walk on the trail for 5–10 minutes feeling the wind in your face and the varied surfaces under your walking shoes.
9. Stop and perform partial push-ups against a tree or an elevated log.
10. Walk on the trail for 5–10 minutes and see how many types of wildlife you can identify.
11. Stop and pick up a long stick (or use one of your trekking poles). Hold the stick (or pole) with both hands and slowly swing it up and down like you are using a long-handle ax to chop wood for 10 repetitions to engage your core muscles.
12. Walk on the trail for 5–10 minutes thinking about all the things you are grateful for in your life.
13. Perform gentle upper and lower body stretches.
14. End: Hydrate and eat a piece of fruit as you observe the calming scenery and reflect on how you feel.

Notes:

- Focus on your personal safety anytime you are in the wilderness. Do not perform any activity beyond your physical abilities or a movement that may be unsafe.
- Dress appropriately for the season and weather conditions.

- Bring a small backpack with water and an energy bar or fruit (such as a banana or orange). Trekking poles are optional.
- For personal safety, bring a smartphone and tell someone which path you will be taking and what time you expect to return home.
- Ideally, use the "buddy" system and go on the trail circuit with a friend.
- The hiking times mentioned in the circuit may be adjusted to shorter or longer lengths depending on your fitness level and goals.

Self-Care Handout 10.7: Garden Meditation

You can meditate or create calming and relaxing thoughts anywhere. You can use your backyard or even your balcony garden as a place to relax. Here is a sample meditation routine:

1. Sit in a comfortable chair in your backyard or balcony garden. Find a sunny area if you wish (unless you are sun sensitive).
2. Start to breathe slowly using belly breathing (or diaphragmatic breathing).
3. Focus on a flower, plant, or tree. See if you notice the leaves gently blowing in the wind.
4. As you belly breathe, see if you can smell the aroma of the flowers or plants.
5. Next, see if you can hear any birds or leaves rustling.
6. Notice the sun's warmth on your skin or the wind gently touching your face.
7. Close your eyes at this point if you wish. Continue belly breathing and think about the happy moments in your life and the goals you want to accomplish.

Note: You can stay at each step for 1–3 minutes or as long as you wish. Try different timeframes to see which one makes you feel best.

Self-Care Handout 10.8: Nature at Work

Here are some ideas for including nature in your workplace or office:

- Place a small indoor plant on the corner of your desk.
- Place larger indoor plants near your desk.
- Place a small Zen garden kit (consisting of a bamboo tray, sand, rake, and rocks) near your desk as an active meditation tool.
- Place photos of natural scenery in front of your desk.
- Use a computer screen saver that uses images of nature.
- Use a smartphone screen saver that uses images of nature.
- If you use a wall calendar, obtain one with natural scenery.
- Eat lunch outside near a tree.

Self-Management Activities: Explore Nature

The following online resources can help patients/clients, healthcare providers, and health/fitness professionals to manage stress and anxiety by exploring nature.

Nature Apps

- The Audubon Bird Guide App provides a fun way to walk, hike, and explore nature by tracking and identifying birds: www.audubon.org/app
- The iNaruralist site provides a fun way to interact with nature: www.inaturalist.org
- The Leafsnap App provides a fun way to walk, hike, and explore nature by taking a photo of a plant and then identifying it: https://leafsnap.app
- The National Geographic app provides a fun way to explore the world: www.nationalgeographic.com/pages/topic/nat-geo-app
- The NatureTime app, founded by Iris Rosin, provides a connection with nature to reduce stress and improve overall health: https://naturetimeapp.com

Virtual Hikes

- Consider searching YouTube for various virtual hikes. For example, search for a famous park or trail and see if there is a recorded hike for that region.

Classroom and Lab Activities

- Identify common local nature-oriented areas that are available in most communities.
- Create simple, fun, and cost-effective nature-based activities for families.
- Determine which plants are ideal for indoor use.

Useful Clinical Resources

Organizations

Environment

- Circadian, www.circadian.life
- Environmental Physiotherapy Association (Founder: Filip Maric, Ph.D.), http://environmentalphysio.com
- Environmental Working Group, www.ewg.org
- United States Environmental Protection Agency, www.epa.gov

Nature and Green Spaces

- American Horticultural Society, https://ahsgardening.org
- American Horticultural Therapy Association, www.ahta.org
- Association of Nature and Forest Therapy, www.natureandforesttherapy.earth
- Bioneers, https://bioneers.org
- Children & Nature Network, www.childrenandnature.org
- EcoMedicine, www.drjohnlapuma.com/ecomedicine
- International Living Future Institute, https://living-future.org
- International Nature and Forest Therapy Alliance, https://infta.net
- National Park Service, www.nps.gov/index.htm
- Therapeutic Landscapes Network, https://healinglandscapes.org

Light Therapy

- American Academy of Ophthalmology, www.aao.org
- Center for Circadian Biology—UC San Diego, http://ccb.ucsd.edu
- Center for Environmental Therapeutics, https://cet.org
- Centre for Chronobiology—University of Basel, www.chronobiology.ch
- Icahn School of Medicine at Mount Sinai—Mount Sinai Light and Health Research Center, https://icahn.mssm.edu/research/light-health
- International Society for Affective Disorders, www.isad.org.uk
- Lighting Research Center, www.lrc.rpi.edu/healthyliving
- National Institute of Mental Health, www.nimh.nih.gov (search for seasonal affective disorder)
- National Lighting Bureau, https://nlb.org
- Society for Light Treatment and Biological Rhythms, https://sltbr.org

Soundscape

- Soundscapes (sounds of nature and the wild), www.soundscapes-app.com

Apps

- AllTrails: Hike, Bike & Run, https://apps.apple.com/us/app/alltrails-hike-bike-run/id405075943
- D Minder Pro (track and manage vitamin D), https://apps.apple.com/us/app/d-minder-pro/id547102495
- NatureQuant, www.naturequant.com/naturedose
- NatureTime (Founder: Iris Rosin), https://naturetimeapp.com

Outdoor Fitness Courts and Equipment

- GameTime, www.gametime.com
- Greenfields Outdoor Fitness, https://gfoutdoorfitness.com
- National Fitness Campaign, https://nationalfitnesscampaign.com
- Zoom Recreation, www.zoomrecreation.com

Products

- Beurer (light therapy products), www.beurer.com/web/us
- Carex (light therapy products), https://carex.com
- Coolibar (sun protective clothing), www.coolibar.com
- Northern Light Technologies (light therapy products), https://northernlighttechnologies.com
- REI—trekking poles (fitness walking poles), www.rei.com/c/trekking-poles
- Solumbra by Sun Precautions (sun protective clothing), www.sunprecautions.com
- Sunbox Company (light therapy products), www.sunbox.com
- Verilux (light therapy products), https://verilux.com

Outcome Measures

- *Morningness-Eveningness Questionnaire*
  Horne JA, Ostberg O. A self-assessment questionnaire to determine morningness-eveningness in human circadian rhythms. *Int J Chronobiol.* 1976;4(2):97–110.
- *Munich Chronotype Questionnaire*
  Roenneberg T, Wirz-Justice A, Merrow M. Life between clocks: daily temporal patterns of human chronotypes. *J Biol Rhythms.* 2003;18(1):80–90.
- *Seasonal Health Questionnaire*
  Thompson C, Cowan A. The Seasonal Health Questionnaire: a preliminary validation of a new instrument to screen for seasonal affective disorder. *J Affect Disord.* 2001;64(1):89–98.
- *Seasonal Pattern Assessment Questionnaire*
  Mersch PP, Vastenburg NC, Meesters Y, *et al.* The reliability and validity of the Seasonal Pattern Assessment Questionnaire: a comparison between patient groups. *J Affect Disord.* 2004;80(2–3):209–219.
  Murray G. The Seasonal Pattern Assessment Questionnaire as a measure of mood seasonality: a prospective validation study. *Psychiatry Res.* 2003;120(1):53–59.

Rosenthal N, Bradt G, Wehr T. *Seasonal Pattern Assessment Questionnaire (SPAQ)*. Bethesda, MD: National Institute of Mental Health; 1984.

References

Aldahan AS, Shah VV, Mlacker S, Nouri K. Sun exposure in history. *JAMA Dermatol.* 2016;152(8):896.

Altug Z. *Integrative Healing: Developing Wellness in the Mind and Body.* Springville, UT: Cedar Fort, Inc; 2018.

Altug Z. Exercise, dance, tai chi, Pilates, and Alexander technique. In: Ishak WW, ed. *The Handbook of Wellness Medicine*. Cambridge, United Kingdom: Cambridge University Press; 2020.

Ambrosi C, Zaiontz C, Peragine G, Sarchi S, Bona F. Randomized controlled study on the effectiveness of animal-assisted therapy on depression, anxiety, and illness perception in institutionalized elderly. *Psychogeriatrics*. 2019;19(1):55–64.

Amichai B, Grunwald MH, Davidovici B, Shemer A. "Sunlight is said to be the best of disinfectants": The efficacy of sun exposure for reducing fungal contamination in used clothes. *Isr Med Assoc J*. 2014;16(7):431–433.

An M, Colarelli SM, O'Brien K, Boyajian ME. Why we need more nature at work: effects of natural elements and sunlight on employee mental health and work attitudes. *PLoS One*. 2016;11(5):e0155614.

Baggerly CA, Cuomo RE, French CB, *et al.* Sunlight and vitamin D: necessary for public health. *J Am Coll Nutr*. 2015;34(4):359–365.

Baloch RMM, Maesano CN, Christoffersen J, *et al.* Daylight and school performance in European schoolchildren. *Int J Environ Res Public Health*. 2020;18(1):258.

Barbiero G, Berto R. Biophilia as evolutionary adaptation: an onto- and phylogenetic framework for biophilic design. *Front Psychol.* 2021;12:700709

Baruki SB, DE Lima Montebello MI, Pazzianotto-Forti EM. Physical training in outdoor fitness gym improves blood pressure, physical fitness, and quality of life of hypertensive patients: a randomized controlled trial. *J Sports Med Phys Fitness*. 2022;62(7):997–1005.

Bauer A, White ND. Time in nature: a prescription for the prevention or management of hypertension. *American Journal of Lifestyle Medicine*. 2023. Online publication ahead of print.

Birnbaum MH. Nearpoint visual stress: a physiological model. *Journal of the American Optometric Association.* 1984;55(11):825–835.

Birnbaum MH. Nearpoint visual stress: clinical implications. *Journal of the American Optometric Association.* 1985;56(6):480–490.

Blasche G, deBloom J, Chang A, Pichlhoefer O. Is a meditation retreat the better vacation? Effect of retreats and vacations on fatigue, emotional well-being, and acting with awareness. *PLoS One*. 2021;16(2):e0246038.

Boubekri M, Cheung IN, Reid KJ, Wang CH, Zee PC. Impact of windows and daylight exposure on overall health and sleep quality of office workers: a case-control pilot study. *J Clin Sleep Med*. 2014;10(6):603–611.

Boubekri M, Lee J, MacNaughton P, *et al.* The impact of optimized daylight and views on the sleep duration and cognitive performance of office workers. *Int J Environ Res Public Health*. 2020;17(9):3219.

Britton E, Kindermann G, Domegan C, Carlin C. Blue care: a systematic review of blue space interventions for health and wellbeing. *Health Promot Int*. 2020;35(1):50–69.

Bullo V, Gobbo S, Vendramin B, *et al.* Nordic walking can be incorporated in the exercise prescription to increase aerobic capacity, strength, and quality of life for elderly: a systematic review and meta-analysis. *Rejuvenation Res*. 2018;21(2):141–161.

Burgess HJ, Park M, Ong JC, Shakoor N, Williams DA, Burns J. Morning versus evening bright light treatment at home to improve function and pain sensitivity for women with fibromyalgia: a pilot study. *Pain Med*. 2017;18(1):116–123.

Burns AC, Saxena R, Vetter C, Phillips AJK, Lane JM, Cain SW. Time spent in outdoor light is associated with mood, sleep, and circadian rhythm-related outcomes: a cross-sectional and longitudinal study in over 400,000 UK Biobank participants. *J Affect Disord*. 2021;295:347–352.

Cerwén G, Pedersen E, Pálsdóttir AM. The role of soundscape in nature-based rehabilitation: a patient perspective. *Int J Environ Res Public Health*. 2016;13(12):1229.

Chan YT, Lau HY, Chan WY, *et al.* Adventure therapy for child, adolescent, and young adult cancer patients: a systematic review. *Support Care Cancer*. 2021;29(1):35–48.

Chaudhury P, Banerjee D. "Recovering with nature": a review of ecotherapy and implications for the COVID-19 pandemic. *Front Public Health*. 2020;8:604440.

Choukroun J, Geoffroy PA. Light therapy in mood disorders: a brief history with physiological insights. *Chronobiol Med*. 2019;1(1):3–8.

Cohen ET, Huser S, Barone K, Barone DA. Trekking poles to aid multiple sclerosis walking impairment: an exploratory comparison of the effects of assistive devices on psychosocial impact and walking. *Int J MS Care*. 2021;23(3):135–141.

Coventry PA, Brown JE, Pervin J, *et al.* Nature-based outdoor activities for mental and physical health: systematic review and meta-analysis. *SSM Popul Health*. 2021;16:100934.

Danilenko KV, Mustafina SV, Pechenkina EA. Bright light for weight loss: results of a controlled crossover trial. *Obes Facts*. 2013;6(1):28–38.

Dasgupta P. *The Economics of Biodiversity: The Dasgupta Review*. London, United Kingdom: HM Treasury; 2021. https://assets.publishing.service.gov.uk/government/uploads/system/uploads/attachment_data/file/962785/The_Economics_of_Biodiversity_The_Dasgupta_Review_Full_Report.pdf

de Boer B, Hamers JP, Zwakhalen SM, Tan FE, Beerens HC, Verbeek H. Green care farms as innovative nursing homes, promoting activities and social interaction for people with dementia. *J Am Med Dir Assoc*. 2017;18(1):40–46.

de Keijzer C, Tonne C, Basagaña X, *et al.* Residential surrounding greenness and cognitive decline: a 10-year follow-up of the Whitehall II cohort. *Environ Health Perspect*. 2018;126(7):077003.

Ellingsen-Dalskau LH, de Boer B, Pedersen I. Comparing the care environment at farm-based and regular day care for people with dementia in Norway: an observational study. *Health Soc Care Community*. 2021;29(2):506–514.

Engineer A, Ida A, Sternberg EM. Healing spaces: designing physical environments to optimize health, wellbeing, and performance. *Int J Environ Res Public Health*. 2020;17(4):1155.

Espiritu RC, Kripke DF, Ancoli-Israel S, *et al.* Low illumination experienced by San Diego adults: association with atypical depressive symptoms. *Biol Psychiatry*. 1994;35(6):403–407.

Even C, Schröder CM, Friedman S, Rouillon F. Efficacy of light therapy in nonseasonal depression: a systematic review. *J Affect Disord*. 2008;108(1–2):11–23.

Fahimipour AK, Hartmann EM, Siemens A, *et al.* Daylight exposure modulates bacterial communities associated with household dust. *Microbiome*. 2018;6(1):175.

Feng Y, Lin Y, Zhang N, Jiang X, Zhang L. Effects of animal-assisted therapy on hospitalized children and teenagers: a systematic review and meta-analysis. *J Pediatr Nurs*. 2021;60:11–23.

Figueiro MG, Nagare R, Price L. Non-visual effects of light: how to use light to promote circadian entrainment and elicit alertness. *Light Res Technol*. 2018;50(1):38–62.

Figueiro MG, Plitnick BA, Lok A, *et al.* Tailored lighting intervention improves measures of sleep, depression, and agitation in persons with Alzheimer's disease and related dementia living in long-term care facilities. *Clin Interv Aging*. 2014;9:1527–1537.

Figueiro MG, Rea MS. Lack of short-wavelength light during the school day delays dim light melatonin onset (DLMO) in middle school students. *Neuro Endocrinol Lett*. 2010;31(1):92–96.

Figueiro MG, Sahin L, Kalsher M, Plitnick B, Rea MS. Long-term, all-day exposure to circadian-effective light improves sleep, mood, and behavior in persons with dementia. *J Alzheimers Dis Rep*. 2020;4(1):297–312.

Figueiro MG, Steverson B, Heerwagen J, *et al.* The impact of daytime light exposures on sleep and mood in office workers. *Sleep Health*. 2017;3(3):204–215.

Gatto NM, Martinez LC, Spruijt-Metz D, Davis JN. LA sprouts randomized controlled nutrition, cooking and gardening programme reduces obesity and metabolic risk in Hispanic/Latino youth. *Pediatr Obes*. 2017;12(1):28–37.

Giorgini P, Rubenfire M, Bard RL, Jackson EA, Ferri C, Brook RD. Air pollution and exercise: a review of the cardiovascular implications for health care professionals. *J Cardiopulm Rehabil Prev*. 2016;36(2):84–95.

Gray T, Birrell C. Are biophilic-designed site office buildings linked to health benefits and high performing occupants? *Int J Environ Res Public Health*. 2014;11(12):12204–12222.

Grigoletto A, Mauro M, Maietta Latessa P, *et al.* Impact of different types of physical activity in green urban space on adult health and behaviors: a systematic review. *Eur J Investig Health Psychol Educ*. 2021;11(1):263–275.

Haber MA, Gaviola GC, Mann JR, *et al.* Reducing burnout among radiology trainees: a novel residency retreat curriculum to improve camaraderie and personal wellness: 3 strategies for success. *Curr Probl Diagn Radiol*. 2020;49(2):89–95.

Hahn IH, Grynderup MB, Dalsgaard SB, *et al.* Does outdoor work during the winter season protect against depression and mood difficulties? *Scand J Work Environ Health*. 2011;37(5):446–449.

He M, Xiang F, Zeng Y, *et al.* Effect of time spent outdoors at school on the development of myopia among children in China: a randomized clinical trial. *JAMA*. 2015;314(11):1142–1148.

Hermann C. Bonsai as a group art therapy intervention among traumatized youth in KwaZulu-Natal. *Psych J*. 2021;10(2):177–186.

Hermann C, Edwards SD. Practitioners' experiences of the influence of bonsai art on health. *Int J Environ Res Public Health*. 2021;18(6):2894.

Hobday RA, Cason JW. The open-air treatment of pandemic influenza. *Am J Public Health*. 2009;(Suppl 2):S236–S242.

Hobday RA, Dancer SJ. Roles of sunlight and natural ventilation for controlling infection: historical and current perspectives. *J Hosp Infect*. 2013;84(4):271–282.

Holick MF. Sunlight and vitamin D for bone health and prevention of autoimmune diseases, cancers, and cardiovascular disease. *Am J Clin Nutr*. 2004;80(6 Suppl):1678S–88S.

Holick MF. *The Vitamin D Solution*. New York, NY: Plume; 2010.

Holick MF. Biological effects of sunlight, ultraviolet radiation, visible light, infrared radiation and vitamin D for health. *Anticancer Res*. 2016;36(3):1345–1356.

Howarth M, Brettle A, Hardman M, Maden M. What is the evidence for the impact of gardens and gardening on health and well-being: a scoping review and evidence-based logic model to guide healthcare strategy decision making on the use of gardening approaches as a social prescription. *BMJ Open*. 2020;10(7):e036923.

Huber D, Grafetstätter C, Proßegger J, *et al.* Green exercise and Mg-Ca-SO_4 thermal balneotherapy for the treatment of non-specific chronic low back pain: a randomized controlled clinical trial. *BMC Musculoskelet Disord*. 2019;20(1):221.

Huntsman DD, Bulaj G. Healthy dwelling: design of biophilic interior environments fostering self-care practices for people living with migraines, chronic pain, and depression. *Int J Environ Res Public Health*. 2022;19(4):2248.

Ideno Y, Hayashi K, Abe Y, *et al.* Blood pressure-lowering effect of Shinrin-yoku (forest bathing): a systematic review and meta-analysis. *BMC Complement Altern Med*. 2017;17(1):409.

Johnson EG, Davis EB, Johnson J, Pressley JD, Sawyer S, Spinazzola J. The effectiveness of trauma-informed wilderness therapy with adolescents: a pilot study. *Psychol Trauma*. 2020;12(8):878–887.

Johnson JA, Garland SN, Carlson LE, *et al.* Bright light therapy improves cancer-related fatigue in cancer survivors: a randomized controlled trial. *J Cancer Surviv*. 2018;12(2):206–215.

Joschko L, Pálsdóttir AM, Grahn P, Hinse M. Nature-based therapy in individuals with mental health disorders, with a focus on mental well-being and connectedness to nature—a pilot study. *Int J Environ Res Public Health*. 2023;20(3):2167.

Juster-Horsfield HH, Bell SL. Supporting "blue care" through outdoor water-based activities: practitioner perspectives. *Qualitative Research in Sport, Exercise and Health*. 2022;14(1):137–150.

Kellert SR. *Nature by Design: The Practice of Biophilic Design*. New Haven, CT: Yale University Press; 2018.

Kellert SR, Heerwagen JH, Mador ML, eds. *Biophilic Design: The Theory, Science, and Practice of Bringing Buildings to Life*. Hoboken, NJ; Wiley; 2008.

Kent ST, McClure LA, Crosson WL, Arnett DK, Wadley VG, Sathiakumar N. Effect of sunlight exposure on cognitive function among depressed and non-depressed participants: a REGARDS cross-sectional study. *Environ Health*. 2009;8:34.

Khoury B, Knäuper B, Schlosser M, Carrière K, Chiesa A. Effectiveness of traditional meditation retreats: a systematic review and meta-analysis. *J Psychosom Res*. 2017;92:16–25.

Klompmaker JO, Laden F, Browning MHEM, *et al.* Associations of greenness, parks, and blue space with neurodegenerative disease hospitalizations among older US adults. *JAMA Netw Open*. 2022;5(12):e2247664.

Lacharité-Lemieux M, Brunelle JP, Dionne IJ. Adherence to exercise and affective responses: comparison between outdoor and indoor training. *Menopause*. 2015;22(7):731–740.

Lahart I, Darcy P, Gidlow C, Calogiuri G. The effects of green exercise on physical and mental wellbeing: a systematic review. *Int J Environ Res Public Health*. 2019;16(8):1352.

Lam C, Chung MH. Dose-response effects of light therapy on sleepiness and circadian phase shift in shift workers: a meta-analysis and moderator analysis. *Sci Rep*. 2021;11(1):11976.

Lee I, Choi H, Bang KS, Kim S, Song M, Lee B. Effects of forest therapy on depressive symptoms among adults: a systematic review. *Int J Environ Res Public Health*. 2017;14(3):321.

Lee JLC, Lo TLT, Ho RTH. Understanding outdoor gyms in public open spaces: a systematic review and integrative synthesis of qualitative and quantitative evidence. *Int J Environ Res Public Health*. 2018;15(4):590.

Lehrl S, Gerstmeyer K, Jacob JH, *et al.* Blue light improves cognitive performance. *J Neural Transm (Vienna)*. 2007;114(4):457–460.

Leichtfried V, Matteucci Gothe R, Kantner-Rumplmair W, *et al.* Short-term effects of bright light therapy in adults with chronic nonspecific back pain: a randomized controlled trial. *Pain Med*. 2014;15(12):2003–2012.

Li H, Zhang X, Bi S, Cao Y, Zhang G. Can residential greenspace exposure improve pain experience? A comparison between physical visit and image viewing. *Healthcare (Basel)*. 2021;9(7):918.

Li WHC, Ho KY, Lam KKW, *et al.* Adventure-based training to promote physical activity and reduce fatigue among childhood cancer survivors: a randomized controlled trial. *Int J Nurs Stud*. 2018;83:65–74.

Lindqvist PG, Epstein E, Nielsen K, Landin-Olsson M, Ingvar C, Olsson H. Avoidance of sun exposure as a risk factor for major causes of death: a competing risk analysis of the Melanoma in Southern Sweden cohort. *J Intern Med.* 2016;280(4):375–387.

Lu LC, Lan SH, Hsieh YP, Yen YY, Chen JC, Lan SJ. Horticultural therapy in patients with dementia: a systematic review and meta-analysis. *Am J Alzheimers Dis Other Demen.* 2020;35:1533317519883498.

Malenbaum S, Keefe FJ, Williams ACC, Ulrich R, Somers TJ. Pain in its environmental context: implications for designing environments to enhance pain control. *Pain.* 2008;134(3):241–244.

Mateen FJ, Vogel AC, Kaplan TB, *et al.* Light therapy for multiple sclerosis-associated fatigue: a randomized, controlled phase II trial. *J Neurol.* 2020;267(8):2319–2327.

McCullough PJ, Lehrer DS. Vitamin D, cod liver oil, sunshine, and phototherapy: safe, effective and forgotten tools for treating and curing tuberculosis infections: a comprehensive review. *J Steroid Biochem Mol Biol.* 2018;177:21–29.

Miller JM, Sadak KT, Shahriar AA, *et al.* Cancer survivors exercise at higher intensity in outdoor settings: the GECCOS trial. *Pediatr Blood Cancer.* 2021;68(5):e28850.

Nguyen PY, Astell-Burt T, Rahimi-Ardabili H, Feng X. Effect of nature prescriptions on cardiometabolic and mental health, and physical activity: a systematic review. *Lancet.* 2023;7(4):e313–e328.

Pálsdóttir AM, Spendrup S, Mårtensson L, Wendin K. Garden smellscape-experiences of plant scents in a nature-based intervention. *Front Psychol.* 2021;12:667957.

Penders TM, Stanciu CN, Schoemann AM, Ninan PT, Bloch R, Saeed SA. Bright light therapy as augmentation of pharmacotherapy for treatment of depression: a systematic review and meta-analysis. *Prim Care Companion CNS Disord.* 2016;18(5):10.4088/PCC.15r01906.

Pjrek E, Friedrich ME, Cambioli L, *et al.* The efficacy of light therapy in the treatment of seasonal affective disorder: a meta-analysis of randomized controlled trials. *Psychother Psychosom.* 2020;89(1):17–24.

Pun TB, Phillips CL, Marshall NS, *et al.* The effect of light therapy on electroencephalographic sleep in sleep and circadian rhythm disorders: a scoping review. *Clocks Sleep.* 2022;4(3):358–373.

Reuben A, Rutherford GW, James J, Razani N. Association of neighborhood parks with child health in the United States. *Prev Med.* 2020;141:106265.

Rosenthal NE. *Winter Blues: Everything You Need to Know to Beat Seasonal Affective Disorder,* 4th ed. New York, NY: The Guilford Press; 2013.

Ryu J, Jung JH, Kim J, *et al.* Outdoor cycling improves clinical symptoms, cognition and objectively measured physical activity in patients with schizophrenia: a randomized controlled trial. *J Psychiatr Res.* 2020;120:144–153.

Savoie-Roskos MR, Wengreen H, Durward C. Increasing fruit and vegetable intake among children and youth through gardening-based interventions: a systematic review. *J Acad Nutr Diet.* 2017;117(2):240–250.

Schuit M, Gardner S, Wood S, *et al.* The influence of simulated sunlight on the inactivation of influenza virus in aerosols. *J Infect Dis.* 2020;221(3):372–378.

Selby S, Hayes C, O'Sullivan N, O'Neil A, Harmon D. Facilitators and barriers to green exercise in chronic pain. *Ir J Med Sci.* 2019;188(3):973–978.

Sit DK, McGowan J, Wiltrout C, *et al.* Adjunctive bright light therapy for bipolar depression: a randomized double-blind placebo-controlled trial. *Am J Psychiatry.* 2018;175(2):131–139.

Song C, Ikei H, Nara M, Takayama D, Miyazaki Y. Physiological effects of viewing bonsai in elderly patients undergoing rehabilitation. *Int J Environ Res Public Health.* 2018;15(12):2635.

Sternberg EM. *Healing Spaces: The Science of Place and Well-being.* Cambridge, MA: The Belknap Press of Harvard University Press; 2009.

Sundermann M, Chielli D, Spell S. Nature as medicine: the 7th (unofficial) pillar of lifestyle medicine. *American Journal of Lifestyle Medicine.* 2023. First published online May 31, 2023.

Szczepańska-Gieracha J, Cieślik B, Serweta A, Klajs K. Virtual therapeutic garden: a promising method supporting the treatment of depressive symptoms in late-life: a randomized pilot study. *J Clin Med.* 2021;10(9):1942.

Tainio M, Jovanovic Andersen Z, Nieuwenhuijsen MJ, *et al.* Air pollution, physical activity and health: a mapping review of the evidence. *Environ Int.* 2021;147:105954.

Tang L, Liu M, Ren B, *et al.* Sunlight ultraviolet radiation dose is negatively correlated with the percent positive of SARS-CoV-2 and four other common human coronaviruses in the U.S. *Sci Total Environ.* 2021;751:141816.

Tekin BH, Corcoran R, Gutiérrez RU. A systematic review and conceptual framework of biophilic design parameters in clinical environments. *HERD.* 2023;16(1):233–250.

Terman M, McMahan I. *Chronotherapy: Resetting Your Inner Clock to Boost Mood, Alertness and Quality Sleep.* New York, NY: Avery; 2012.

Terman M, Terman JS. Light therapy for seasonal and nonseasonal depression: efficacy, protocol, safety, and side effects. *CNS Spectr.* 2005;10(8):647–672.

Terman M, Terman JS, Ross DC. A controlled trial of timed bright light and negative air ionization for treatment of winter depression. *Arch Gen Psychiatry.* 1998;55(10):875–882.

Thompson Coon J, Boddy K, Stein K, Whear R, Barton J, Depledge MH. Does participating in physical activity in outdoor natural environments have a greater effect on physical and mental wellbeing than physical activity indoors? A systematic review. *Environ Sci Technol*. 2011;45(5):1761–1772.

Turner PL, Mainster MA. Circadian photoreception: ageing and the eye's important role in systemic health. *Br J Ophthalmol*. 2008;92(11):1439–1444.

Turunen AW, Halonen J, Korpela K, *et al.* Cross-sectional associations of different types of nature exposure with psychotropic, antihypertensive and asthma medication. *Occup Environ Med*. 2023;80(2):111–118.

Twohig-Bennett C, Jones A. The health benefits of the great outdoors: a systematic review and meta-analysis of greenspace exposure and health outcomes. *Environ Res*. 2018;166:628–637.

van Maanen A, Meijer AM, van der Heijden KB, Oort FJ. The effects of light therapy on sleep problems: a systematic review and meta-analysis. *Sleep Med Rev*. 2016;29:52–62.

Venes D. ed. *Taber's Cyclopedic Medical Dictionary*, 24th ed. Philadelphia, PA: FA Davis; 2021.

Vibholm AP, Christensen JR, Pallesen H. Occupational therapists and physiotherapists experiences of using nature-based rehabilitation. *Physiother Theory Pract*. 2023;39(3):529–539.

Victorson D, Luberto C, Koffler K. Nature as medicine: mind, body, and soil. *J Altern Complement Med*. 2020;26(8):658–662.

Videnovic A, Klerman EB, Wang W, Marconi A, Kuhta T, Zee PC. Timed light therapy for sleep and daytime sleepiness associated with Parkinson disease: a randomized clinical trial. *JAMA Neurol*. 2017;74(4):411–418.

Wacker M, Holick MF. Sunlight and vitamin D: a global perspective for health. *Dermatoendocrinol*. 2013;5(1):51–108.

Walch JM, Rabin BS, Day R, Williams JN, Choi K, Kang JD. The effect of sunlight on postoperative analgesic medication use: a prospective study of patients undergoing spinal surgery. *Psychosom Med*. 2005;67(1):156–163.

Wirz-Justice A, Benedetti F, Terman M. *Chronotherapeutics for Affective Disorders: A Clinician's Manual for Light and Wake Therapy*, 2nd ed. Basel: Karger, Switzerland; 2013.

Wu PC, Chen CT, Lin KK, *et al.* Myopia prevention and outdoor light intensity in a school-based cluster randomized trial. *Ophthalmology*. 2018;125(8):1239–1250.

Youngstedt SD, Leung A, Kripke DF, Langer RD. Association of morning illumination and window covering with mood and sleep among post-menopausal women. *Sleep Biol Rhythms*. 2004;2(3):174–183.

Zhang X, Zhang Y, Zhai J, Wu Y, Mao A. Waterscapes for promoting mental health in the general population. *International Journal of Environmental Research and Public Health*. 2021;18(22):11792.

Zhao Y, Zhan Q, Xu T. Biophilic design as an important bridge for sustainable interaction between humans and the environment: based on practice in Chinese healthcare space. *Comput Math Methods Med*. 2022:8184534.

Zhou TY, Yuan XM, Ma XJ. Can an outdoor multisurface terrain enhance the effects of fall prevention exercise in older adults? A randomized controlled trial. *Int J Environ Res Public Health*. 2020;17(19):7023.

Additional Reading

Astell-Burt T, Pritchard T, Francois M, Ivers R, Olcoń K, Davidson PM, Feng X. Nature prescriptions should address motivations and barriers to be effective, equitable, and sustainable. *Lancet Planet Health*. 2023;7(7):e542–e543.

Atkins S, Snyder M. *Nature-Based Expressive Arts Therapy: Integrating the Expressive Arts and Ecotherapy*. London, United Kingdom: Jessica Kingsley Publishers; 2018.

Butler CW, Richardson M. Nature Connected Organisations Handbook: A guide for connecting organizations with nature for sustainable futures and workplace wellbeing. United Kingdom. 2023. https://findingnatureblog.files.wordpress.com/2022/04/the-nature-connection-handbook.pdf

Courtney JA, Langley JL, Wonders LL, Heiko R, LaPiere R, eds. *Nature-Based Play and Expressive Therapies: Interventions for Working with Children, Teens, and Families*. New York, NY: Routledge; 2022.

Gascon M, Triguero-Mas M, Martínez D, *et al.* Residential green spaces and mortality: a systematic review. *Environ Int*. 2016;86:60–67.

Haller RL, Kennedy KL, Capra CL, eds. *The Profession and Practice of Horticultural Therapy*. Boca Raton, FL: CRC Press; 2019.

Han JW, Choi H, Jeon YH, Yoon CH, Woo JM, Kim W. The effects of forest therapy on coping with chronic widespread pain: physiological and psychological differences between participants in a forest therapy program and a control group. *Int J Environ Res Public Health*. 2016;13(3):255.

Harper N, Rose K, Segal D. *Nature-Based Therapy: A Practitioner's Guide to Working Outdoors with Children, Youth, and Families*. Gabriola Island, BC, Canada: New Society Publishers; 2019.

Harper NJ, Dobud WW, eds. *Outdoor Therapies: An Introduction to Practices, Possibilities, and Critical Perspectives*. New York, NY: Routledge; 2021.

Hurtado-Soler A, Marín-Liébana P, Martínez-Gallego S, Botella-Nicolás AM. The garden and landscape as an interdisciplinary resource between experimental science and artistic-musical expression: analysis of competence development in student teachers. *Front Psychol*. 2020;11:2163.

Kolster A, Heikkinen M, Pajunen A, Mickos A, Wennman H, Partonen T. Targeted health promotion with guided nature walks or group exercise: a controlled trial in primary care. *Frontiers in Public Health*. 2023;11:1–12.

Kotte D, Li Q, Shin WS, Michalsen A, eds. *International Handbook of Forest Therapy*. Newcastle upon Tyne, United Kingdom: Cambridge Scholars Publishing; 2021.

Li H, Zhang X, Wang H, *et al*. Access to nature via virtual reality: a mini-review. *Front Psychol*. 2021;12:725288.

Marcus CC, Barnes M. *Healing Gardens: Therapeutic Benefits and Design Recommendations (Wiley Series in Healthcare and Senior Living Design)*. Hoboken, NJ: John Wiley & Sons; 1999.

Marcus CC, Sachs N. *Therapeutic Landscapes: An Evidenced Approach to Designing Healing Gardens and Restorative Outdoor Spaces*. Hoboken, NJ: John Wiley & Sons; 2014.

Menardo E, Di Marco D, Ramos S, *et al*. Nature and mindfulness to cope with work related stress: a narrative review. *Int J Environ Res Public Health*. 2022;19(10):5948.

Oh KH, Shin WS, Khil TG, Kim DJ. Six-step model of nature-based therapy process. *Int J Environ Res Public Health*. 2020;17(3):685.

Owens M, Bunce HLI. Nature-based meditation, rumination and mental wellbeing. *Int J Environ Res Public Health*. 2022;19(15):9118.

Rosenthal NE. Defeating SAD (Seasonal Affective Disorder): A Guide to Health and Happiness Through All Seasons. New York, NY: Gildan Media; 2023.

Selby S, Hayes C, O'Sullivan N, O'Neil A, Harmon D. Facilitators and barriers to green exercise in chronic pain. *Ir J Med Sci*. 2019;188(3):973–978.

Stanhope J, Breed MF, Weinstein P. Exposure to greenspaces could reduce the high global burden of pain. *Environ Res*. 2020;187:109641.

Sturm VE, Datta S, Roy ARK, *et al*. Big smile, small self: awe walks promote prosocial positive emotions in older adults. *Emotion*. 2022;22(5):1044–1058.

Timko Olson ER, Olson AA, Driscoll M, Vermeesch AL. Nature-based interventions and exposure among cancer survivors: a scoping review. *Int J Environ Res Public Health*. 2023;20(3):2376.

Verra ML, Angst F, Beck T, *et al*. Horticultural therapy for patients with chronic musculoskeletal pain: results of a pilot study [published correction appears in *Altern Ther Health Med*. 2012 Nov–Dec;18(6):79]. *Altern Ther Health Med*. 2012;18(2):44–50.

Vujcic M, Tomicevic-Dubljevic J, Grbic M, Lecic-Tosevski D, Vukovic O, Toskovic O. Nature based solution for improving mental health and well-being in urban areas. *Environ Res*. 2017;158:385–392.

Wagenfeld A, Marder S. *Nature-Based Allied Health Practice*. London, United Kingdom: Jessica Kingsley Publishers; 2023.

White MP, Alcock I, Grellier J, *et al*. Spending at least 120 minutes a week in nature is associated with good health and wellbeing. *Sci Rep*. 2019;9(1):7730.

Winterbottom D, Wagenfeld A. *Therapeutic Gardens: Design for Healing Spaces*. Portland, OR: Timber Press; 2015.

CHAPTER 11

Expressive Therapies and the Healing Arts

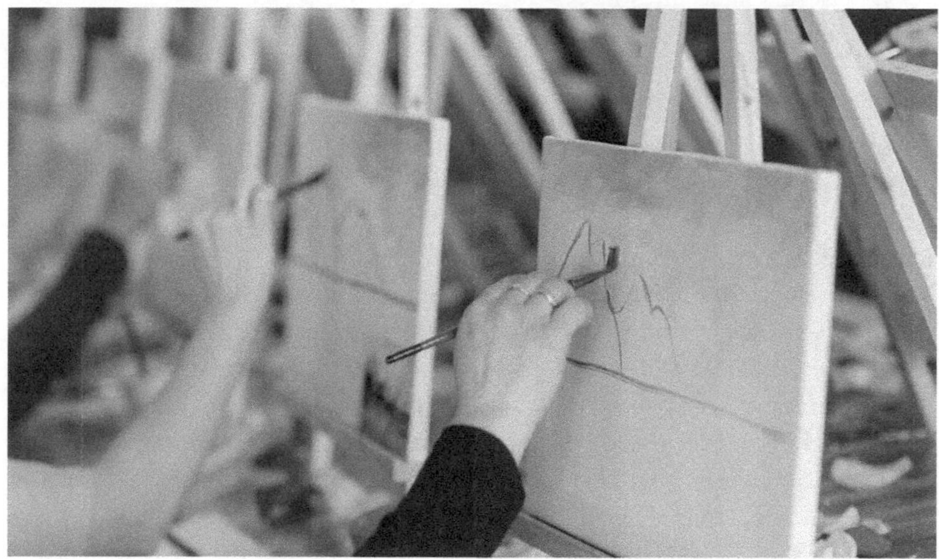

Artistic expression is a form of relaxation

Learning Objectives

- Understand the basic research for expressive therapies and art-based therapies.
- Recognize expressive therapies for practical pain management.

Chapter Highlights

- Key Concept: Benefits of Creative Arts Therapies
- Clinical Tip: Gratitude Journal
- Clinical Tip: Juggling and Neuroplasticity

- Featured Topic 11.1: Online Relaxation Resources for the Creative Arts
- Featured Topic 11.2: Creative Arts for Preventing Burnout Among Healthcare Providers
- Featured Topic 11.3: Case Vignette—Pottery for Hand Pain and Stress Reduction
- Self-Care Handout 11.1: Basic Lifestyle and Pain Tracker and Journal
- Self-Care Handout 11.2: Basic Data Analytics Tracker for Health Monitoring
- Self-Management Activities
- Classroom and Lab Activities
- Useful Clinical Resources
- References
- Additional Reading

Lifestyle Matters*: Criticize less; create more.*

Introduction

Aristotle, a Greek philosopher, said, "The aim of art is not to represent the outward appearance of things, but their inward significance." Practitioners from various healthcare and fitness professions would benefit from an understanding of the expressive and art-based therapy disciplines. Engaging in interprofessional collaborations with creative arts therapists may help provide potential adjuncts to conventional therapy and rehabilitation programs for managing pain, stress, anxiety, and depression.

The focus of this chapter is to provide an overview of the creative arts and expressive therapies. Creative arts therapists (CATs) work in art, music, dance, drama, and poetry therapies. The CAT may be used in addiction treatment programs, mental health centers, nursing homes, schools, hospitals, community art centers, museums, prisons, and homeless shelters (Reed *et al.* 2020). Also, art therapy (Campbell *et al.* 2016), dance therapy (Steinberg-Oren *et al.* 2016), drama therapy (Wasmuth and Pritchard 2016), expressive writing (Sayer *et al.* 2015), music therapy (Vaudreuil *et al.* 2020), and poetry therapy (Deshpande and Recon 2010) may be helpful for military service members.

The following figure outlines the various disciplines of creative arts and expressive therapies.

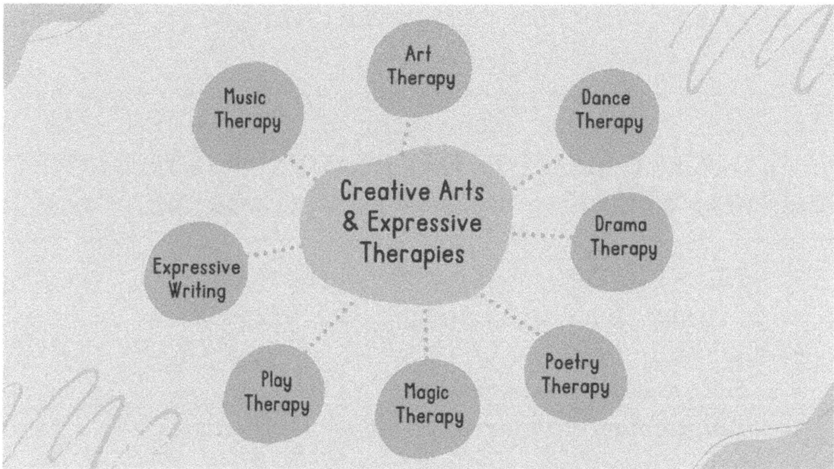

Creative arts and expressive therapies

The National Coalition of Creative Arts Therapies Associations (2023) defines CATs as:

> human service professionals who use distinct arts-based methods and creative processes for the purpose of ameliorating disability and illness and optimizing health and wellness. Treatment outcomes include, for example, improving communication and expression, and increasing physical, emotional, cognitive and/or social functioning.

A review in the *Physical Therapy* journal (Brown *et al.* 2022, p.1) indicates:

> Findings demonstrate that combining the arts with physical therapist practice amplifies not only psychomotor but affective and cognitive outcomes as well. The arts have applicability across broad populations (e.g., chronic pain, neurologic dysfunction, respiratory conditions). This study supports that physical therapist education and practice should embrace the arts as a collaborative modality to promote enhanced psychomotor, affective, and cognitive outcomes.

Studies show that creative arts and expressive therapies may, for example, be helpful for anxiety, depression, and sleep problems among individuals undergoing bone marrow transplantation (Sertbaş *et al.* 2023), children and adolescents exposed to traumatic events (Morison *et al.* 2022), depression in older adults (Dunphy *et al.* 2019), mindfulness-based arts interventions in older adults with mild cognitive impairment (Zhao *et al.* 2018), psychological distress in health care professionals (Moss *et al.* 2022), quality of life and wellness in individuals with cancer (Rieger *et al.* 2021), stress management (Gelatti *et al.* 2020; Martin *et al.* 2018), and stroke survivors (Lo *et al.* 2018).

KEY CONCEPT: BENEFITS OF CREATIVE ARTS THERAPIES

The following are some benefits of creative arts therapies (de Witte *et al.* 2021):

- Help individuals express feelings and emotions.
- Help individuals work through issues and problems.
- Build self-confidence.
- Improve social connections.
- Build emotional resilience.
- Help manage pain.
- Help manage stress and anxiety.

Introduction to Art Therapy

The American Art Therapy Association (2023) defines art therapy as "an integrative mental health and human services profession that enriches the lives of individuals, families, and communities through active art-making, creative process, applied psychological theory, and human experience within a psychotherapeutic relationship." Art therapy may include drawing, filmmaking, illustrating, painting, photography, and/or sculpting.

Art therapy may, for example, be helpful for chronic pain (Koebner *et al.* 2019), reduce the sense of loneliness and hopelessness in older adults (Aydın and Kutlu 2021), improve quality of life in people with dementia (Schall *et al.* 2018), improve cognitive function in the elderly with mild neurocognitive disorder (Mahendran *et al.* 2018), improve mood and quality of life in individuals with mild Alzheimer's disease (Pongan *et al.* 2017), improve depressive and anxiety symptoms in older women (Ciasca *et al.* 2018), improve self-esteem, hope, and social support of those living with multiple sclerosis (Fraser and Keating 2014), improve visual-cognitive skills and general motor function in individuals with Parkinson's (Cucca *et al.* 2021), and provide mood enhancement (Babouchkina and Robbins 2015).

In addition, a study in the *Pain Medicine* journal (Wiercioch-Kuzianik and Bąbel 2019, p.1955) concluded that "participants rated pain stimuli preceded by red as being more painful compared with pain stimuli preceded by other colors, especially green and blue." What is the potential practical application of this information? For example, could the color of a practitioner's work clothing, the colors in the clinic, or the color of educational handouts influence pain treatment outcomes?

The image below shows outdoor painting as a form of art therapy.

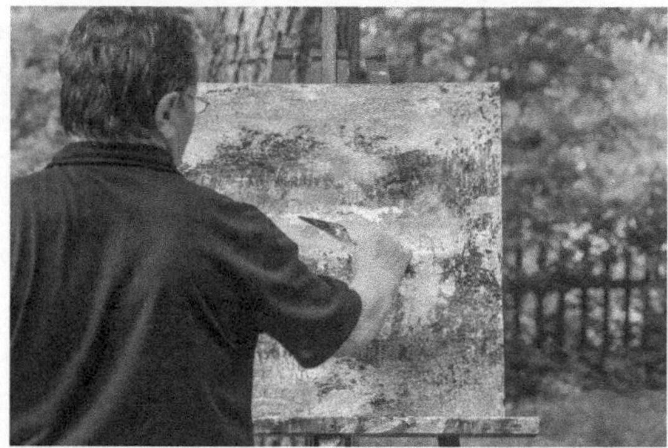

Painting in an outdoor environment for wellness

One practical application of art therapy is to use a coloring book for adults. The image below shows a sample.

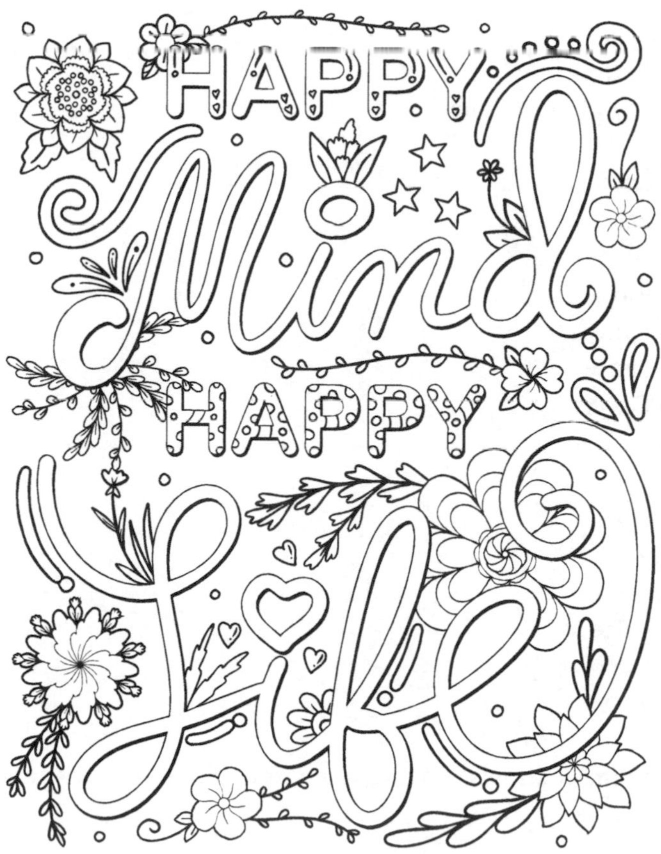

Coloring for relaxation

Introduction to Dance Therapy

The American Dance Therapy Association (2023) defines dance and movement therapy as "the psychotherapeutic use of movement to promote emotional, social, cognitive and physical integration of the individual." Dance therapy may include dance styles, therapeutic movements, mirroring techniques, jumping rhythms, and/or movement metaphors.

Dance therapy may, for example, be helpful for back pain (Castrillon *et al.* 2017), decreasing fall risk in healthy older adults (Mattle *et al.* 2020), fatigue and physical capacity in individuals with multiple sclerosis (Van Geel *et al.* 2020), improving resilience and pain intensity in individuals with chronic pain (Shim *et al.* 2017), improving motor parameters of Parkinson's (Dos Santos Delabary *et al.* 2018), managing stress in individuals with breast cancer undergoing radiotherapy (Ho *et al.* 2016), and rehabilitation of adults with neurologic conditions (Patterson *et al.* 2018).

The following is a list of various dance styles:

- Ballet
- Cha Cha
- Charleston
- Country western dance
- Disco
- Flamenco
- Folk dance
- Foxtrot
- Hip hop
- Irish dance
- Line dance
- Paso Doble
- Rumba
- Salsa
- Samba
- Swing
- Tango
- Tap dance
- Waltz
- Zumba

The following image shows dancing as a part of physical activity and wellness.

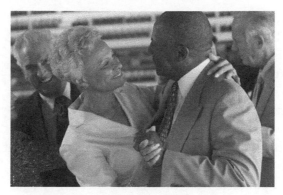

Dancing for wellness

Introduction to Music Therapy

The American Music Therapy Association (2023) defines music therapy as "the clinical and evidence-based use of music interventions to accomplish individualized goals within a therapeutic relationship by a credentialed professional who has completed an approved music therapy program." Music therapy may include listening to music, creating music, singing and vocal activities, and/or playing a musical instrument.

Music therapy may, for example, be helpful for back pain (Guétin *et al.* 2005), be used as an adjunct for chronic pain management (Garza-Villarreal *et al.* 2017; Low *et al.* 2020), enhance conventional cognitive rehabilitation in individuals with multiple sclerosis (Impellizzeri *et al.* 2020) and motor and cognitive problems, and quality of life in individuals with Parkinson's (Pereira *et al.* 2019), reduce anxiety in critically ill patients (Umbrello *et al.* 2019), reduce pain and anxiety during a colonoscopy (Çelebi *et al.* 2020), help reduce blood pressure during a primary care visit (Volkov and Volkova 2023), and relieve postoperative pain (Lin *et al.* 2020).

The following lists include various music that may be used in wellness and fitness settings. Of course, the ideal music is the one that the patient or client selects.

If a patient/client enjoys classical music, the following may be added to a playlist to help with relaxation, stress, and anxiety reduction.

- Johann Sebastian Bach
  - "Air on the G String"
  - "Brandenburg Concertos"
  - "Goldberg Variations"
  - "Suite for Solo Cello No. 1 in G major"
- Ludwig van Beethoven

  - "Bagatelle No. 25 in A minor (Für Elise)"
  - "Ode to Joy"
- Frédéric François Chopin
  - "Nocturne in E-flat major, Op. 9, No. 2"
  - "Waltz in A minor"
  - "Waltz in C-sharp minor, Op. 64, No. 2"
- Wolfgang Amadeus Mozart
  - "Piano Concerto No. 21 in C major, K. 467, II. Andante"
  - "Violin Concerto No. 3 in G major, K. 216, II. Adagio"
  - "Violin Concerto No. 5 in A major, K. 219, II. Adagio"
- Pyotr Ilyich Tchaikovsky
  - "Dance of the Sugar Plum Fairy"
  - "Piano Concerto No. 1 in B-flat minor, Op. 23"

The following music may also be added to a relaxation music playlist to help patients/clients with various needs (the songs listed are only examples).

- Music for happiness
  - "Dancing Queen"—Abba
  - "Good Vibrations"—The Beach Boys
  - "I'm Happy Just to Dance with You"—The Beatles
  - "Girls Just Wanna Have Fun"—Cyndi Lauper
  - "Sunshine, Lollipops, and Rainbows"—Lesley Gore
  - "What a Wonderful World"—Louis Armstrong
  - "It's a Good Day"—Peggy Lee
  - "Don't Stop Me Now"—Queen
- Music for excitement
  - "Beat It"—Michael Jackson
  - "Eye of the Tiger"—Survivor
- Music for slower exercise
  - "Twist and Shout"—The Beatles
  - "Return to Sender"—Elvis Presley
- Music for faster exercise
  - "The Twist"—Chubby Checker
  - "At the Hop"—Danny & the Juniors
  - "I Want You Back"—The Jackson 5
- Music for meditation
  - "Smile"—Charlie Chaplin
  - "Canon in D major"—Johann Pachelbel
  - "Meditation from Thais"—Jules Massenet
- Music for tai chi/qigong

- "Cloud Hands"—Silk Orchestra/Pat Clemence
- "Her Graceful Heart"—Silk Orchestra/Pat Clemence
- "White Crane" (slow form)—Silk Orchestra/Pat Clemence

The image below shows that music may be a social activity and include activities such as a drum circle or group singing.

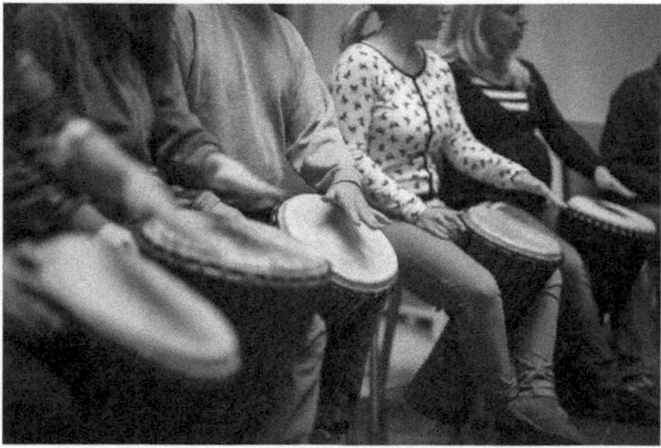

Music for socialization and wellness

Introduction to Drama Therapy and Psychodrama

The North American Drama Therapy Association (2023) defines drama therapy as:

> an active, experiential approach to facilitating change. Through storytelling, projective play, purposeful improvisation, and performance, participants are invited to rehearse desired behaviors, practice being in relationship, expand and find flexibility between life roles, and perform the change they wish to be and see in the world.

Drama therapy may include storytelling, role-playing, improvisational techniques, group games, and/or puppetry.

An article in the *PLos One* journal (Orkibi and Feniger-Schaal 2019, p.3) tries to draw some distinctions between psychodrama and drama therapy. The authors state that in psychodrama:

> clients typically use role-play to enact themselves, parts of themselves, or significant others in their real lives, and hence work more directly on reality-based issues. In contrast, drama therapy is more fantasy-based, and clients typically use role-play to enact fictional and symbolic roles, use storytelling, puppetry, masks, and miniature objects to work more indirectly and with greater dramatic distance from their issues.

Drama therapy may, for example, be helpful for social anxiety disorder (Abeditehrani *et al.* 2020), improving activities of daily living measures in individuals with Parkinson's (Bega *et al.* 2017), and establishing positive attitudes in overweight teenagers (Demir Acar and Bayat 2019).

The image below shows how drama may be a fun social activity for learning skills such as communication, confidence, teamwork, leadership, and empathy.

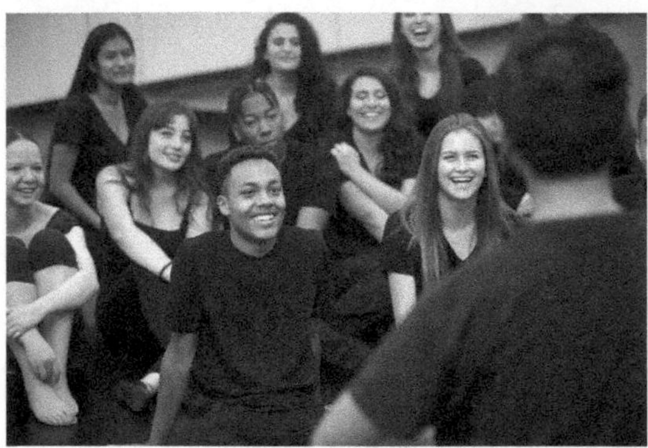

Drama class for social engagement, learning, and wellness

The images below show the mirror game, a fun activity used in drama therapy and classes for non-verbal movement patterns to promote coordination, cooperation, social connectedness, and relaxation, and also improve cognitive performance (Feniger-Schaal *et al.* 2018; Gueugnon *et al.* 2016; Keisari *et al.* 2022). In the mirror game one person is the leader and the other person follows their movements, facial expressions, and mannerisms. The mirror game exercise could be used, for example, in stroke rehabilitation or other neurologic conditions to improve coordination. It may also be used to mimic sports skills. Have patients/clients try it at home with friends and family or use it in the clinic/fitness setting.

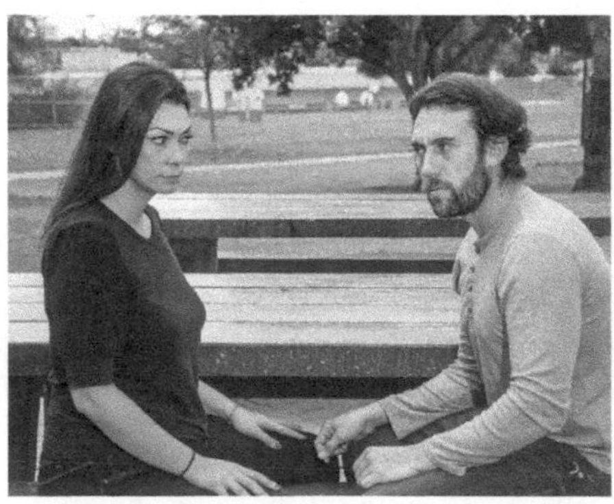

Mirror game—follow the leader in sitting

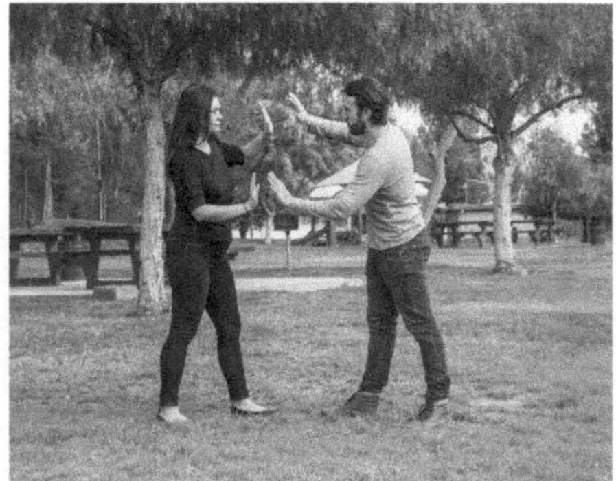

Mirror game—follow the leader in standing

Mirror game as a part of drama therapy

Introduction to Expressive Writing

In the *Journal of Affective Disorders* (Baikie *et al.* 2012, p.310), the authors define expressive writing as "writing about traumatic, stressful or emotional events—often leads to improvements in physical and psychological health in non-clinical and clinical populations." Expressive writing may include diaries, journals, memoirs, opinion pieces, songs, and/or poetry.

Expressive writing may, for example, be helpful for improving post-traumatic stress disorder (PTSD) symptoms (Gerger *et al.* 2021), improving lung function in individuals with asthma (Smith *et al.* 2015), improving wound healing in older adults (Koschwanez *et al.* 2013), reducing musculoskeletal pain (Pepe *et al.* 2014), and reducing stress in individuals undergoing chemotherapy for breast cancer (Wang *et al.* 2022).

The image below shows expressive writing being used as an effective part of psychological wellness.

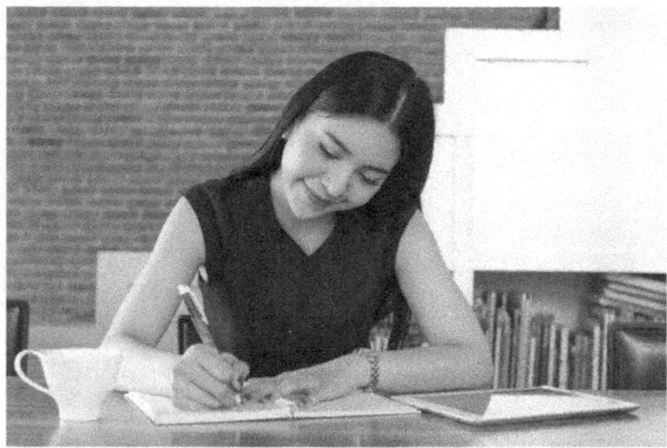

Expressive writing for wellness

A personal journal may help a person find the root cause of chronic pain and help manage symptoms. For example, individuals with pain may track their lifestyle through an app, small notebook or journal, wall calendar, electronic calendar, or personal blog.

The following figure outlines a sample journaling format to track various aspects of lifestyle and pain. See Self-Care Handout 11.1 for a blank version of this journal.

Date: October 31, 2024

Sleep: 9 pm–5 am = 8 hours (restful)

Exercise:

Morning: walk—20 minutes outdoors before work

Lunch: walk—10 minutes

Evening: yoga—15 minutes

Nutrition:

Breakfast: a bowl of oatmeal with blueberries, nuts, and honey. Oat milk and veggie/fruit smoothie.

Lunch: a vegetable and hummus sandwich, veggie salad, banana, water, and/or tea.

Dinner: salmon, veggie salad, fresh fruit salad, water, and/or tea.

Snacks: water throughout the day, nuts/seeds, fruit, veggies.

Stress: Moderate stress level day. Meditated 2 x 5 minutes during the day.

Back symptoms: Pain 1–6/10 (1 is best; 10 worst). Pain is best in the morning.

Sitting at work is worse. Moving around is best.

Diary: I am grateful I finished my project today. Tonight, I'm going to a concert with friends.

Sample lifestyle and pain tracker and journal format

CLINICAL TIP: GRATITUDE JOURNAL

Gratitude interventions may help build positive emotions, enhance life satisfaction, improve happiness, and reduce stress and anxiety. A gratitude list or journal could be kept, for example, in a paper journal/diary, app, or web-based platform. A person could also send themselves a weekly text or email with three things they are grateful for in their life and periodically reflect on the items during the week (Cunha *et al.* 2019; Redwine *et al.* 2016).

Introduction to Poetry Therapy

The National Association for Poetry Therapy (2023) defines poetry therapy as the:

> use of language, symbol, and story in therapeutic, education, growth, and community-building capacities. It relies upon the use of poems, stories, song lyrics, imagery, and metaphor to facilitate personal growth, healing, and greater self-awareness. Bibliotherapy, narrative, journal writing, metaphor, storytelling, and ritual are all within the realm of poetry therapy.

In a review article in *Anesthesiology Clinics* (Shafer 2022), the author indicates that physicians, healthcare workers, and patients can benefit from reading, writing, and reflecting on poetry.

Poetry therapy may, for example, be helpful for oncologic pain relief (Arruda *et al.* 2016), improving complex linguistic abilities (Zimmermann *et al.* 2014), improving communication confidence in individuals with multiple sclerosis (Balchin *et al.* 2020), reducing stress in nursing students (Park *et al.* 2022), and reducing fear, sadness, anger, worry, and fatigue in pediatric patients (Delamerced *et al.* 2021).

Poetry may be used in a wellness program to connect individuals to nature and also to the past, present, and future.

The following are two sample inspirational poems.

THINKING

By Walter D. Wintle

If you think you are beaten, you are;
If you think you dare not, you don't.
If you'd like to win, but you think you can't,
It is almost a certain – you won't.

If you think you'll lose, you've lost;
For out in this world we find
Success begins with a fellow's will
It's all in the state of mind.

If you think you're outclassed, you are;
You've got to think high to rise.
You've got to be sure of yourself before
You can ever win the prize.

Life's battles don't always go
To the stronger or faster man;
But sooner or later the man who wins
Is the one who thinks he can!

LIFE

By Henry van Dyke

Let me but live my life from year to year,
With forward face and unreluctant soul;
Not hurrying to, nor turning from the goal;
Not mourning for the things that disappear
In the dim past, nor holding back in fear

From what the future veils; but with a whole
And happy heart, that pays its toll
To Youth and Age, and travels on with cheer.

So let the way wind up the hill or down,
O'er rough or smooth, the journey will be joy:
Still seeking what I sought when but a boy,
New friendship, high adventure, and a crown,
My heart will keep the courage of the quest,
And hope the road's last turn will be the best.

Introduction to Play Therapy

The Association for Play Therapy (2023) defines play therapy as "the systematic use of a theoretical model to establish an interpersonal process wherein trained play therapists use the therapeutic powers of play to help clients prevent or resolve psychosocial difficulties and achieve optimal growth and development." Play therapy may include storytelling, puppets, music, dance, drama, painting, and/or games.

Play therapy may, for example, help decrease body fat among children 8–12 years old (Sánchez-López *et al.* 2020), improve social, emotional, and behavioral skills in preschool children (Sezici *et al.* 2017), improve psychological well-being in older adults (Tse *et al.* 2016), and provide pain relief in children (Mohan *et al.* 2015).

The following image shows how play may enhance social connections as part of a wellness program.

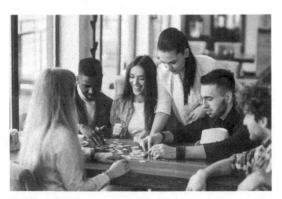

Play for enhancing social connections

The following figure shows a sample fun labyrinth puzzle for relaxation and play. See if you can trace your way out of the puzzle!

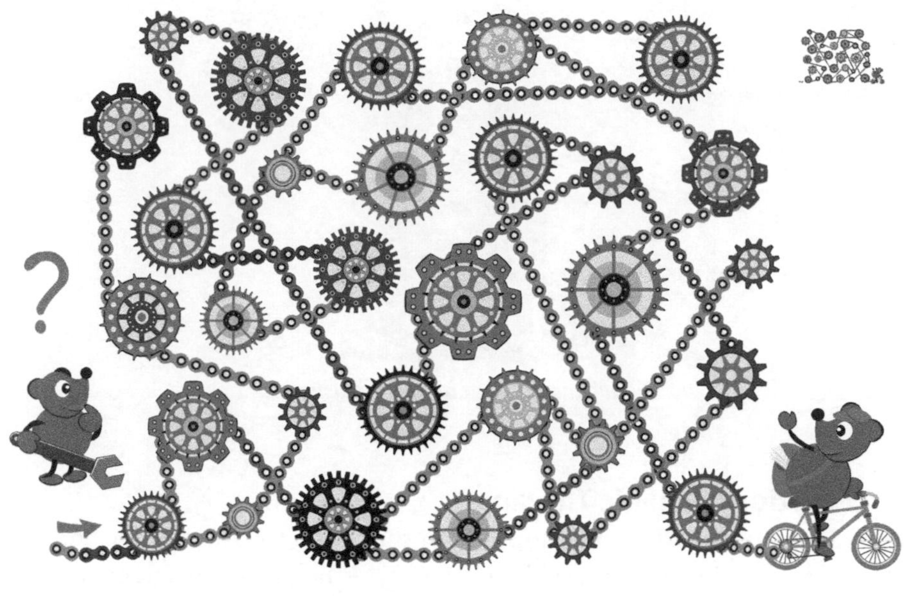
?
Logic puzzle game with labyrinth
Find the way between the gears to turn the bike wheel.

Find your way out of the fun labyrinth puzzle for relaxation

The Sandplay Therapists of America® (2023) defines sandplay therapy as "'hand-on' psychological work, and is an adjunct to talk therapy. It is a powerful therapeutic method that facilitates the psyche's natural capacity for healing." *Psychology Today* (2023) goes on to say, "Sandplay therapy is a nonverbal, therapeutic intervention that makes use of a sandbox, toy figures, and sometimes water, to create scenes of miniature worlds that reflect a person's inner thoughts, struggles, and concerns."

Sandplay therapy is a form of play therapy developed by Dora Kalff (1904–1990), a Swiss analytical psychologist (Tan *et al.* 2021). It is a method based on the foundations of Jungian psychology (Ammann 2022). Sandplay therapy can, for example, reduce anxiety and behavioral problems in school-age children with chronic diseases (Tan *et al.* 2021), slow development of anxiety and depression in children with childhood-onset systemic lupus erythematosus (Li *et al.* 2022), and improve sleep quality and social interactions of preschool children with autism spectrum disorder (Liu *et al.* 2023). In addition, sandplay therapy may be used with adults (Doyle and Magor-Blatch 2017).

CLINICAL TIP: JUGGLING AND NEUROPLASTICITY

Juggling is one form of sensorimotor task that may be used to improve neuroplasticity (Malik *et al.* 2022). Give it a try!

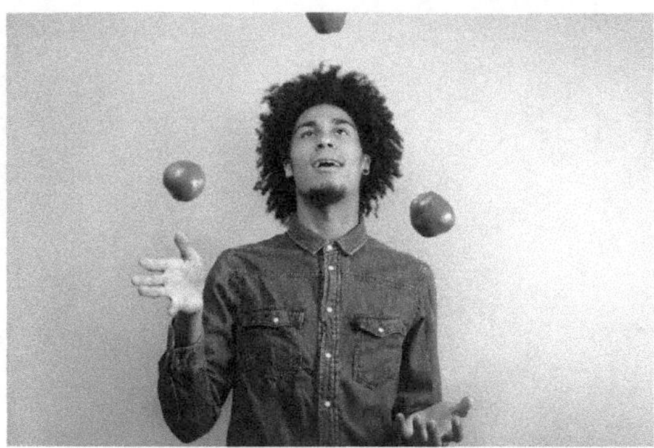

Juggling for fun and neuroplasticity

Introduction to Magic Therapy

Kevin Spencer, Ph.D. (Spencer 2023), an authority on the therapeutic and educational application of magic tricks, indicates, "A therapeutic magic camp is one that incorporates the learning and performing of carefully selected magic tricks using an organized, theme-based approach" (Spencer *et al.* 2021, p.16).

Magic therapy may, for example, help enhance social skills, improve fine and gross movements, and raise self-esteem (Wiseman *et al.* 2021), enhance self-esteem in children with attention-deficit/hyperactivity disorder (Yuen *et al.* 2021), and improve a hand therapy program (Harte and Spencer 2014).

Card tricks in magic therapy may be used to improve hand coordination and as a fun therapeutic tool.

Introduction to Graphic Medicine

Graphic Medicine is "a field at the intersection of comics and health care..." (Maatman *et al.* 2022, p.113).

The National Library of Medicine (2023) indicates that Graphic Medicine is "the use of comics to tell personal stories of illness and health" and has an exhibition along with educational resources. The *Graphic Medicine Review* (2023) website publishes works relevant to the medium of comics (such as comic books, graphic novels, and manga) and healthcare, medicine, and wellness. The *European Journal of Clinical Investigation* (Alemany-Pagès *et al.* 2022) indicates that comics may be a way to communicate information about disease awareness to the general public.

The Graphic Medicine website (Graphic Medicine 2023) is a collection of content relating to comics in medicine.

The following images show cartoon strips from the author of this text that may be used therapeutically to educate children about lifestyle medicine and wellness.

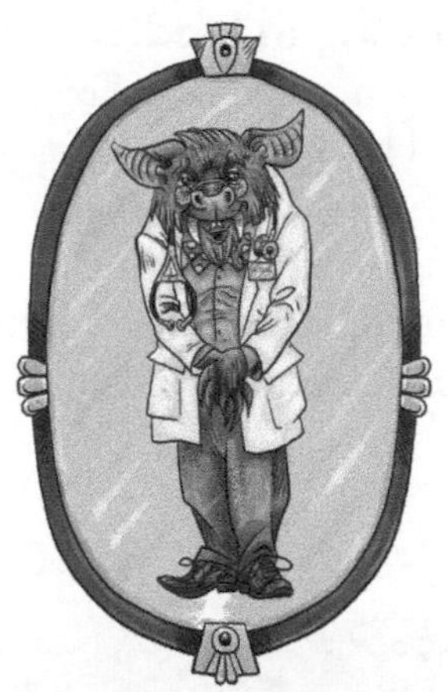

Dr. Fang encourages kids to eat nutritious foods

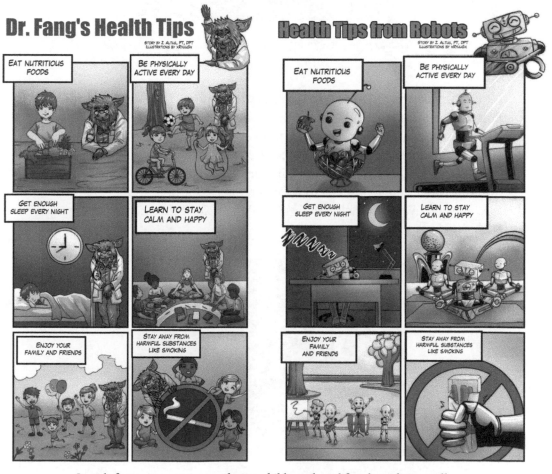

Sample fun cartoon strips to educate children about lifestyle medicine wellness

Introduction to Storytelling in Medicine and Therapy

Fiction books can help parents, teachers, and librarians introduce kids to fitness, wellness, good nutrition, and healthful habits for life. Various research studies open the door for authors to write unique fictional stories that blend entertainment and education. For example, storytelling may help address health behaviors (Bravender *et al.* 2010), promote development and well-being (Pulimeno *et al.* 2020), and reduce anxiety in children (Brondani and Pedro 2019).

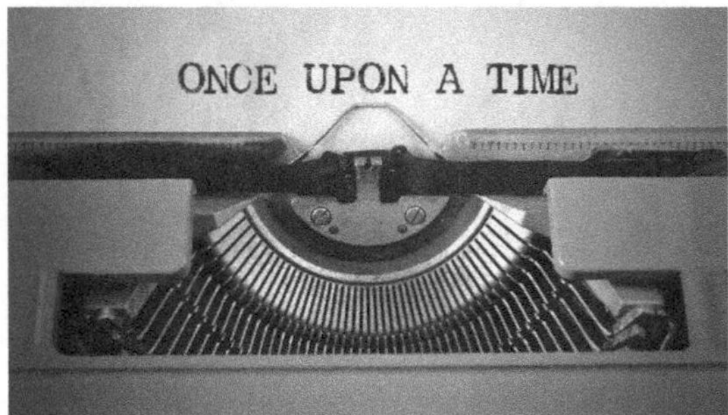

Fiction books play a role in introducing children to wellness concepts

Introduction to Filmmaking in Medicine and Therapy

Filmmaking may be used as a therapeutic approach to help patients/clients tell their individual stories about trauma, recovery, and healing. The Patton Veterans Project (2023) helps veterans reduce social isolation and cope with posttraumatic stress through therapeutic filmmaking or video-based therapy. For information on using filmmaking as a tool for veterans, see the studies in *Frontiers in Psychology* (Tuval-Mashiach *et al.* 2018) and *Psychological Services* (Drebing *et al.* 2022).

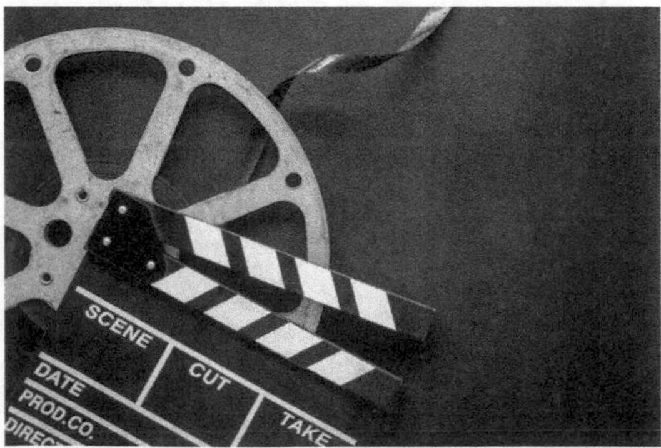

Filmmaking plays a role in video-based therapy and rehabilitation

Featured Topics

Featured Topic 11.1 lists online relaxation resources that use the creative arts. Consider trying each resource to see how it may be used to help patients/clients overcome anxiety or manage stress or pain.

Featured Topic 11.2 looks at how various creative arts may help prevent burnout among healthcare providers.

Featured Topic 11.3 outlines a case vignette of a surgeon who uses pottery to manage her hand pain and stress.

■ Featured Topic 11.1: Online Relaxation Resources Using the Creative Arts

Music	Art
• NYU Music Experience Design, https://musedlab.org • Dot Piano, https://dotpiano.com • Plink, https://plink.in • Online Pianist, www.onlinepianist.com/virtual-piano • BandLab, www.bandlab.com • GarageBand, www.apple.com/ios/garageband • Soundtrap, www.soundtrap.com	• Lake, www.lakecoloring.com • Color Therapy, www.colortherapy.app • Pigment—Adult Coloring Book, https://apps.apple.com/us/app/pigment-coloring-book-for/id1062006344 • Sketchbook, www.sketchbook.com • Astropad, https://astropad.com • Draw for Free, www.davidporterapps.com • Tayasui Sketches, www.tayasui.com • Quick, Draw!, https://quickdraw.withgoogle.com
Poetry	**Dance**
• Poetry Creator, http://tiny-mobile.com/poetry-creator-verses • Poetry Foundation, www.poetryfoundation.org	• STEEZY—Learn How to Dance, www.steezy.co • Pocket Salsa, www.addicted2salsa.com/pocketsalsa • Koros, https://gokoros.com • CLI Studios, www.clistudios.com • Learn To Dance, www.learntodance.com • Arthur Murray International, https://arthurmurray.com
Pottery	**Games**
• Let's Create! Pottery, https://apps.apple.com/us/app/lets-create-pottery-2/id1476378632 • Pottery.ly, https://apps.apple.com/us/app/pottery-ly-3d-ceramic-maker/id1449834010 • Sculpd, https://sculpd.com	• Pac-Man, https://freepacman.org • Pong Game, www.ponggame.org • Space Invaders, www.crazygames.com • Tetris, https://tetris.com

■ Featured Topic 11.2: Creative Arts for Preventing Burnout Among Healthcare Providers

Art-based therapies such as art, music, dance, drama, and poetry therapy may serve as a strategy to help reduce burnout and build resilience among healthcare professionals (Moss *et al.* 2022; Reed *et al.* 2020). For example, healthcare providers might engage in various weekday or weekend hobbies to learn how to paint, make pottery, play a musical instrument, write stories or poetry, or take a dance or acting class, to help manage psychological stress, build community, increase socialization, and improve happiness.

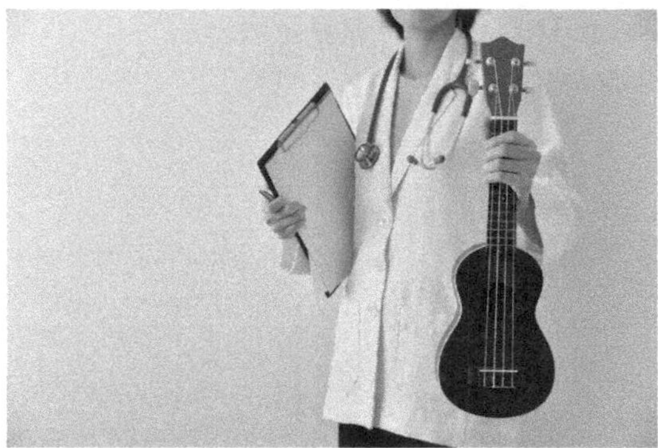

Try art-related hobbies to help reduce burnout

■ Featured Topic 11.3: Case Vignette—Pottery for Hand Pain and Stress Reduction

Katherine, a 45-year-old orthopedic surgeon at a large hospital, notices that she is experiencing more hand stiffness and pain after she performs surgery. Also, the surgeon is looking for activities to help manage her stress levels due to her heavy caseload. A colleague recommends she see an occupational therapist (OT) specializing in hand therapy. After four weeks of hand therapy with the OT, the surgeon has significant pain relief. As a home program, the OT recommends the surgeon try some pottery classes for stress management and as a gentle form of exercise to keep her hands mobile and pain-free. Katherine enrolls in a local pottery class and finds that she really enjoys the activities, and it helps prevent hand pain. She enjoys the eight-week pottery program at the studio so much that she decides to purchase a home pottery wheel and other appropriate equipment. First, Katherine redesigns the shed in her backyard so it serves as her home hobby studio. She ensures the new shed includes plenty of large windows for bright light and sunshine. The surgeon also plants a vegetable and flower garden around her shed and bird feeders to attract songbirds. Katherine finds that after finishing her work, this is her happy place for pottery, reading, and listening to music. The only problem Katherine now faces is that almost every surgeon at her hospital wants her to help them design a hobby shed for their home!

Self-Care Education Guides

See **Self-Care Handout 11.1: Basic Lifestyle and Pain Tracker and Journal** for a simple way for patients/clients to document their symptoms and track their health.

Data analytic trackers via paper journals, desktop trackers, spreadsheets, or apps may be incorporated into clinical practice to track and analyze data, help improve motivation, enhance self-care, and improve outcomes. Trackers may be used by patients/clients to determine if there is a lifestyle correlation to their condition and how it may be modified. The style of the tracker is based on the individual's preference.

See **Self-Care Handout 11.2: Basic Data Analytics Tracker for Health Monitoring** for a simple way for patients/clients to track daily variables to help understand and manage weekly fluctuations in pain and/or symptoms. Practitioners may add or subtract variables based on the needs of their patients/clients.

Self-Care Handout 11.1: Basic Lifestyle and Pain Tracker and Journal

Date: ....

Sleep: ....

Exercise:

Morning: ....

Lunch: ....

Evening: ....

Nutrition:

Breakfast: ....

....

Lunch: ....

....

Dinner: ....

....

Snacks: ....

Stress: ....

Symptoms: ....

Diary: ....

....

Self-Care Handout 11.2: Basic Data Analytics Tracker for Health Monitoring

Variables	Scale	Daily Patient Record						
		Monday	Tuesday	Wednesday	Thursday	Friday	Saturday	Sunday
Pain level	0 to 10[1]							
Sleep scale	0 to 10[2]							
Stress scale	0 to 10[3]							
Exercise soreness scale	0 to 10[4]							
Exercise	minutes per day or number of steps per day							
Heart rate	bpm							
Blood pressure	mm Hg							
Fruit/vegetable servings	number per day							
Blood sugar	mg/dL							
Body weight	lb or kg							
Risky substances (smoking, alcohol, caffeine)	yes/no							
Socialization	yes/no							
Work	hours							
Day off/vacation	yes/no							
Constipation	yes/no							

[1] Pain level: 0 means no pain, 5 is moderate pain, 10 is the worst imaginable pain.

[2] Sleep scale: 0 means no difficulty with sleep, 5 is moderate difficulty, 10 is marked difficulty.

[3] Stress scale: 0 means no mental stress, 5 is moderate stress, 10 is severe stress.

[4] Exercise soreness scale: 0 means no soreness, 5 is moderate soreness, 10 is severe soreness.

Self-Management Activities: Explore Dancing, Poetry, and Sketching

The following online resources can help patients/clients, healthcare providers, and health/fitness professionals to manage stress and anxiety by exploring dance, poetry, and sketching.

Explore Dancing

- The CLI Studios site provides fun, on-demand dance classes: www.clistudios.com
- The Learn To Dance site provides a fun way to learn dance moves: www.learntodance.com
- The Pocket Salsa app provides salsa dance lessons: www.addicted2salsa.com/pocketsalsa

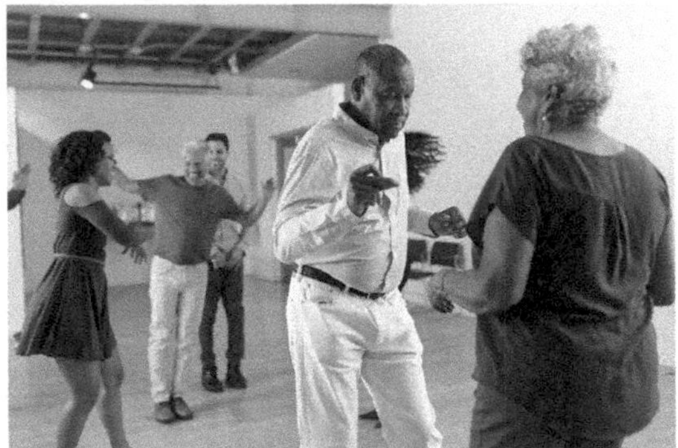

Take a community dance class

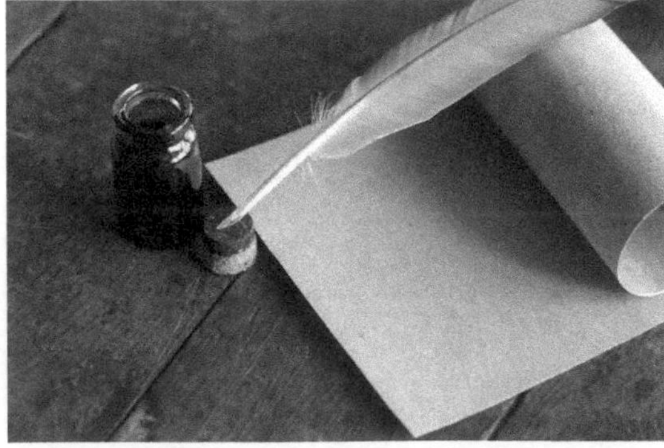

Get creative for overall well-being

Explore Poetry

- The Poetry Foundation site provides a platform to find, read, and enjoy poetry. For example, search for famous poets such as William Shakespeare, Robert Frost, or Maya Angelou: www.poetryfoundation.org

Explore Sketching

- Get a piece of blank paper and test your artistic skills by sketching the following image.

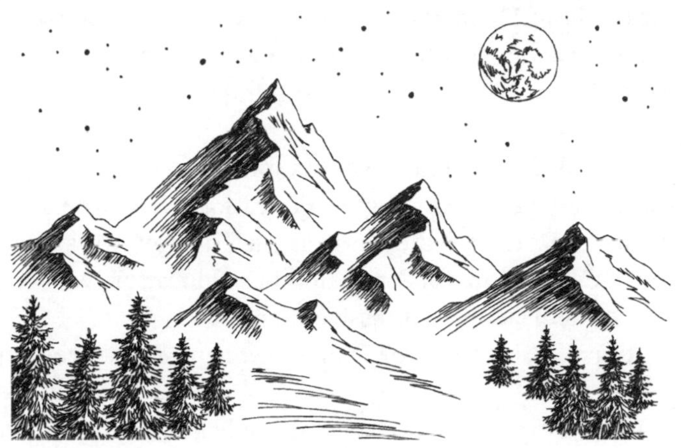

Mountain landscape sketching for adults

- Sketching apps:
  - The Sketchbook app provides a platform to create sketches, drawings, and cartoons: www.sketchbook.com
  - The Astropad app provides a platform to create sketches and drawings: https://astropad.com
  - The David Porter apps provide a platform to doodle and engage in an interactive coloring experience: www.davidporterapps.com
  - The Tayasui Sketches app provides a platform to draw, sketch, doodle, and try calligraphy: www.tayasui.com

Classroom and Lab Activities

- Try singing as a group or listening to various styles of soothing music. Which one is the most relaxing?
- Try a drum circle. What are the benefits?

- What is the difference between singing, listening to music, and playing a musical instrument? How might these variations help a person with pain?
- What are the best sounds of nature for relaxation? For example, consider the sounds of birds, water, wind, and leaves rustling.

Useful Clinical Resources

Organizations

- American Art Therapy Association, https://arttherapy.org
- American Dance Therapy Association, www.adta.org
- American Music Therapy Association, www.musictherapy.org
- American Psychological Association, www.apa.org
- American Society of Group Psychotherapy and Psychodrama, https://asgpp.org
- Association for Play Therapy, www.a4pt.org
- Association for Theatre in Higher Education, www.athe.org
- European Association Dance Movement Therapy, https://eadmt.com
- European Consortium for Arts Therapies Education, www.ecarte.info
- Expressive Media, www.expressivemedia.org
- International Association for Dance Medicine & Science, https://iadms.org
- International Association for Music & Medicine, https://iammonline.com
- International Expressive Arts Therapy Association, www.ieata.org
- International Federation for Biblio/Poetry Therapy, https://ifbpt.org
- International Society for Sandplay Therapy, www.isst-society.com
- Magic Therapy, https://magictherapy.com
- Music Mends Minds, www.musicmendsminds.org
- National Association for Poetry Therapy, https://poetrytherapy.org
- National Center for Complementary and Integrative Health, www.nccih.nih.gov (search for music and health)
- National Coalition of Creative Arts Therapies Associations, Inc, www.nccata.org
- North American Drama Therapy Association, www.nadta.org
- Patton Veterans Project, https://pattonveteransproject.org
- Performing Arts Medicine Association, www.artsmed.org
- Poetry Foundation, www.poetryfoundation.org
- Project Magic, https://projectmagic.org
- Sandplay Therapists of America, www.sandplay.org
- Theater Veder, www.theaterveder.nl/nl/english
- UCLA Arts and Healing, https://uclartsandhealing.org

Journals and Trackers

- Habit Nest (The Morning Sidekick Journal), www.habitnest.com
- Intelligent Change, Inc. (The Five-Minute Journal), www.intelligentchange.com
- Moleskine, www.moleskine.com

Online Trackers

- Curable, www.curablehealth.com
- Fitbit, www.fitbit.com
- Kaia Health, https://kaiahealth.com
- PainScale—Pain Diary, www.painscale.com
- SuperBetter, www.superbetter.com

Outcome Measure

- *Self-expression and Emotion Regulation in Art Therapy Scale*
  Haeyen S, van Hooren S, van der Veld WM, Hutschemaekers G. Measuring the contribution of art therapy in multidisciplinary treatment of personality disorders: the construction of the Self-expression and Emotion Regulation in Art Therapy Scale (SERATS). *Personal Ment Health*. 2018;12(1):3–14.

References

Abeditehrani H, Dijk C, Sahragard Toghchi M, Arntz A. Integrating cognitive behavioral group therapy and psychodrama for social anxiety disorder: an intervention description and an uncontrolled pilot trial. *Clin Psychol Eur*. 2020;2(1):e2693.

Alemany-Pagès M, Azul AM, Ramalho-Santos J. The use of comics to promote health awareness: a template using nonalcoholic fatty liver disease. *Eur J Clin Invest*. 2022;52(3):e13642.

American Art Therapy Association. 2023. https://arttherapy.org

American Dance Therapy Association. 2023. www.adta.org

American Music Therapy Association. 2023. www.musictherapy.org

Ammann R. Sandplay: traces in the sand—traces in the brain. *J Anal Psychol*. 2022;67(4):962–978.

Arruda MA, Garcia MA, Garcia JB. Evaluation of the effects of music and poetry in oncologic pain relief: a randomized clinical trial. *J Palliat Med*. 2016;19(9):943–948.

Association for Play Therapy. 2023. www.a4pt.org

Aydın M, Kutlu FY. The effect of group art therapy on loneliness and hopelessness levels of older adults living alone: a randomized controlled study. *Florence Nightingale J Nurs*. 2021;29(3):271–284.

Babouchkina A, Robbins SJ. Reducing negative mood through mandala creation: a randomized controlled trial. *Art Ther*. 2015;32:34–39.

Baikie KA, Geerligs L, Wilhelm K. Expressive writing and positive writing for participants with mood disorders: an online randomized controlled trial. *Journal of Affective Disorders*. 2012;136(3):310–319.

Balchin R, Hersh D, Grantis J, Godfrey M. "Ode to confidence": poetry groups for dysarthria in multiple sclerosis. *International Journal of Speech Language Pathology*. 2020;22(3):347–358.

Bega D, Palmentera P, Wagner A, *et al.* Laughter is the best medicine: the Second City® improvisation as an intervention for Parkinson's disease. *Parkinsonism and Related Disorders.* 2017;34:62–65.

Bravender T, Russell A, Chung RJ, Armstrong SC. A "novel" intervention: a pilot study of children's literature and healthy lifestyles. *Pediatrics.* 2010;125(3):e513–e517.

Brondani JP, Pedro ENR. The use of children's stories in nursing care for the child: an integrative review. *Rev Bras Enferm.* 2019;72(Suppl 3):333–342.

Brown EL, Gannotti ME, Veneri DA. Including arts in rehabilitation enhances outcomes in the psychomotor, cognitive, and affective domains: a scoping review. *Phys Ther.* 2022;102(4):pzac003.

Campbell M, Decker KP, Kruk K, Deaver SP. Art therapy and cognitive processing therapy for combat-related PTSD: a randomized controlled trial. *Art Ther (Alex).* 2016;33(4):169–177.

Castrillon T, Hanney WJ, Rothschild CE, Kolber MJ, Liu X, Masaracchio M. The effects of a standardized belly dance program on perceived pain, disability, and function in women with chronic low back pain. *J Back Musculoskelet Rehabil.* 2017;30(3):477–496.

Çelebi D, Yılmaz E, Şahin ST, Baydur H. The effect of music therapy during colonoscopy on pain, anxiety and patient comfort: a randomized controlled trial. *Complementary Therapies in Clinical Practice.* 2020;38:101084.

Ciasca EC, Ferreira RC, Santana CLA, *et al.* Art therapy as an adjuvant treatment for depression in elderly women: a randomized controlled trial. *Braz J Psychiatry.* 2018;40(3):256–263.

Cucca A, Di Rocco A, Acosta I, *et al.* Art therapy for Parkinson's disease. *Parkinsonism Relat Disord.* 2021;84:148–154.

Cunha LF, Pellanda LC, Reppold CT. Positive psychology and gratitude interventions: a randomized clinical trial. *Front Psychol.* 2019;10:584.

de Witte M, Orkibi H, Zarate R, *et al.* From therapeutic factors to mechanisms of change in the creative arts therapies: a scoping review. *Front Psychol.* 2021;12:678397.

Delamerced A, Panicker C, Monteiro K, Chung EY. Effects of a poetry intervention on emotional wellbeing in hospitalized pediatric patients. *Hosp Pediatr.* 2021;11(3):263–269.

Demir Acar M, Bayat M. The effect of diet-exercise trainings provided to overweight and obese teenagers through creative drama on their knowledge, attitude, and behaviors. *Childhood Obesity.* 2019;15(2):93–104.

Deshpande A. Recon mission: familiarizing veterans with their changed emotional landscape through poetry therapy. *Journal of Poetry Therapy.* 2010;23(4):239–251.

Dos Santos Delabary M, Komeroski IG, Monteiro EP, Costa RR, Haas AN. Effects of dance practice on functional mobility, motor symptoms and quality of life in people with Parkinson's disease: a systematic review with meta-analysis. *Aging Clinical and Experimental Research.* 2018;30(7):727–735.

Doyle K, Magor-Blatch LE. "Even adults need to play": sandplay therapy with an adult survivor of childhood abuse. *International Journal of Play Therapy.* 2017;26(1):12–22.

Drebing CE, Mamon D, Calixte RM, *et al.* Pilot outcomes of a filmmaking intervention designed to enhance treatment entry and social reintegration of veterans [published online ahead of print, 2022 Feb 21]. *Psychol Serv.* 2022;10.1037/ser0000618.

Dunphy K, Baker FA, Dumaresq E, *et al.* Creative arts interventions to address depression in older adults: a systematic review of outcomes, processes, and mechanisms. *Front Psychol.* 2019;9:2655.

Feniger-Schaal R, Hart Y, Lotan N, Koren-Karie N, Noy L. The body speaks: using the mirror game to link attachment and non-verbal behavior. *Front Psychol.* 2018;9:1560.

Fraser C, Keating M. The effect of a creative art program on self-esteem, hope, perceived social support, and self-efficacy in individuals with multiple sclerosis: a pilot study. *J Neurosci Nurs.* 2014;46(6):330–336.

Garza-Villarreal EA, Pando V, Vuust P, Parsons C. Music-induced analgesia in chronic pain conditions: a systematic review and meta-analysis. *Pain Physician.* 2017;20(7):597–610.

Gelatti F, Viganò C, Borsani S, Conistabile L, Bonetti L. Efficacy of live versus recorded harp music in reducing preoperative stress and fear related to minor surgery: a pilot study. *Altern Ther Health Med.* 2020;26(3):10–15.

Gerger H, Werner CP, Gaab J, Cuijpers P. Comparative efficacy and acceptability of expressive writing treatments compared with psychotherapy, other writing treatments, and waiting list control for adult trauma survivors: a systematic review and network meta-analysis [published online ahead of print, 2021 Feb 26]. *Psychol Med.* 2021;1–13.

Graphic Medicine. 2023. www.graphicmedicine.org

Graphic Medicine Review. 2023. https://graphicmedicinereview.com

Guétin S, Coudeyre E, Picot MC, *et al.* Intérêt de la musicothérapie dans la prise en charge de la lombalgie chronique en milieu hospitalier (Etude contrôlée, randomisée sur 65 patients) [Effect of music therapy among hospitalized patients with chronic low back pain: a controlled, randomized trial]. *Ann Readapt Med Phys*. 2005;48(5):217–224.

Gueugnon M, Salesse RN, Coste A, Zhao Z, Bardy BG, Marin L. The acquisition of socio-motor improvisation in the mirror game. *Hum Mov Sci*. 2016;46:117–128.

Harte D, Spencer K. Sleight of hand: magic, therapy and motor performance. *J Hand Ther*. 2014;27(1):67–69.

Ho RT, Fong TC, Cheung IK, Yip PS, Luk MY. Effects of a short-term dance movement therapy program on symptoms and stress in patients with breast cancer undergoing radiotherapy: a randomized, controlled, single-blind trial. *Journal of Pain and Symptom Management*. 2016;51(5):824–831.

Impellizzeri F, Leonardi S, Latella D, *et al.* An integrative cognitive rehabilitation using neurologic music therapy in multiple sclerosis: a pilot study. *Medicine (Baltimore)*. 2020;99(4):e18866.

Keisari S, Feniger-Schaal R, Palgi Y, Golland Y, Gesser-Edelsburg A, Ben-David B. Synchrony in old age: playing the mirror game improves cognitive performance. *Clin Gerontol*. 2022;45(2):312–326.

Koebner IJ, Fishman SM, Paterniti D, *et al.* The art of analgesia: a pilot study of art museum tours to decrease pain and social disconnection among individuals with chronic pain. *Pain Med*. 2019;20(4):681–691.

Koschwanez HE, Kerse N, Darragh M, Jarrett P, Booth RJ, Broadbent E. Expressive writing and wound healing in older adults: a randomized controlled trial. *Psychosom Med*. 2013;75(6):581–590.

Li J, Shi Y, Zhou W. Sandplay therapy could be a method to decrease disease activity and psychological stress in children with systemic lupus erythematosus. *Lupus*. 2022;31(2):212–220.

Lin CL, Hwang SL, Jiang P, Hsiung NH. Effect of music therapy on pain after orthopedic surgery: a systematic review and meta-analysis. *Pain Pract*. 2020;20(4):422–436.

Liu G, Chen Y, Ou P, *et al.* Effects of Parent-Child Sandplay Therapy for preschool children with autism spectrum disorder and their mothers: a randomized controlled trial [published online ahead of print, 2023 Mar 20]. *J Pediatr Nurs*. 2023;71:6–13.

Lo TLT, Lee JLC, Ho RTH. Creative arts-based therapies for stroke survivors: a qualitative systematic review [published correction appears in *Front Psychol*. 2019 Jul 2;10:1538]. *Front Psychol*. 2018;9:1646.

Low MY, Lacson C, Zhang F, Kesslick A, Bradt J. Vocal music therapy for chronic pain: a mixed methods feasibility study. *J Altern Complement Med*. 2020;26(2):113–122.

Maatman T, Green MJ, Noe MN. Graphic medicine in graduate medical education. *J Grad Med Educ*. 2022;14(1):113–114.

Mahendran R, Gandhi M, Moorakonda RB, *et al.* Art therapy is associated with sustained improvement in cognitive function in the elderly with mild neurocognitive disorder: findings from a pilot randomized controlled trial for art therapy and music reminiscence activity versus usual care. *Trials*. 2018;19(1):615.

Malik J, Stemplewski R, Maciaszek J. The effect of juggling as dual-task activity on human neuroplasticity: a systematic review. *Int J Environ Res Public Health*. 2022;19(12):7102.

Martin L, Oepen R, Bauer K, *et al.* Creative arts interventions for stress management and prevention: a systematic review. *Behav Sci (Basel)*. 2018;8(2):28.

Mattle M, Chocano-Bedoya PO, Fischbacher M, *et al.* Association of dance-based mind-motor activities with falls and physical function among healthy older adults: a systematic review and meta-analysis [published correction appears in *JAMA Netw Open*. 2021 Jan 4;4(1):e2037105]. *JAMA Netw Open*. 2020;3(9):e2017688.

Mohan S, Nayak R, Thomas RJ, Ravindran V. The effect of Entonox, play therapy and a combination on pain relief in children: a randomized controlled trial. *Pain Management Nursing*. 2015;16(6):938–943.

Morison L, Simonds L, Stewart SF. Effectiveness of creative arts-based interventions for treating children and adolescents exposed to traumatic events: a systematic review of the quantitative evidence and meta-analysis. *Arts Health*. 2022;14(3):237–262.

Moss M, Edelblute A, Sinn H, *et al.* The effect of creative arts therapy on psychological distress in health care professionals. *Am J Med*. 2022;135(10):1255–1262.e5.

National Association for Poetry Therapy. 2023. https://poetrytherapy.org

National Coalition of Creative Arts Therapies Associations. 2023. www.nccata.org

National Library of Medicine. Graphic medicine; 2023. www.nlm.nih.gov/exhibition/graphicmedicine/index.html

North American Drama Therapy Association. 2023. www.nadta.org

Orkibi H, Feniger-Schaal R. Integrative systematic review of psychodrama psychotherapy research: trends and methodological implications. *PLoS One*. 2019;14(2):e0212575.

Park JH, Kim JY, Kim HO. Effects of a group poetry therapy program on stress, anxiety, ego-resilience, and psychological well-being of nursing students. *Arch Psychiatr Nurs*. 2022;41:144–152.

Patterson KK, Wong JS, Prout EC, Brooks D. Dance for the rehabilitation of balance and gait in adults with neurological conditions other than Parkinson's disease: a systematic review. *Heliyon.* 2018;4(3):e00584.

Patton Veterans Project. 2023. https://pattonveteransproject.org

Pepe L, Milani R, Di Trani M, Di Folco G, Lanna V, Solano L. A more global approach to musculoskeletal pain: expressive writing as an effective adjunct to physiotherapy. *Psychol Health Med.* 2014;19(6):687–697.

Pereira APS, Marinho V, Gupta D, Magalhães F, Ayres C, Teixeira S. Music therapy and dance as gait rehabilitation in patients with Parkinson's disease: a review of evidence. *J Geriatr Psychiatry Neurol.* 2019;32(1):49–56.

Pongan E, Tillmann B, Leveque Y, *et al.* Can musical or painting interventions improve chronic pain, mood, quality of life, and cognition in patients with mild Alzheimer's disease? Evidence from a randomized controlled trial. *Journal of Alzheimer's Disease.* 2017;60(2):663–677.

Psychology Today. Sandplay therapy; 2023. www.psychologytoday.com/us/therapy-types/sandplay-therapy

Pulimeno M, Piscitelli P, Colazzo S. Children's literature to promote students' global development and wellbeing. *Health Promot Perspect.* 2020;10(1):13–23.

Redwine LS, Henry BL, Pung MA, *et al.* Pilot randomized study of a gratitude journaling intervention on heart rate variability and inflammatory biomarkers in patients with stage B heart failure. *Psychosom Med.* 2016;78(6):667–676.

Reed K, Cochran KL, Edelblute A, *et al.* Creative arts therapy as a potential intervention to prevent burnout and build resilience in health care professionals. *AACN Adv Crit Care.* 2020;31(2):179–190.

Rieger KL, Lobchuk MM, Duff MA, *et al.* Mindfulness-based arts interventions for cancer care: a systematic review of the effects on wellbeing and fatigue. *Psychooncology.* 2021;30(2):240–251.

Sánchez-López AM, Menor-Rodríguez MJ, Sánchez-García JC, Aguilar-Cordero MJ. Play as a method to reduce overweight and obesity in children: an RCT. *International Journal of Environmental Research and Public Health.* 2020;17(1):346.

Sandplay Therapists of America®. 2023. www.sandplay.org

Sayer NA, Noorbaloochi S, Frazier PA, *et al.* Randomized controlled trial of online expressive writing to address readjustment difficulties among U.S. Afghanistan and Iraq war veterans. *J Trauma Stress.* 2015;28(5):381–390.

Schall A, Tesky VA, Adams AK, Pantel J. Art museum-based intervention to promote emotional well-being and improve quality of life in people with dementia: the ARTEMIS project. *Dementia (London).* 2018;17(6):728–743.

Sertbaş G, Ok E, Unver V. Effects of creative arts intervention on anxiety, depression and sleep quality among bone marrow transplantation patients during protective isolation. *Cancer Nurs.* 2023;46(1):e1–e10.

Sezici E, Ocakci AF, Kadioglu H. Use of play therapy in nursing process: a prospective randomized controlled study. *J Nurs Scholarsh.* 2017;49(2):162–169.

Shafer A. Poetry and medicine. *Anesthesiol Clin.* 2022;40(2):359–372.

Shim M, Johnson RB, Gasson S, Goodill S, Jermyn R, Bradt J. A model of dance/movement therapy for resilience-building in people living with chronic pain. *Eur J Integr Med.* 2017;9:27–40.

Smith HE, Jones CJ, Hankins M, *et al.* The effects of expressive writing on lung function, quality of life, medication use, and symptoms in adults with asthma: a randomized controlled trial. *Psychosom Med.* 2015;77(4):429–437.

Spencer K. Kevin Spencer Live; 2023. http://kevinspencerlive.com

Spencer K, Yuen HK, Jenkins GR, Kirklin K, Vogtle LK, Davis D. The "magic" of magic camp from the perspective of children with hemiparesis. *J Exerc Rehabil.* 2021;17(1):15–20.

Steinberg-Oren SL, Krasnova M, Krasnov IS, Baker MR, Ames D. Let's dance: a holistic approach to treating veterans with posttraumatic stress disorder. *Fed Pract.* 2016;33(7):44–49.

Tan J, Yin H, Meng T, Guo X. Effects of sandplay therapy in reducing emotional and behavioural problems in school-age children with chronic diseases: a randomized controlled trial. *Nurs Open.* 2021;8(6):3099–3110.

Tse MM, Ng SS, Lee PH, *et al.* Play activities program to relieve chronic pain and enhance functional mobility and psychological well-being for frail older adults: a pilot cluster randomized controlled trial. *Journal of the American Geriatrics Society.* 2016;64(10):e86–e88.

Tuval-Mashiach R, Patton BW, Drebing C. "When you make a movie, and you see your story there, you can hold it": qualitative exploration of collaborative filmmaking as a therapeutic tool for veterans. *Front Psychol.* 2018;9:1954.

Umbrello M, Sorrenti T, Mistraletti G, Formenti P, Chiumello D, Terzoni S. Music therapy reduces stress and anxiety in critically ill patients: a systematic review of randomized clinical trials. *Minerva Anestesiologica.* 2019;85(8):886–898.

Van Geel F, Van Asch P, Veldkamp R, Feys P. Effects of a 10-week multimodal dance and art intervention program leading to a public performance in persons with multiple sclerosis: a controlled pilot-trial. *Mult Scler Relat Disord*. 2020;44:102256.

Vaudreuil R, Langston DG, Magee WL, Betts D, Kass S, Levy C. Implementing music therapy through telehealth: considerations for military populations [published online ahead of print, 2020 Jul 1]. *Disabil Rehabil Assist Technol*. 2020;1–10.

Volkov R, Volkova N. Effects of listening to music during blood pressure check in primary care clinic settings. *American Journal of Lifestyle Medicine*. 2023. Online publication ahead of print.

Wang R, Li L, Xu J, *et al.* Effects of structured expressive writing on quality of life and perceived self-care self-efficacy of breast cancer patients undergoing chemotherapy in central China: a randomized controlled trial. *Healthcare (Basel)*. 2022;10(9):1762.

Wasmuth S, Pritchard K. Theater-based community engagement project for veterans recovering from substance use disorders. *Am J Occup Ther*. 2016;70(4):7004250020.

Wiercioch-Kuzianik K, Bąbel P. Color hurts. The effect of color on pain perception. *Pain Medicine*. 2019;20(10):1955–1962.

Wiseman R, Wiles A, Watt C. Conjuring up creativity: the effect of performing magic tricks on divergent thinking. *PeerJ*. 2021;9:e11289.

Yuen HK, Spencer K, Kirklin K, Edwards L, Jenkins GR. Contribution of a virtual magic camp to enhancing self-esteem in children with ADHD: a pilot study. *Health Psychol Res*. 2021;9(1):26986.

Zhao J, Li H, Lin R, Wei Y, Yang A. Effects of creative expression therapy for older adults with mild cognitive impairment at risk of Alzheimer's disease: a randomized controlled clinical trial. *Clin Interv Aging*. 2018;13:1313–1320.

Zimmermann N, Netto TM, Amodeo MT, Ska B, Fonseca RP. Working memory training and poetry-based stimulation programs: are there differences in cognitive outcome in healthy older adults? *NeuroRehabilitation*. 2014;35(1):159–170.

Additional Reading

Carson S. *Your Creative Brain: Seven Steps to Maximize Imagination, Productivity, and Innovation in Your Life*. San Francsisco: Jossey-Bass; 2010.

Chaiklin S, Wengrower H, eds. *The Art and Science of Dance/Movement Therapy: Life is Dance,* 2nd ed. New York, NY: Routledge; 2016.

Golden TL, Bantham A, Mason K, Sonke J, Swaback K, Kuge MN, Lokuta AM, Caven J, Shan M, Clinesmith R, Keene K, Manhas N. *Arts on Prescription: A Field Guide for US Communities*. Mass Cultural Council: University of Florida Center for Arts in Medicine. 2023. https://massculturalcouncil.org/documents/arts_on_prescription_field_guide.pdf

Jennings S. *Dramatherapy: Theory and Practice 2*. London, United Kingdom: Routledge; 1992.

Johnson DR, Pendzik S, Snow S, eds. *Assessment in Drama Therapy*. Springfield, IL: Charles C Thomas Publishers; 2012.

King JL, ed. *Art Therapy, Trauma, and Neuroscience: Theoretical and Practical Perspectives.* New York, NY: Routledge; 2016.

Malchiodi CA, ed. *Expressive Therapies*. New York, NY: The Guilford Press; 2005.

Malchiodi CA, ed. *The Handbook of Art Therapy,* 2nd ed. New York, NY: Guilford Press; 2012.

Malchiodi CA. *Trauma and Expressive Arts Therapy: Brain, Body, & Imagination in the Healing Process*. New York, NY: Guilford Press; 2020.

Mazza N. *Poetry Therapy: Theory and Practice,* 2nd ed. New York, NY: Routledge; 2017.

Pennebaker JW, Evans JF. *Expressive Writing: Words That Heal*. Enumclaw, WA: Idyll Arbor; 2014.

Rajendran N, Mitra TP, Shahrestani S, Coggins A. Randomized controlled trial of adult therapeutic coloring for the management of significant anxiety in the emergency department. *Acad Emerg Med*. 2020;27(2):92–99.

Rosenthal NE. Poetry Rx. *How 50 Inspiring Poems Can Heal and Bring Joy to Your Life*. New York, NY: Gildan Media; 2021.

Schaefer CE, ed. *Foundations of Play Therapy,* 2nd ed. Hoboken, NJ: John Wiley & Sons; 2011.

Spencer K. Hocus Focus: magic as a creative art therapy. In: Bailey S, ed. *Creative Arts Therapy Careers: Succeeding as a Creative Professional*. New York, NY: Routledge/Taylor and Francis; 2021.

Støre SJ, Jakobsson N. The effect of mandala coloring on state anxiety: a systematic review and meta-analysis. *Art Therapy*. 2022;39(4):173–181.

Thaut MH, Hoemberg V, eds. *Handbook of Neurologic Music Therapy*. Oxford, UK: Oxford University Press; 2014.

CHAPTER 12

Self-Care Strategies

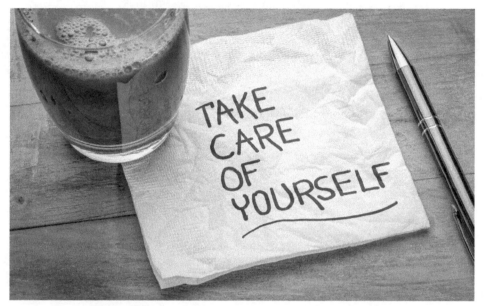

Self-care strategies are a part of person-centered medicine

Learning Objectives

- Understand the basic research for conventional and integrative therapies.
- Apply conventional and integrative therapies for practical pain management.

Chapter Highlights

- Key Concept: Self-Care Healthcare
- Clinical Tip: Change Posture and Position
- Featured Topic 12.1: Acupressure and Back Pain
- Featured Topic 12.2: Managing Constipation

- Featured Topic 12.3: Office Stretch and Movement Breaks
- Featured Topic 12.4: Aromatherapy
- Featured Topic 12.5: Reducing Home Pollution and Chemical Use
- Featured Topic 12.6: Eastern Approaches to Manual Therapy
- Featured Topic 12.7: Back Supports and Back Pain
- Featured Topic 12.8: Improving Medication Adherence
- Self-Care Handout 12.1: Suggested Office Break Movements
- Self-Care Handout 12.2: Suggested Creative Office Break Solutions
- Self-Care Handout 12.3: Joint Protection Techniques
- Self-Care Handout 12.4: Activity Pacing/Energy Conservation Techniques
- Self-Care Handout 12.5: Improved Body Mechanics with Daily Activities
- Self-Care Handout 12.6: Shoe Fit and Selection Guidelines
- Self-Care Handout 12.7: Optimizing Brain Health
- Self-Care Handout 12.8: Improving Quality of Life with Assistive Devices
- Self-Care Handout 12.9: Fall Prevention Guidelines
- Self-Care Handout 12.10: Personal Safety Checklist
- Self-Management Activities
- Classroom and Lab Activities
- Useful Clinical Resources
- References
- Additional Reading

Lifestyle Matters: *Train to be grateful.*

Introduction

Self-care interventions in rehabilitation tend to focus on pain management and activities of daily living skills such as dressing, bathing, food preparation, and cooking. Self-care also includes actions to maintain good health, prevent disease, and cope with disability and illness (Kongsted *et al.* 2021). Home management training may require educating the patient/client and caregiver in adaptive equipment and/or assistive technology (e.g., using a cane, crutches, walker, wheelchair, braces, or splints). Research shows that self-care and self-management strategies may be used for back pain (Du *et al.* 2017; French *et al.* 2019; Lim *et al.* 2019; Snook 2004) and other conditions.

KEY CONCEPT: SELF-CARE HEALTHCARE

For the purpose of this book, self-care and self-management interventions may include providing patients/clients with strategies such as:

- activity pacing or energy conservation techniques
- body-mechanics guidelines (e.g., proper lifting, carrying, pushing, pulling, reaching)
- fall-prevention guidelines
- flare-up management strategies
- home exercise program guidelines
- joint-protection techniques
- pain neuroscience education
- physical modality use (e.g., heat or cold application)
- proper application of taping (e.g., kinesiotaping)
- proper use and selection of transcutaneous electrical nerve stimulation (TENS) unit
- proper use of over-the-counter topical analgesics
- self-acupressure strategies
- self-massage strategies.

Self-care interventions to improve the overall quality of life for patients/clients may include strategies such as:

- guidelines on avoidance of risky substance use (e.g., quitting smoking)
- exercise and physical activity guidelines
- nature-based activity guidelines (e.g., help reduce anxiety and depression)
- nutrition optimization guidelines to help promote healing and reduce inflammation
- sleep hygiene and optimization guidelines
- socialization and community involvement guidelines
- stress management guidelines.

Note: Many of the pain management strategies outlined in this chapter use back pain as an example. For this reason, the healthcare provider and professional must adapt techniques and strategies as needed for other conditions.

Sample Self-Care for Healthcare Professionals

This section illustrates basic concepts that may be used by dentists, nurses, therapists, and physicians. Each medical and nonmedical profession needs specific lifestyle, ergonomic, and wellness guidelines.

Dentists

A randomized study in the *International Archives of Occupational and Environmental Health* (Letafatkar *et al.* 2020) found that specific therapeutic exercises (e.g., performing various wall slides using the arms while facing the wall or with the back to the wall) helped alleviate chronic neck pain in dentists. A study in the *Journal of Physical Therapy Science* (Gaowgzeh *et al.* 2015) indicates that dentists may potentially benefit from stretching and exercise breaks and utilizing more assistive tools for performing work-related tasks. From a patient perspective, a dentist in a physical therapy session told the author, "After suffering for years with back pain, I found dancing with all the varying movements to be the best form of activity to manage my pain."

Nurses

A randomized study in the *Journal of Clinical Nursing* (Járomi *et al.* 2018) found that a Spine Care for Nurses program reduced chronic nonspecific low back pain and improved patient lifting technique. From a patient perspective, a nurse in a physical therapy session told the author, "Doing a quick yoga session at lunch keeps me focused for the second half of my shift. I also find swimming several days per week helps me to decompress mentally and physically."

Physical Therapists/Physiotherapists

A review article in the *Journal of Integrative Medicine* (Gyer *et al.* 2018) indicated that hand injuries were common in physical therapists and other manual therapy professionals. A systematic review (Gorce and Jacquier-Bret 2023) found that the most common musculoskeletal injuries in physiotherapists worldwide were in the lower back, neck, thumb, and shoulder regions. Many physiotherapists indicated that using light instrument-assisted soft-tissue mobilization techniques and tools helped to prevent excess strain to the hands. Manual therapy professionals can consider using tools and instruments such as those seen with the Graston Technique, gua sha, and cupping.

Surgeons

A literature review in *Plastic and Reconstructive Surgery Global Open* (Winters *et al.* 2020) provides educational exercise videos embedded in the article that may be used by surgeons as a part of a wellness program. A systematic review in *Acta Neurochirurgica* (Lavé *et al.* 2020) indicates that neurosurgeons and spine surgeons may need to adjust their weekly schedules, include exercise, and practice better ergonomics strategies during surgery to prevent back pain and other musculoskeletal disorders. From a patient perspective, a surgeon in a physical therapy session told the author, "What helped me most is doing pottery to keep my hands and mind nimble and periodically standing erect while I'm doing surgery."

CLINICAL TIP: CHANGE POSTURE AND POSITION

Change sitting, standing, and work postures and positions periodically to reduce strain.

Professor Stuart McGill, Ph.D., in his book *Low Back Disorders* (McGill 2016, p.195), states that "tissue loads must be migrated from tissue to tissue to minimize the risk of any single tissue's accumulating microtrauma. This is accomplished by changing posture."

Practical Self-Care Strategies

The following are practical self-care strategies that may be used to help patients/clients manage pain.

Self-Care with Self-Massage

Some individuals may find periodic self-massages to their low back throughout the day a helpful strategy to manage pain. For example, a randomized study in the *Journal of Bodywork and Movement Therapies* (Buttagat *et al.* 2020) found that self-massage and home stretching exercises may help manage chronic low back pain. The images below show upper and lower back self-massage options.

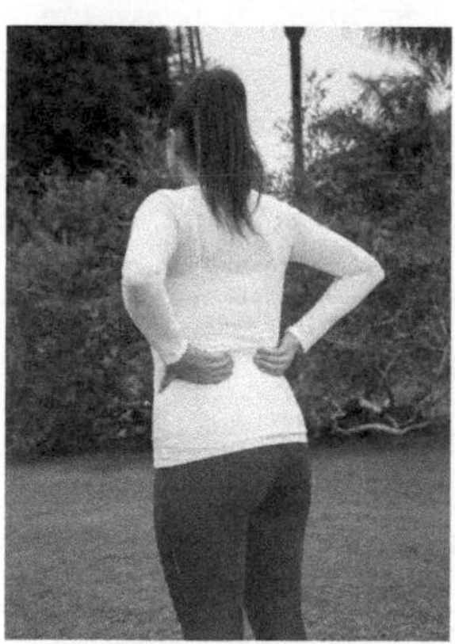

Self-massage to the back using the hands

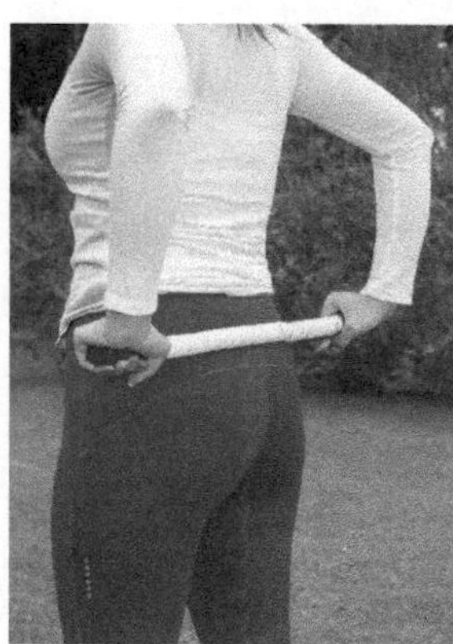

Self-massage to the back using The Stick massage apparatus

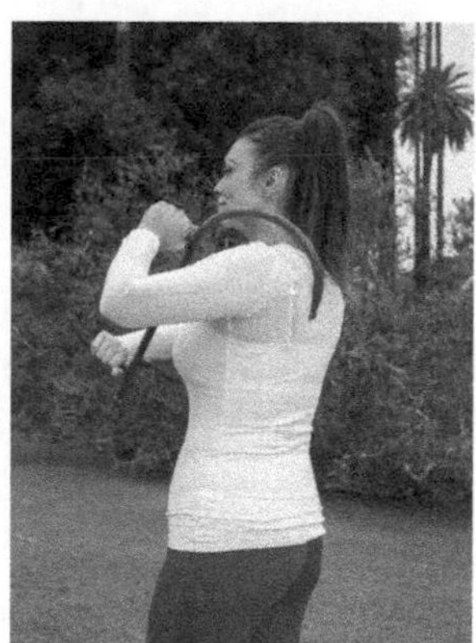

Self-massage to the upper back using the Thera Cane apparatus

Self-Care with Sleep and Relaxation Products

Some individuals who sleep on their side may benefit from special pillows to help improve the quality of sleep. Others may find a weighted blanket a useful strategy to relax and reduce anxiety. The images below show self-care comfort products.

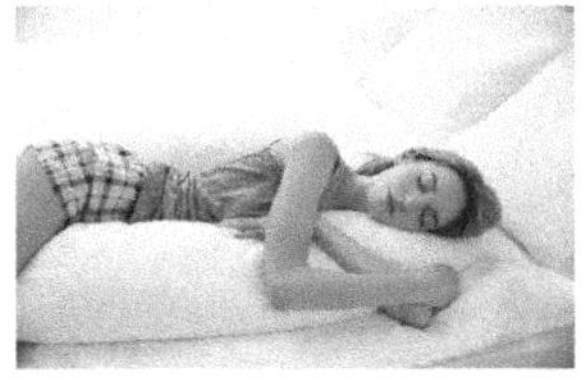

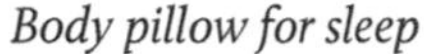

Body pillow for sleep

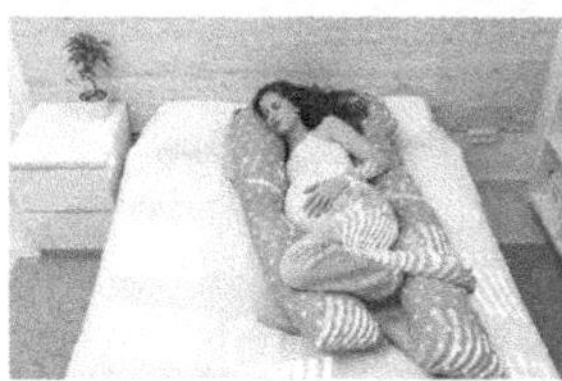

U-shaped pillow for sleep

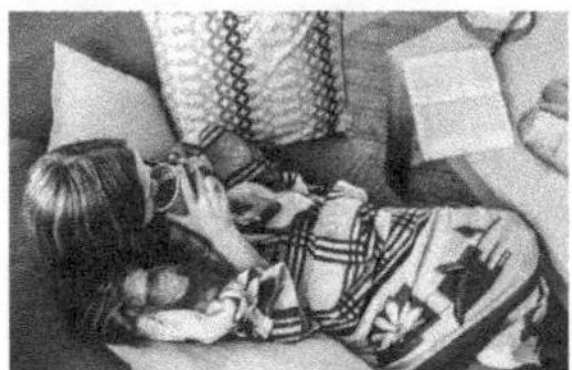

Weighted blanket for relaxation

Self-Care with Relaxation Positions

Supine lying and reclining positions may be used for 5–10 minutes after a person returns home from work to physically and mentally decompress and unwind. The images below show self-care relaxation positions.

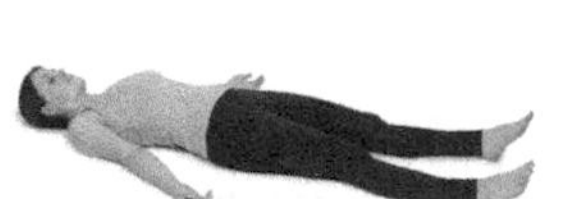

Supine lying (with or without a pillow under the knees)

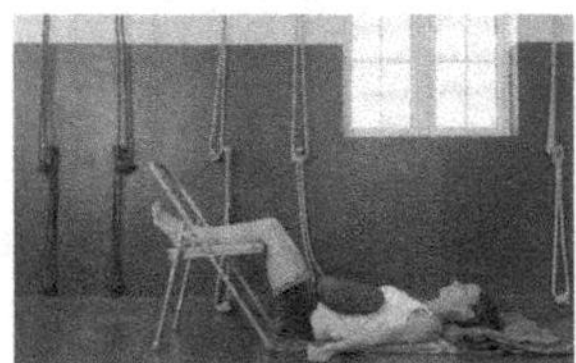

Supine lying with legs elevated

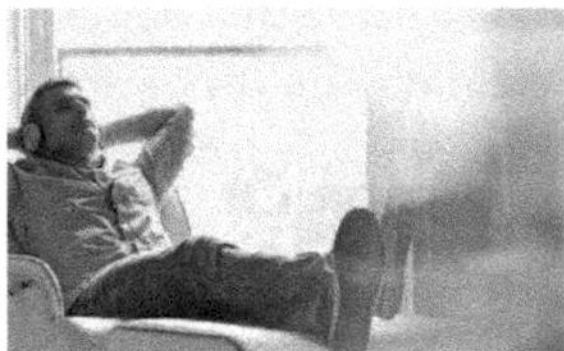

Reclining for relaxation

Self-Care with a Personal Comfort Kit

Individuals with chronic pain may want to consider creating a personalized comfort kit, which is similar to a first aid kit or an emergency preparedness kit. It can contain strategies they have found to be effective for reducing and managing pain. An article in *Pain Management Nursing* (Blackburn *et al.* 2019) found that using a comfort kit benefits adult cancer pain management. Also, a study in the *Journal of Alternative and Complementary Medicine* (Stoerkel *et al.* 2018) used a similar approach of creating a self-care toolkit for patients with breast cancer who were undergoing surgery.

These creative and practical concepts may be adapted to suit the needs of other patients/clients. A personalized pain management comfort kit for the home (and a variation for work) may include the following:

- Essential oils for aromatherapy (e.g., lavender)
- Green tea packet (for reducing stress and improving sleep) (Unno *et al.* 2017)
- Guided imagery audiotapes
- Heating pad or cold pack
- Pre-cut kinesiotape strips (Sheng *et al.* 2019)
- Pre-selected music playlist for relaxation
- Self-massage tools
- Topical analgesics (e.g., containing capsaicin)
- Transcutaneous electrical nerve stimulation (TENS) unit

Self-Care with a Flare-Up Management Plan

Pain flare-ups impact the lives of individuals with back pain (Suri *et al.* 2012; Suri *et al.* 2018; Tan *et al.* 2019) and other chronic pain conditions. For this reason, flare-up management must be addressed by healthcare providers. For example, a study in the *Journal of Orthopaedic and Sports Physical Therapy* (Bartholdy *et al.* 2016) used a "rescue" exercise program of predefined exercises for flare-ups in patients with knee osteoarthritis. The flare-up management concept may be adapted for patients with other types of chronic pain.

A flare-up pain management plan for individuals in chronic pain may include teaching patients/clients the following strategies:

- Learn to identify potential triggers to avoid flare-ups or manage the symptoms earlier.
- Learn to identify early changes in symptoms such as swelling, stiffness, or reduced functional ability (e.g., pain moving from sitting to standing). This way, the person may minimize provoking factors and start using their comfort kit and predefined modified exercise program until the flare-up subsides.

Training in Proper Body Mechanics

A randomized study in the *International Journal of Caring Sciences* (Akca *et al.* 2017) showed that body mechanics training may help manage back pain. For this reason, teaching patients/clients safe body mechanics for various functional daily activities such as lifting, carrying, pushing, and pulling may help reduce the risk of back pain and help with recovery. For optimal results, lifting and other body mechanics guidelines need to be personalized according to a person's strength, flexibility, coordination, and the demands of the task or job. For example, a person may have weakness in their legs, pain, or limited range of motion in their knee which prevents them from bending their knees while lifting a box or package. For this reason, other lifting strategies may need to be addressed. The following image shows one strategy for lifting an item (such as groceries or a box) from the floor.

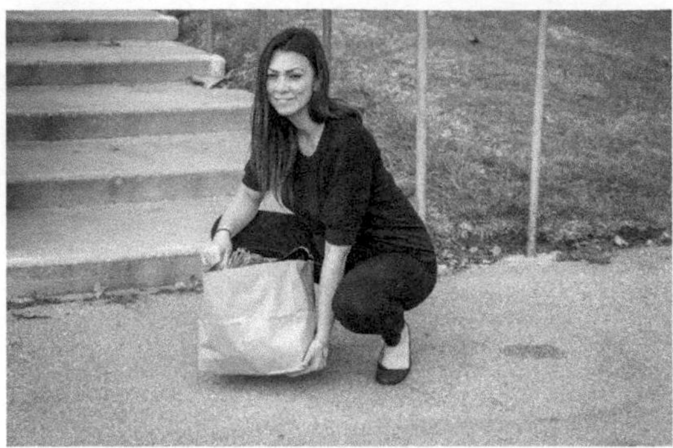

One strategy for lifting a grocery bag from the ground

Motor Skill Training

Motor skill training is one strategy that may be used for managing back pain (Lanier *et al.* 2019; van Dillen *et al.* 2021). Motor skill training interventions for an individual with back pain may consist of the following:

- To increase standing tolerance, the person gradually progresses from 10 minutes to 60 minutes with graded exposure to tasks such as:
  - cooking a meal (e.g., using a small bowl, then larger bowls) and washing the dishes (e.g., placing objects on the countertop, then to lower and higher shelves) (see the image below)
  - shopping
  - yardwork (e.g., watering the plants, raking the leaves)
  - housework (e.g., dusting, mopping, sweeping).
- To increase sitting tolerance, the person gradually progresses from 10 minutes to 45 minutes with graded exposure to tasks such as:
  - working on the computer
  - answering phone calls and taking notes
  - donning/doffing shoes and socks.

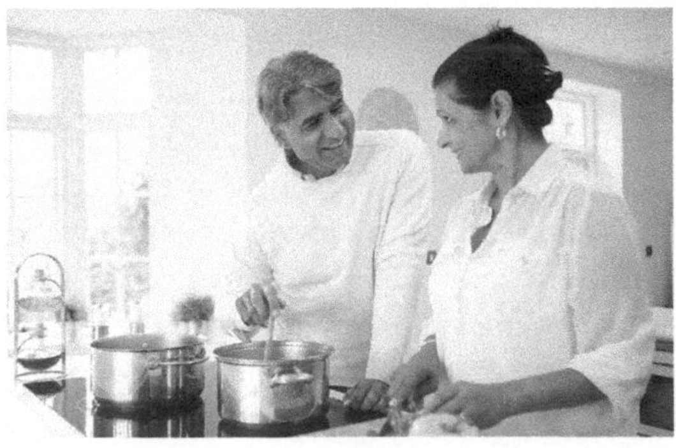

Cooking an enjoyable meal at home

Work Wellness Strategies

According to Venes (2021), ergonomics is the science of fitting a job to a person's physiological, anatomical, and psychological needs to enhance well-being and efficiency. Studies show that microbreaks, vacations, and the effects of working long hours can affect work-related wellness (Hruska *et al.* 2020; Kivimäki *et al.* 2015; Luger *et al.* 2019; McLean *et al.* 2001; Park *et al.* 2017; Rivera *et al.* 2020; Virtanen *et al.* 2009a; Virtanen *et al.* 2009b; Virtanen *et al.* 2011). For this reason, every person needs to find the optimal rest and break timeframe. Consider the following:

- **Microbreaks**: How often (e.g., every 30 or 60 minutes) and for how long (e.g., 20–60 seconds) should a person take a microbreak from their tasks for optimal mental and physical health? These need to be determined for the individual, occupation, and job task. For example, an office worker performing seated tasks may benefit from standing up every 30 minutes and stretching for 30 seconds. Also, there is some evidence to suggest that computer users should consider taking visual breaks to help prevent eyestrain and eye fatigue (Blehm *et al.* 2005; Toomingas *et al.* 2014). However, ideal visual break lengths have not been identified and may depend on individual needs. One practical solution may be for an individual to take a short visual break every 10–20 minutes to gaze off into the distance and then have the impact of this assessed. The key is not to take a vision break from the computer and then do more close-up work such as writing or checking phone messages. Each computer user should gaze into the distance during their vision break (Coles-Brennan *et al.* 2019). Ideally, each office worker should have a window nearby so they can gaze out into the distance to see nature (such as trees, birds, and clouds).
- **Macrobreaks**: How many hours (e.g., 6-, 8-, 10-, or 12-hour shifts) should a person work in one day, and how many consecutive days (e.g., 3, 4, or 5 days) can this person tolerate for optimal mental and physical health? Once again, these need to be determined for the individual, occupation, and job task.
- **Vacations**: How often should a person take a vacation for optimal mental or physical health? Is the ideal vacation one long break once a year, or is it better to take a mini vacation once every three months by spreading out allotted vacation days from the employer? Again, these factors must be determined for the individual and occupation.

Featured Topics

Featured Topic 12.1 outlines various acupressure points that may be used for back pain in conjunction with other treatments.

Featured Topic 12.2 outlines various strategies that may be used to manage constipation.

Featured Topic 12.3 outlines various office stretch and movement breaks.

Featured Topic 12.4 outlines some of the benefits of aromatherapy.

Featured Topic 12.5 outlines strategies that may be used to reduce home pollution and chemical use.

Featured Topic 12.6 outlines various Eastern approaches to manual therapy, which includes cupping, gua sha, and tuina.

Featured Topic 12.7 outlines the use of lumbar back supports in industrial workers and practical injury prevention tips for the workplace.

Featured Topic 12.8 outlines selected strategies to help patients improve medication adherence.

■ Featured Topic 12.1: Acupressure and Back Pain

Rekha Lund, DAOM, MPT, Dipl.O.M., LAc.

Acupuncture is a technique for treating pain based on the principles used in Traditional Chinese Medicine. The following are self-care acupressure points that may be used by acupuncturists to help manage low back pain (Chou *et al.* 2017; Godley and Smith 2020; Murphy *et al.* 2019; Qaseem *et al.* 2017; Xiang *et al.* 2020; Yuan *et al.* 2015). Perform a circular motion for 60 to 90 seconds at each point.

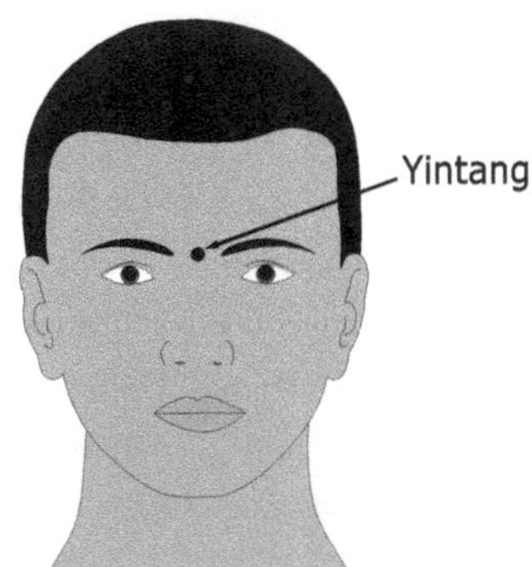

Acupressure point: Yintang

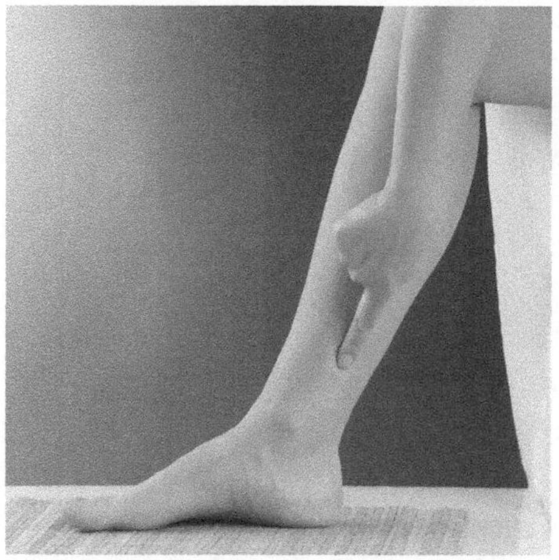

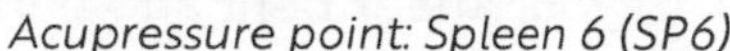

Acupressure point: Spleen 6 (SP6)

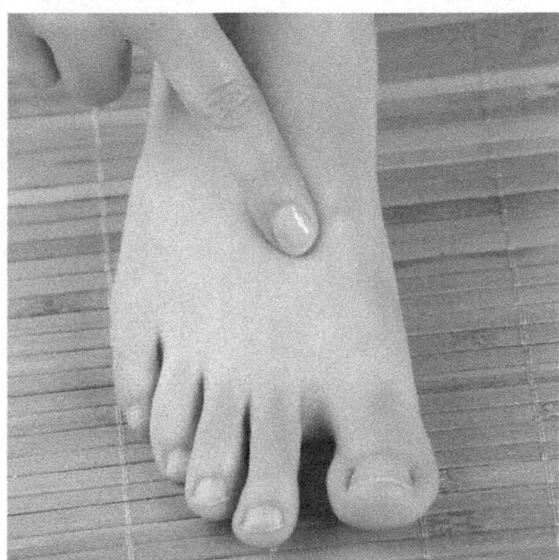

Acupressure point: Liver 3 (LIV3)

Created by Rekha Lund, DAOM, MPT, Dipl.O.M., LAc. She is a Doctor of Acupuncture & Herbal Medicine and licensed physical therapist who lives in Los Angeles, California. www.rekhalund.com

Used with permission from Rekha Lund, DAOM, MPT, Dipl.O.M., LAc.

■ Featured Topic 12.2: Managing Constipation

Constipation should be managed and prevented for overall good health. Constipation may be seen in individuals with, for example, back pain, hypothyroidism, multiple sclerosis, Parkinson's, and stroke, as well as individuals using opioids for pain. Moreover, constipation may be linked to anxiety and depression. Furthermore, a study in the *Stroke* journal found that "straining for defecation" may be one of the eight trigger factors for an aneurysmal rupture (Vlak *et al.* 2011).

The following are some practical solutions for preventing and managing constipation:

- Ritualize bowel habits (such as a morning bowel movement).
- Drink enough fluids.
- Eat enough fiber (vegetables, fruits, whole grains).
- Consider adding foods such as figs, kiwis, druid plums, or prune juice.
- Obtain enough probiotics from food sources (such as sauerkraut, kimchi).
- Engage in an exercise program. Consider walking, yoga, or tai chi.
- Consider using a toilet posture modification device such as the

Squatty Potty (www.squattypotty.com) to help reduce straining during a bowel movement.

- Speak with your acupuncturist to learn self-acupressure techniques.
- Speak with your physical therapist and healthcare provider to learn self-massage, aromatherapy massage, and diaphragmatic breathing (or belly breathing) techniques.

The following are some immediate strategies you may try based on your healthcare provider's recommendations. For example, your provider may advise against certain techniques based on your medical history or limitations.

- **Level 1**: Try lying on your back with your knees bent and perform diaphragmatic breathing for 2–3 minutes.

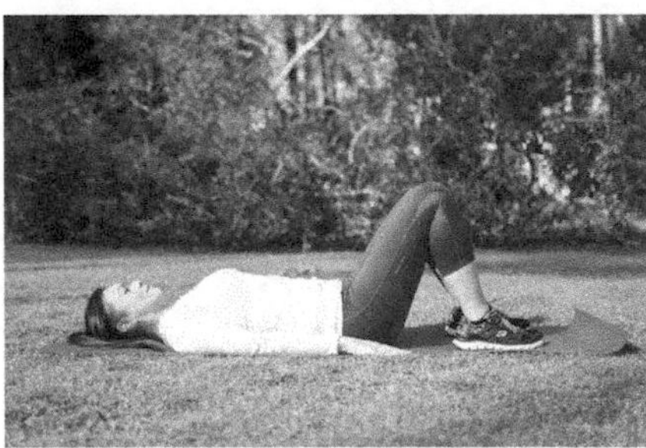

Diaphragmatic breathing

- **Level 2**: If level 1 does not provide relief, select one or two of the exercises below.

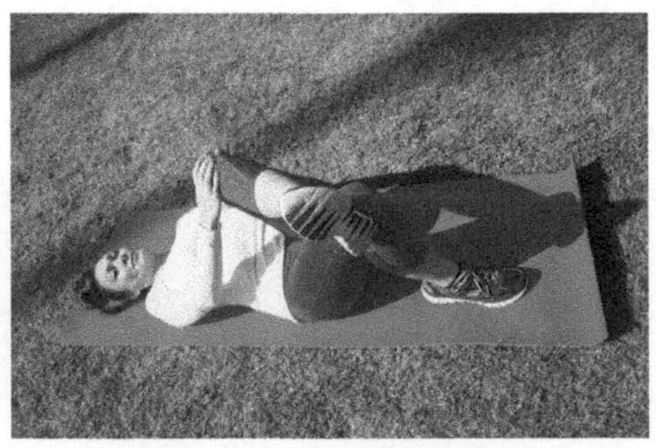

If tolerated, perform repeated single knee to the chest movements for 10–15 repetitions

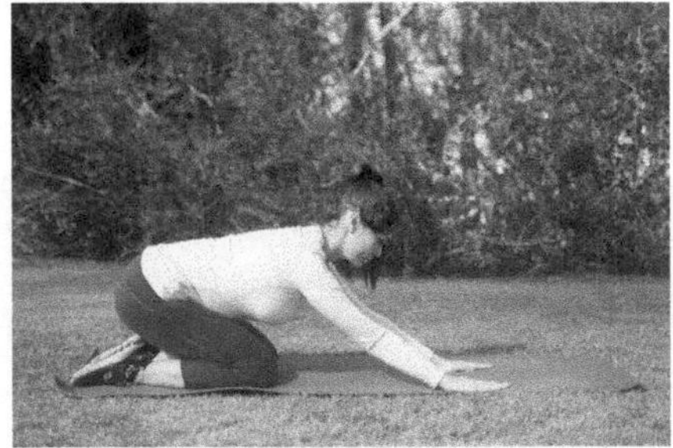

If tolerated, perform repeated hands and knees position to heel sit movements for 10–15 repetitions

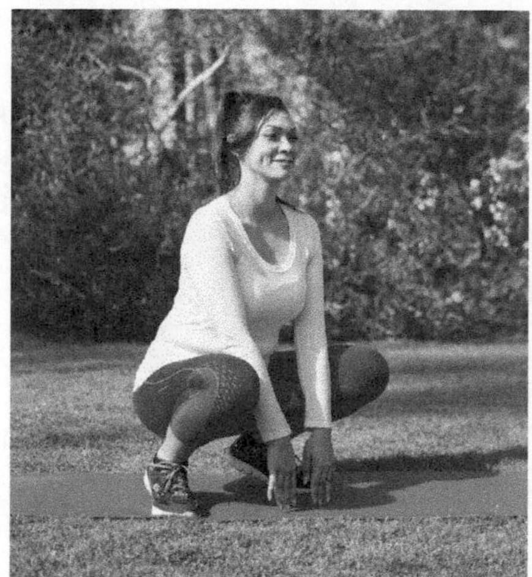
If tolerated, get into a squat stretch position for 10–15 seconds (hold on to a solid object if needed)

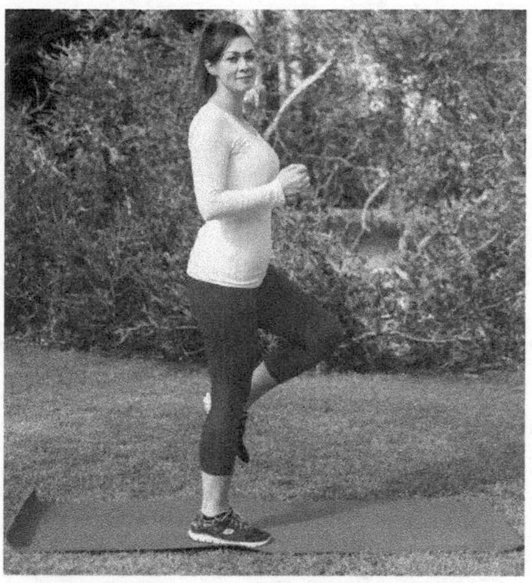
If tolerated, try marching in place (and hold on to a solid object for balance if needed) for 30 seconds

- **Level 3**: If levels 1 and 2 do not provide relief, try the following gentle abdominal massage sequence.

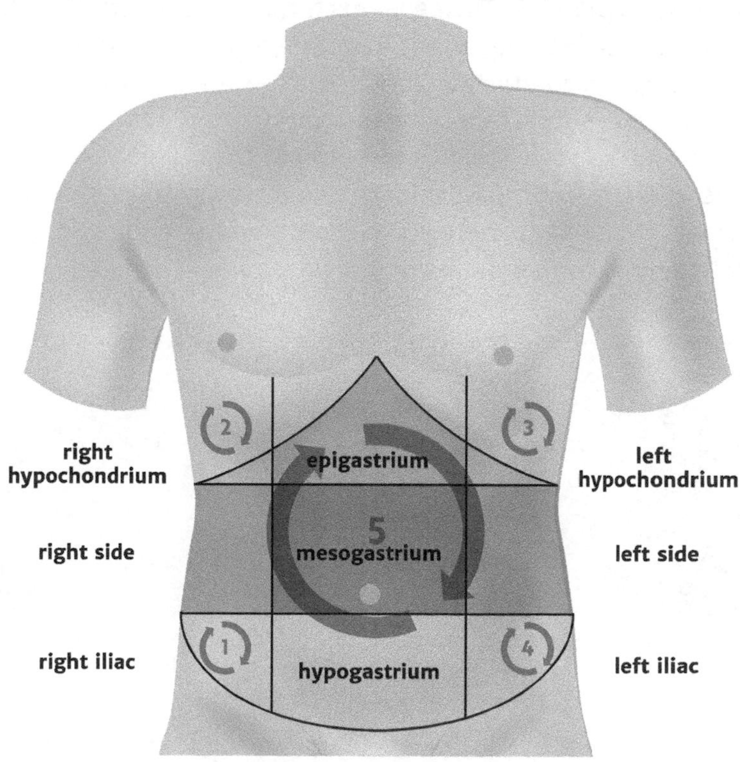

Abdominal massage

1. Start by lying on your bed with your knees bent and your feet on the mattress.
2. Start with 10 slow and small clockwise massage circles using gentle pressure to your right lower abdomen.
3. Repeat the above sequence in each of the outer four frames in the image.
4. Finally, perform 10 slow and large clockwise massage circles using gentle pressure covering all four outer frames.

From Abbott et al. 2015; Altug 2016; Aydinli and Karadağ 2022; Chey et al. 2021; Doğan et al. 2022; Durmuş İskender and Çalışkan 2022; Gao et al. 2019; George and Borello-France 2017; Harrington and Haskvitz 2006; Ho et al. 2020a; Ishiyama et al. 2019; Kalkdijk et al. 2022; Koyama et al. 2022; Li et al. 2017; Li et al. 2022; Modi et al. 2019; Müller-Lissner et al. 2017; Sadler et al. 2022; Silva and Motta 2013; Singh et al. 2022; Stocchi and Torti 2017; Sundbøll et al. 2020; Vlak et al. 2011; Yildirim et al. 2022; Zhang et al. 2020; Zhou et al. 2019; Zivkovic et al. 2012.

■ Featured Topic 12.3: Office Stretch and Movement Breaks

Standing-up several times throughout the workday to perform the overhead reach stretch is a good way to stretch the shoulders and upper back region to help relieve muscle tension from prolonged sitting.

Standing-up several times throughout the workday to perform the overhead reach with a partial lunge is a good way to stretch not only the shoulders and upper back region, but also the hips and calf to help relieve muscle tension from prolonged sitting.

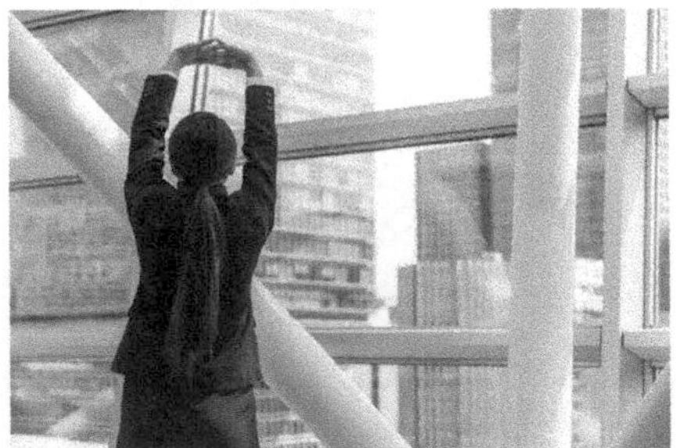

Stand-up overhead reach stretch

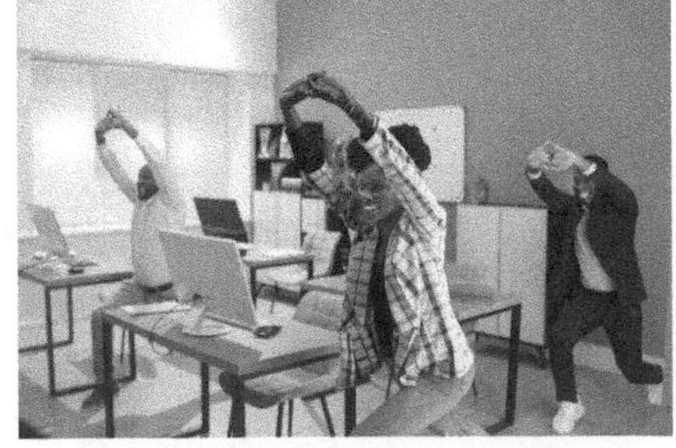

Stand-up overhead reach with partial lunge for hip stretch

Standing up several times throughout the workday to perform partial squats is a good way to increase circulation and add some easy physical activity.

Consider transforming seated meetings into some walking meetings at work to help increase productivity, improve mood, and add physical activity (Kling *et al.* 2021). When feasible, try walking outdoors near the workplace for fresh air, natural light, and exposure to nature.

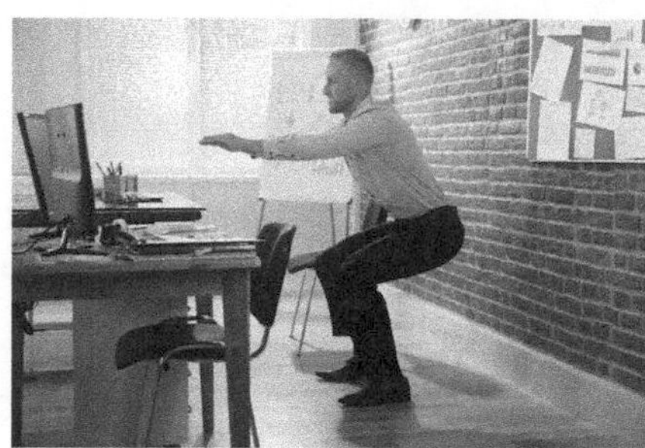

Partial squats for circulation

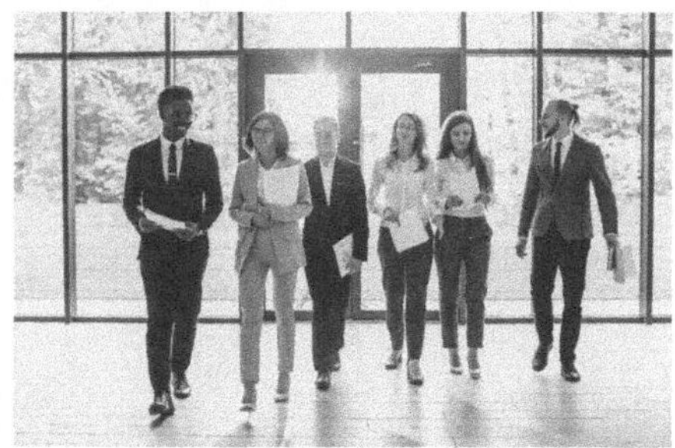

Use a walking meeting to stimulate creativity and enhance wellness

Featured Topic 12.4: Aromatherapy

Aromatherapy is the therapeutic use of essential oils derived from plants and used in massage, baths, or inhalants to help manage anxiety, stress, and depression (Venes 2021). The following are examples of uses for aromatherapy:

- **Bergamot** may reduce preoperative anxiety (Ni *et al.* 2013).
- **Chamomile** may decrease depression, anxiety, and stress in older adults (Ebrahimi *et al.* 2022).
- **Lavender** may decrease depression, anxiety, and stress levels in older adults (Ebrahimi *et al.* 2022) and dental anxiety in children (Ghaderi and Solhjou 2020).
- **Lemon** may decrease nausea in palliative care (Kreye *et al.* 2022) and in pregnant women (Nassif *et al.* 2022).
- **Peppermint** may reduce the severity of nausea in cancer patients undergoing chemotherapy (Efe Ertürk *et al.* 2021) and improve alertness (Hoult *et al.* 2019; Moss *et al.* 2008).
- **Rose** may reduce pain and anxiety after cesarean section (C-section) (Abbasijahromi *et al.* 2020) and increase sleep quality, and decrease anxiety in patients in a cardiac care unit (Jodaki *et al.* 2021).

Resources

- Alliance of International Aromatherapists, www.alliance-aromatherapists.org

- International Federation of Aromatherapists, www.ifaroma.org
- Tisserand Institute, https://tisserandinstitute.org
- Book: Tisserand R, Young R. *Essential Oil Safety: A Guide for Health Care Professionals*, 2nd ed. London, United Kingdom: Elsevier; 2014.

Featured Topic 12.5: Reducing Home Pollution and Chemical Use

Certain products or strategies in the home may create health risks and medical problems for some individuals, such as respiratory or cardiovascular illness.

Potential Alternatives
Instead of using chemicals to freshen the air in the home, consider opening the windows regularly for fresh air and opening the curtains for sunshine to enter.
Instead of using harsh chemicals in the home, consider using white vinegar for cleaning floors and kitchen countertops. Keep small areas ventilated.
If needed, use a water filter on the sink to rinse fruits and vegetables.
To help reduce indoor air pollution, use range hoods and open windows to ventilate.
To help reduce indoor air pollution, print fewer documents, save documents as PDFs instead of printing, and use a printer near an open window for ventilation.
If needed, use a shower filter to help filter out excess chlorine and other chemicals that may irritate the skin.
Create a smoke-free home environment by encouraging family members, friends, and guests to smoke outside.
Consider replacing wall-to-wall carpeting with hardwood or ceramic tile floors if there are individuals in the home who have various airborne sensitivities.
If changing wall-to-wall carpeting is not feasible, consider wearing shoes only meant for indoors and remove shoes that are worn outdoors. It may be especially important for healthcare workers to remove work shoes before entering their home.
To keep the interior of your car air fresh, consider airing out the inside of the car by opening windows at the beginning of each trip, avoiding smoking in the car (ideally don't smoke at all), using the car air filters in heavy traffic, and, if possible, using less congested roads to minimize automobile exhaust.

From Becher et al. 2018; Dymond et al. 2021; Kanwar et al. 2019; Lebel et al. 2022; Lindberg et al. 2021; Meesters et al. 2018; Meesters et al. 2022; Salonen et al. 2018; Shi et al. 2015; Tang et al. 2012; Vardoulakis et al. 2020; Zulauf et al. 2019.

■ Featured Topic 12.6: Eastern Approaches to Manual Therapy

The following are some Eastern approaches to manual therapy that may be used in rehabilitation.

Acupressure is "a non-invasive treatment in which pressure is applied to specific body points" (Waits *et al.* 2018, p.24). Acupressure may be used to reduce arthritic symptoms (Guo *et al.* 2022), postpartum low back pain (Cheng *et al.* 2020), cancer-related fatigue (Hsieh *et al.* 2021), nausea in pregnant women (Tara *et al.* 2020), pain (He *et al.* 2020), premenstrual symptoms (Simsek Kücükkelepce and Timur Tashan 2021), and other symptoms.

Cupping is the "application to the skin of a glass or bamboo vessel from which air has been withdrawn by heat or of a special suction apparatus in order to draw blood to the surface" (Venes 2021, p.606). Dry cupping may be used to treat carpal tunnel syndrome (Mohammadi *et al.* 2019), nonspecific low back pain (Salemi *et al.* 2021), chronic pain (Cramer *et al.* 2020), chronic fatigue syndrome (Meng *et al.* 2020), chronic nonspecific neck pain (Saha *et al.* 2017), myofascial pain dysfunction syndrome (Sajedi *et al.* 2022), plantar fasciitis (Ge *et al.* 2017), and other conditions.

Gua sha is "an instrument-assisted 'pressure-stroking' of a lubricated area of the body surface" (Saha *et al.* 2019, p.64). Gua sha may be used to treat chronic neck and low back pain (Lauche *et al.* 2012), perimenopausal symptoms (Meng *et al.* 2017), and other conditions.

Tuina (also tui na or tui-na) is "a traditional method of Chinese massage in which the body is lifted, squeezed, and pushed to improve circulation and enhance disease resistance" (Venes 2021, p.2458). Tuina may be used for knee osteoarthritis (Xu *et al.* 2022), chronic neck pain (Pach *et al.* 2018), tension-type headache (Fan *et al.* 2021), and other conditions.

■ Featured Topic 12.7: Back Supports and Back Pain

The incidence of back pain varies among different occupations, and it is a serious concern in industrial workers. Some specialists have proposed the use of lumbar supports. However, there is no overwhelming evidence for recommending industrial workers wear lumbar back supports (or back belts) as a part of regular work tasks to prevent back injuries (National Institute for Occupational Safety and Health 2023; Roelofs *et al.* 2007; van Duijvenbode *et al.* 2008). However, practitioners may make specific recommendations depending on an individual worker's needs.

Key factors for injury prevention include ensuring that:

- workers collaborate with managers to keep the work environment and job tasks safe
- adequate breaks are a part of job demands
- workers are instructed to use good body mechanics
- work-specific conditioning exercises and healthy lifestyle choices are encouraged.

■ Featured Topic 12.8: Improving Medication Adherence

A review in the *American Journal of the Medical Sciences* indicates, "Medication nonadherence leads to poor outcomes, increasing healthcare service utilization and overall healthcare costs" (Brown *et al.* 2016, p.388). The following are some practical strategies to enhance medication adherence (Marcum *et al.* 2017; Palacio *et al.* 2016):

- Have the patient bring medications to an appointment and review each medication.
- Provide individualized patient education regarding medical conditions and the purpose of each medication.
- Establish a trusting relationship.
- Address patients' beliefs, fears, and values.
- Engage family members for support.
- Use motivational interviewing.
- Use screening tools.
- Use technology (e.g., apps, phone call reminders).

Screening Tool

- Morisky Medication Adherence Scale

Self-Care Education Guides

See **Self-Care Handout 12.1: Suggested Office Break Movements** for office break movements.

See **Self-Care Handout 12.2: Suggested Creative Office Break Solutions** for ideas for employers to consider keeping workers active for increased well-being and improved job satisfaction, and to help reduce job burnout. Some of the strategies may be used during breaks or lunchtime. However, many of the strategies may not be appropriate for every job, so employees and managers should use alternative methods when appropriate (Xu *et al.* 2023).

Self-Care Handout 12.3: Joint Protection Techniques may be used for individuals with joint pain (Altug 2010; Altug 2018; Coenen *et al.* 2017; Flexner and Hertling 2018; Hammond and Freeman 2004; Hochberg *et al.* 2012; Iversen and Westby 2014; Masiero *et al.* 2007; McGill 2016; Rocabado and Iglarsh 1991; Sheon 1985; Sheon and Orr 1996; Thosar *et al.* 2015).

Self-Care Handout 12.4: Activity Pacing/Energy Conservation Techniques may be used for individuals with pain, fatigue, or weakness (Abonie *et al.* 2020; Altug 2011; Altug 2018; Gerber *et al.* 1987; Iversen and Westby 2014; Mathiowetz *et al.* 2005; Murphy *et al.* 2012; Velloso and Jardim 2006; Young 1991).

Self-Care Handout 12.5: Improved Body Mechanics with Daily Activities may be used to help minimize pain and reduce injury in people who are undergoing therapy and rehabilitation for back pain (Altug 2018; Armstrong and Fischer 2020; Beach *et al.* 2018; McGill 2016; Milhem *et al.* 2016; Rowe and Jacobs 2002).

Self-Care Handout 12.6: Shoe Fit and Selection Guidelines may be used to help patients/clients select shoes for daily activities and fitness (Blazer *et al.* 2018; Cook *et al.* 1985; FootCareMD 2023; Vincent and Vincent 2014; Weatherford and Irwin 2023a; Weatherford and Irwin 2023b).

Self-Care Handout 12.7: Optimizing Brain Health may be used to help patients/clients improve their brain health (Cheatham *et al.* 2022; Chen *et al.* 2019; Chételat *et al.* 2022; Eyre *et al.* 2017; Ho *et al.* 2020b; Huang *et al.* 2022; Hughes *et al.* 2020; Jang *et al.* 2022; Kaddoumi *et al.* 2022; Koch *et al.* 2019; Kolberg *et al.* 2021; Kühn *et al.* 2022; Liu *et al.* 2023; McCurry *et al.* 2011; Nakase *et al.* 2022; Ngandu *et al.* 2015; Penninkilampi *et al.* 2018; Peters *et al.* 2019; Peters *et al.* 2022; Riemersma-van der Lek *et al.* 2008; Styck and George 2022; Valls-Pedret *et al.* 2015; Wang *et al.* 2021; Wang *et al.* 2022; Yen and Chiu 2021; Zhang *et al.* 2022).

Self-Care Handout 12.8: Improving Quality of Life with Assistive Devices may be used to help patients/clients select assistive devices for their needs.

See **Self-Care Handout 12.9: Fall Prevention Guidelines** for an adapted checklist for patients/clients who are at risk of falls (Altug 2018; Camacho *et al.* 2020; Centers for Disease Control and Prevention 2015; Liu-Ambrose *et al.* 2019; Montero-Odasso 2021; Montero-Odasso 2022; Zhou *et al.* 2020).

See **Self-Care Handout 12.10: Personal Safety Checklist** for strategies to keep patients/clients safe.

Self-Care Handout 12.1: Suggested Office Break Movements

Stand and perform any of the following activities throughout the day as a mini break:

- Heel raises 10 times.
- Pinch the shoulder blades together 10 times.
- Easy boxing punches 10 times.
- Gently turn the head right and then left 5 times.
- Open and close hands 10 times.
- March in place 10 times.
- Partially squat up and down 10 times.
- Partial push-ups against a wall 10 times.
- Gently shake the arms like a swimmer before a race for 10 seconds.

Also, consider a standing desk option to vary work positions and obtain relief from prolonged sitting during office work.

Self-Care Handout 12.2: Suggested Creative Office Break Solutions

- **Dartboard**: Install a dartboard.
- **Fitness court or gym**: Create a small indoor or outdoor fitness court or gym at the workplace, using simple features such as pull-ups, push-ups, and plank bars.
- **Fitness trail**: Create an outdoor fitness trail around the workplace using simple features such as pull-ups, push-ups, plank bars, a balance beam, a step-up bench, or parallel bars.
- **Foosball**: Place a foosball table in a break room.
- **Mini-basketball**: Install a small basketball rim on a door.
- **Pedometer pacing**: Download a pedometer app to track steps throughout the day.
- **Stair mail**: Take the stairs to deliver a message to a co-worker instead of always sending an email.
- **Table tennis**: Obtain a mini ping-pong table for the break room.
- **Tai chi break**: Perform a mini 5–10-minute tai chi program during lunchtime.
- **Walk club**: Form an office-wide walking club that meets before and after work or during lunch.
- **Walking meetings**: Hold small group creative meetings while walking.
- **Yoga break**: Perform a mini 5–10-minute yoga program during lunchtime.

Self-Care Handout 12.3: Joint Protection Techniques

General

Consider the following general tips to help reduce stress and strain on your joints. The key is to find strategies that work best for your needs.

- Modify daily tasks (e.g., try different bending strategies when picking up items from the floor).
- Use assistive devices as needed (e.g., use a reacher device to pick up small items from the floor).
- Alter movement patterns (e.g., alter your body position when washing dishes or vacuuming).
- Minimize prolonged positions (e.g., change positions periodically while at work or watching television).

Neck

Consider the following tips to see if they make your neck feel better. Make adjustments as needed.

- Minimize prolonged sitting positions (try no more than 30 minutes and see how that feels). For example, set your smartphone or other soft alarm next to your computer as a reminder to get up.
- Minimize lying on a sofa with your head propped too far forward for prolonged periods.
- Minimize prolonged sleeping on your stomach.
- Minimize clenching your jaw at rest. Make sure you have a relaxed "neutral" jaw position. In other words, your mouth should be closed lightly, with the lips together and teeth not touching. Rest the upper part of the tip of your tongue against the hard palate just behind your upper central incisors. This is also a good strategy to use for jaw pain (such as TMJ or temporomandibular joint disorder) or if you grind your teeth (also known as bruxism).
- Minimize prolonged neck bending during tasks such as texting (also known as "text neck"), reading, laptop use, sewing, writing, or any activity involving detailed work with the hands.
- Sleep on your side or back with your arms mostly below chest level.
- Store household items at levels that are not too high or too low.

Back

Consider the following tips to see if they make your back feel better. Make adjustments as needed.

- Minimize prolonged sitting positions (try no more than 30 minutes and see how that feels). For example, try the 30-30 strategy. Get up and move around for at least 30 seconds after 30 minutes of sitting.
- Minimize twisting at the waist when holding a heavy object.
- When lifting heavy items, try to bend at the hips and knees, not the waist.
- When lifting a heavy object, try tightening the abdominal muscles and then lift the item.

Self-Care Handout 12.4: Activity Pacing/ Energy Conservation Techniques

Activity pacing strategies may help you manage pain and fatigue. Consider the following tips to see if they make you feel better in your daily tasks:

- Identify activities that trigger discomfort or pain, and learn how to modify them.
- Determine the easiest and safest way to perform a task. For instance, is it easier to clean your bathtub using longer-handle tools?
- Try doing the most strenuous daily tasks when you have the most energy.
- Try alternating between easy and difficult tasks to help prevent overloading of the muscles and joints.
- Utilize brief rest periods during your daily chores and activities.
- Change the location of household equipment and supplies for easier access.
- Take advantage of labor-saving devices (such as a dishwasher) and tools (such as a power screwdriver).
- Simplify work tasks by planning ahead. For example, create a list to minimize unnecessary trips to the store.
- Use assistive devices (such as a cane or walker), braces, and splints as needed.
- Ask for help, or delegate tasks and chores when needed.

Self-Care Handout 12.5: Improved Body Mechanics with Daily Activities

Every person performs tasks in a slightly different manner. The key is to find the optimal movement strategies for your needs. For this reason, you may need to try several options to arrive at the best solution. Consider the following tips to see if they make you feel better in your daily tasks:

- Find optimal postures for your body and the tasks you need to perform.
- Plan ahead before you lift, carry, push, or pull a heavy item. For example, remove obstructions along your path. Decide how you are going to hold and move the object. Get help if the object is too heavy for you.
- Get a firm hold on an object you are moving so it won't slip. Some individuals find work gloves can be helpful.
- Try bending your knees and hips when lifting to see if this is easier on your back.
- Try keeping heavy objects close to your body.
- Minimize twisting your spine when lifting heavy objects.
- Try to maintain the normal arch in your lower back as you lift and carry. See if this is easier on your back.
- Use tools such as hoists, lifts, and dollies to avoid unnecessary heavy lifting and carrying.

Self-Care Handout 12.6: Shoe Fit and Selection Guidelines

The following are some shoe selection guidelines to help facilitate safe and comfortable exercise and physical activity:

- Have both feet measured at a shoe store for optimal fitting.
- Always try the shoes in the store instead of buying a pair based on the size.
- Consider purchasing shoes later in the day, since the feet may have some "swelling" toward the end of the day.
- Fit the shoes according to the larger foot size.
- The shoe length should be according to the longest toe, and there should be approximately a ½ inch of space between the longest toe and the tip of the shoe.
- Select shoes with a toe box large enough for the width of the foot.
- Match the shoe according to the activity (e.g., walking, running, basketball, cycling, cross-training, or general exercise).
- Change shoes approximately every 300– 500 miles of running or 300 hours of exercise, since the cushioning material in the shoe usually wears down. Track your athletic shoe mileage with an app or exercise journal.

Self-Care Handout 12.7: Optimizing Brain Health

Work with your physician, therapist, or healthcare provider to find, optimize, and individualize the following lifestyle strategies to help improve your quality of life:

- Start with a physical examination with your healthcare provider.
- Control and optimize blood pressure.
- Control and optimize blood sugar.
- Try a Mediterranean diet, or a whole food plant-predominant or plant-based approach.
- Include foods such as fish, blueberries, and olive oil in your diet.
- Engage in physical activities such as walking, dancing, hiking, or biking.
- Engage in resistance training exercises.
- Try mind-body activities such as tai chi, qigong, or yoga.
- Engage in social activities.
- Limit alcohol use (or avoid it altogether).
- Don't smoke.
- Get adequate sleep.
- Manage stress.
- Listen to music.
- Practice meditation.
- Use natural light or light therapy (especially in the morning) to improve mood and sleep.
- Try new activities such as learning a new language, exploring the internet, engaging in social media, learning to play an instrument, painting, drawing, singing, or creative writing.
- Try gardening.
- Try aromatherapy (such as lavender) for relaxation.
- Try virtual reality games.
- Minimize exposure to air pollution.
- Manage and prevent constipation to help reduce stress and anxiety.

Self-Care Handout 12.8: Improving Quality of Life with Assistive Devices

Work with your physician, nurse, physical therapist, or occupational therapist to find the best assistive devices and tools for your needs:

Mobility Aids	Self-Care Aids
• Walking stick (or trekking poles) • Cane • Crutches • Walker (front or four-wheeled walker) • Scooter • Wheelchair • Braces (such as for the knee)	• Electric toothbrush • Electric shaver • Adapted cooking utensils • Devices for dressing (such as for buttoning shirts or putting on shoes and socks)
Personal Safety Aids	**Work and Leisure Aids**
• Grab bars in bathroom • Rails along stairs • Long-handled reachers • Automated pill dispenser • Tub/shower chair • Nonslip bathmat or stickers	• Voice recognition software • Screen magnification software • Closed captioning • Book and paper holders • Pen and pencil grips
Association Resources	**Product Resources**
• American Nurses Association, www.nursingworld.org • American Occupational Therapy Association, www.aota.org • American Physical Therapy Association, www.apta.org • American Speech-Language-Hearing Association, www.asha.org	• School Specialty (physical education and special needs solutions to schools), www.schoolspecialty.com • Orthopedic Physical Therapy Products (OPTP), www.optp.com

Self-Care Handout 12.9: Fall Prevention Guidelines

Use this checklist and instructions from your healthcare provider to help prevent falls.

- ✓ Avoid being in a rush. For example, carry a cellular phone to avoid rushing to answer calls.
- ✓ Stay alert. For example, pay attention to your surroundings to prevent tripping over objects.
- ✓ Widen pathways in your home by rearranging furniture and removing clutter.
- ✓ Space your home furniture to allow comfortable maneuvering.
- ✓ Remove throw rugs that might cause you to slip or trip.
- ✓ Remove electrical cords that extend across the floor.
- ✓ Avoid highly polished floors.
- ✓ Hold on to sturdy handrails when going up and down stairs.
- ✓ Use nonskid mats.
- ✓ Install handrails in bathrooms (especially in the bathtub).
- ✓ Wear sturdy, low-heeled shoes.
- ✓ Ensure adequate lighting in the stairwells, hallways, and entrances.
- ✓ Keep stairs free of clutter.
- ✓ Provide adequate lighting throughout your house.
- ✓ Keep a flashlight in every room and near your bed for emergencies.
- ✓ Don't walk around your house in socks, especially on hardwood or tile floors.
- ✓ Avoid climbing ladders if you are unsteady.
- ✓ Avoid walking with your hands in your pockets.
- ✓ Be careful when carrying large items, like laundry baskets, that prevent you from seeing your walking path.
- ✓ Be careful when wearing long coats, dresses, night garments, or pants.
- ✓ Have your vision and blood pressure checked.
- ✓ Review medications with your physician.
- ✓ Work with a rehabilitation and fitness professional to create an effective home and community program that includes weight-bearing exercise (such as walking), resistance training (such as using bodyweight movements, elastic bands, or dumbbells), and a balance exercise program (such as tai chi, multidirectional stepping, or slow march in place).
- ✓ Include indoor and outdoor multisurface terrain training (such as carpets, wood floors, grass, sidewalk, stairs, and curbs) in your rehabilitation and fitness routine.

Self-Care Handout 12.10: Personal Safety Checklist

Home Safety

- Minimize the use of step stools and step ladders to avoid falls.
- Keep your medications and emergency and medical contacts on your phone and/or in your wallet or purse.

Also, make sure your home has the following:

- Emergency flashlights
- Emergency supplies (such as food, water, and first-aid kits)
- Fire extinguishers
- Smoke detectors

Car Safety

- Don't drink alcohol and drive.
- Don't text while driving.
- Drive courteously.
- Follow speed limit guidelines.
- Always wear your seat belt.
- Minimize horn-honking (unless needed as a safety alert) to avoid potential conflict with other motorists.

Outdoor Fitness Safety

- Wear bright colors when going for a fitness walk or bike ride or exercising at night to make yourself more visible to motorists. Also, carry a flashlight for your evening walk.
- Use the "buddy system" and exercise with a training partner or friend when going into the wilderness or swimming.
- Dress appropriately for weather conditions and bring a smartphone.

Self-Management Activities: Explore Astronomy

The following online resources can help patients/clients, healthcare providers, and health/fitness professionals to manage stress and anxiety by exploring astronomy.

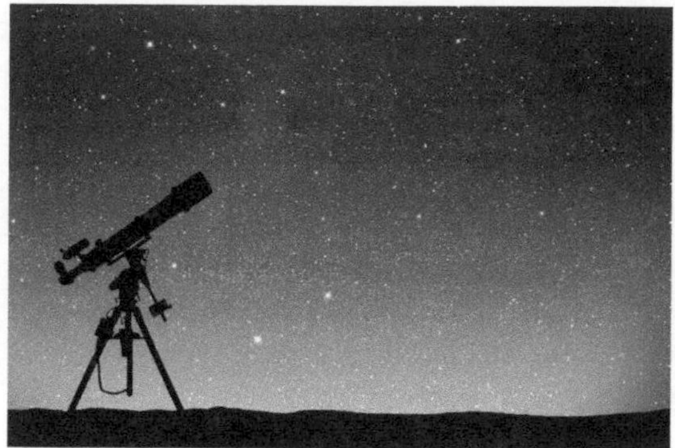

Astronomy for relaxation

- The Astronomy Picture of the Day site provides a different image or photograph every day and serves as an educational and relaxation tool: https://apod.nasa.gov/apod/astropix.html
- The Hubble Space Telescope site provides images and videos to learn about space: https://hubblesite.org
- The NASA app provides images, videos on demand, and news and feature stories to learn about various space missions: www.nasa.gov/nasaapp
- The Night Sky app provides a fun way to learn about space and the night sky: https://nightsky.com
- The SkyView app provides a fun way to learn about space and the night sky: www.terminaleleven.com/skyview/iphone

Classroom and Lab Activities

- Try different supine or seated meditation styles (e.g., body scan meditation, guided imagery, progressive muscle relaxation, self-hypnosis). What are the common characteristics of each style?
- How can each style of meditation be adapted for the clinic, home, and work setting for a person in pain?
- Examine and try various self-massage styles (e.g., acupressure, massage with multiple tools). How can each style be adapted for the home or work setting for a person in pain?
- Analyze different body positions used by various professionals who have

back pain. For example, how would you improve body mechanics for the following professions?
  - Cashier scanning and bagging groceries
  - Construction worker digging
  - Dentist and dental hygienist examining a patient's mouth
  - Nurse getting a patient out of bed
  - Physical therapist transferring a patient from a wheelchair to an exercise table
  - Surgeon standing at an operating room table
- What type of microbreaks would be ideal for various occupations?

Useful Clinical Resources

Therapy-Related Course Information

- Physiopedia, www.physio-pedia.com
- Physiospot, www.physiospot.com
- Plus by Physiopedia, https://members.physio-pedia.com

Selected Physiotherapy Organizations

- American Physical Therapy Association, www.apta.org
- Australian Physiotherapy Association, https://australian.physio
- Canadian Physiotherapy Association, https://physiotherapy.ca
- Chartered Society of Physiotherapy, www.csp.org.uk
- Finnish Association of Physiotherapists, www.suomenfysioterapeutit.fi
- French National Council of Physiotherapists, www.ordremk.fr
- German Association for Physiotherapy, www.physio-deutschland.de
- Indian Association of Physiotherapists, www.physiotherapyindia.org
- Irish Society of Chartered Physiotherapists, www.iscp.ie
- Italian Association of Physiotherapy, https://aifi.net
- Japanese Physical Therapy Association, www.japanpt.or.jp/english
- Nigeria Society of Physiotherapy, www.nsphysio.org
- Order of Physiotherapists, https://ordemdosfisioterapeutas.pt
- Panhellenic Physiotherapists' Association, www.psf.org.gr
- Philippine Physical Therapy Association, www.philpta.org
- Physioswiss, www.physioswiss.ch/de
- Physiotherapists' Association of Brazil, https://world.physio/membership/brazil
- Physiotherapy New Zealand, https://pnz.org.nz
- Royal Dutch Society for Physiotherapy, www.kngf.nl

- South African Society of Physiotherapy, www.saphysio.co.za
- Spanish Association of Physiotherapists, https://aefi.net
- Swedish Association of Physiotherapists, www.fysioterapeuterna.se
- Turkish Physiotherapy Association, www.fizyoterapistler.org.tr
- World Physiotherapy, https://world.physio
- World Physiotherapy (global physiotherapy associations), https://world.physio/our-members

Organizations

- American College of Lifestyle Medicine, https://lifestylemedicine.org
- American College of Sports Medicine, www.acsm.org
- American Nurses Association, www.nursingworld.org
- American Occupational Therapy Association, www.aota.org
- American Speech-Language-Hearing Association, www.asha.org
- International Federations of Aromatherapists, https://ifaroma.org
- National Center for Complementary and Integrative Health, www.nccih.nih.gov
- National Institutes of Health—Division of Occupational Health and Safety, www.ors.od.nih.gov/sr/dohs/Pages/default.aspx
- National Strength and Conditioning Association, www.nsca.com
- United States Department of Labor, Occupational Safety and Health Administration, Ergonomics, www.osha.gov/ergonomics
- World Health Organization, Rehabilitation Resource Repository, https://resources.relabhs.org

Patient Education Information for Therapy and Wellness

- ChoosePT (American Physical Therapy Association), www.choosept.com
- Harvard Health, www.health.harvard.edu
- Mayo Clinic (health information), www.mayoclinic.org
- MedlinePlus, https://medlineplus.gov
- OMNI Self-Care, www.omniself.care
- OrthoInfo (American Academy of Orthopedic Surgeons), https://orthoinfo.aaos.org
- Tame the Beast: It's Time to Rethink Persistent Pain, www.tamethebeast.org
- This Way Up, https://thiswayup.org.au
- UCLA Ergonomics (see "Workstation Setups"), www.ergonomics.ucla.edu
- WebMD, www.webmd.com

Therapy-Related Course Information

- Active Release Techniques, https://activerelease.com
- American Physical Therapy Association Learning Center, https://learningcenter.apta.org
- Barral Institute, Visceral Manipulation, www.barralinstitute.com
- Graston Technique, https://grastontechnique.com
- Gua Sha (Arya Nielsen, Ph.D.), http://guasha.com
- McKenzie Institute, www.mckenzieinstituteusa.org
- Myofascial Cupping (Rocktape), www.rocktape.com
- Myo Fascial Decompression, www.cuptherapy.com
- Myopain Seminars Dry Needling, www.myopainseminars.com
- Physiopedia/Physioplus, www.physio-pedia.com
- Strain Counterstrain, www.jicounterstrain.com
- Therapy Insights, https://therapyinsights.com

Rehabilitation and Therapy Products

- Arnicare Gel (topical pain relief), www.arnicare.com
- Chattanooga (rehabilitation equipment), www.chattanoogarehab.com
- Enovis (braces), www.djoglobal.com
- Helix Cream (topical pain relief), https://helix4pain.com/professional
- Hyperice (self-care massage, recovery, and meditation tools), https://hyperice.com
- Kinesiotape (taping resource center), https://kinesiotape.com
- Medi (orthoses/braces, supports, insoles, compression garments), www.medi.de/en
- Mueller Sports Medicine (sports medicine supplies), www.muellersportsmed.com
- Orthopedic Physical Therapy Products (therapy, rehab, fitness products), www.optp.com
- Össur Braces (braces, supports), www.ossur.com/en-us
- REI (outdoor fitness products), www.rei.com
- Salonpas (pain relief patch), https://us.hisamitsu
- Seca (bodyweight scales), www.seca.com/en_us.html
- Serola Biomechanics (sacroiliac belt), www.serola.net
- Spray and Stretch (Gebauer Company) (topical anesthetic vapocoolant for myofascial pain and trigger point release), www.gebauer.com/sprayandstretch
- Symbyx Biome (for chronic pain, Parkinson's), https://symbyxbiome.com
- Tanita (bodyweight scales), www.tanita.com/en

Pain Management Resources

- Back Doctor/Pain Relief (Robert Watkins, MD) (back exercise guide), https://apps.apple.com/us/app/back-doctor-pain-relief/id1218493415
- Chronic Pain Tracker, http://chronicpaintracker.com
- Curable (pain management), www.curablehealth.com
- Manage My Pain (pain management), https://managemypainapp.com
- My Pain Diary (pain management), http://mypaindiary.com
- Noigroup, www.noigroup.com
- PainScale (pain management), www.painscale.com
- Recognise app (pain management), www.noigroup.com/product/recogniseapp

Integrative Medicine Resources

- Acupuncture Today (acupuncture news), www.acupuncturetoday.com
- Acupuncture.com (acupuncture, cupping, gua sha, massage supplies), www.goacupuncture.com
- Lhasa OMS (acupuncture, cupping, gua sha, massage supplies), www.lhasaoms.com
- UCLA Center for East-West Medicine (professional teaching programs), www.uclahealth.org/locations/center-east-west-medicine

Home Wellness Resources

- Avocado (sleep mattress), www.avocadogreenmattress.com
- Beurer (blood pressure monitors, bodyweight scales, pulse oximeters, TENS units, light therapy products), www.beurer.com/web/us
- Health-o-Meter (bodyweight scales), www.healthometer.com
- OMRON (blood pressure monitors, pedometers, TENS units), https://omronhealthcare.com

Ergonomic Resources

- Ergo Desk (mini reading stands), https://ergodesk.com
- Health by Design (office chairs, desks, and computer accessories), https://healthydesign.com
- HermanMiller (office chairs), www.hermanmiller.com
- Humanscale (seating, standing desks, monitor arms, lighting), www.humanscale.com
- Relax the Back (back wellness products), https://relaxtheback.com

- UCLA Ergonomics (ergonomic information), www.ergonomics.ucla.edu
- US Occupational Safety and Health Department (work safety information), www.osha.gov
- Vari (standing desks), www.vari.com
- The YogaBack Company (adjustable sacral-lower thoracic support), www.yogaback.com

Patient Education and Counseling Information for Healthcare Providers: Sex and Back Pain

- Hebert LA. *Sex and Back Pain*, 3rd ed. Greenville, ME: Impacc USA; 1997.
- Sidorkewicz N, McGill SM. Documenting female spine motion during coitus with a commentary on the implications for the low back pain patient. *Eur Spine J*. 2015;24(3):513–520.
- Sidorkewicz N, McGill SM. Male spine motion during coitus: implications for the low back pain patient. *Spine (Phila Pa 1976)*. 2014;39(20):1633–1639.

References

Abbasijahromi A, Hojati H, Nikooei S, *et al.* Compare the effect of aromatherapy using lavender and Damask rose essential oils on the level of anxiety and severity of pain following C-section: a double-blinded randomized clinical trial. *J Complement Integr Med.* 2020;17(3):10.1515/jcim-2019-0141.

Abbott R, Ayres I, Hui E, Hui KK. Effect of perineal self-acupressure on constipation: a randomized controlled trial. *J Gen Intern Med.* 2015;30(4):434–439.

Abonie US, Edwards AM, Hettinga FJ. Optimising activity pacing to promote a physically active lifestyle in medical settings: a narrative review informed by clinical and sports pacing research. *J Sports Sci.* 2020;38(5):590–596.

Akca NK, Aydin G, Gumus K. Effect of body mechanics brief education in the clinical setting on pain patients with lumbar disc hernia: a randomized controlled trial. *Int J Caring Sci.* 2017;10:1498–1506.

Altug Z. Joint protection guide for older adults. *GeriNotes* (Section on Geriatrics, American Physical Therapy Association). 2010;17(5):11.

Altug Z. Energy conservation guide for older adults. *GeriNotes* (Section on Geriatrics, American Physical Therapy Association). 2011;18(1):8.

Altug Z. Constipation and low back pain in an athlete: a case report. *Orthopaedic Physical Therapy Practice.* 2016;28(3):188–192.

Altug Z. *Integrative Healing: Developing Wellness in the Mind and Body.* Springville, UT: Cedar Fort, Inc; 2018.

Armstrong DP, Fischer SL. Understanding individual differences in lifting mechanics: do some people adopt motor control strategies that minimize biomechanical exposure? *Hum Mov Sci.* 2020;74:102689.

Aydinli A, Karadağ S. Effects of abdominal massage applied with ginger and lavender oil for elderly with constipation: a randomized controlled trial [published online ahead of print, 2022 Aug 20]. *Explore (NY).* 2022;S1550-8307(22)00152-5.

Bartholdy C, Klokker L, Bandak E, Bliddal H, Henriksen M. A standardized "Rescue" exercise program for symptomatic flare-up of knee osteoarthritis: description and safety considerations. *J Orthop Sports Phys Ther.* 2016;46(11):942–946.

Beach TAC, Stankovic T, Carnegie DR, Micay R, Frost DM. Using verbal instructions to influence lifting mechanics: does the directive "lift with your legs, not your back" attenuate spinal flexion? *J Electromyogr Kinesiol.* 2018;38:1–6.

Becher R, Øvrevik J, Schwarze PE, Nilsen S, Hongslo JK, Bakke JV. Do carpets impair indoor air quality and cause adverse health outcomes? A review. *Int J Environ Res Public Health.* 2018;15(2):184.

Blackburn LM, Abel S, Green L, Johnson K, Panda S. The use of comfort kits to optimize adult cancer pain management. *Pain Manag Nurs.* 2019;20(1):25–31.

Blazer MM, Jamrog LB, Schnack LL. Does the shoe fit? Considerations for proper shoe fitting. *Orthop Nurs*. 2018;37(3):169–174.

Blehm C, Vishnu S, Khattak A, Mitra S, Yee RW. Computer vision syndrome: a review. *Surv Ophthalmol*. 2005;50(3):253–262.

Brown MT, Bussell J, Dutta S, Davis K, Strong S, Mathew S. Medication adherence: truth and consequences. *Am J Med Sci*. 2016;351(4):387–399.

Buttagat V, Techakhot P, Wiriya W, Mueller M, Areeudomwong P. Effectiveness of traditional Thai self-massage combined with stretching exercises for the treatment of patients with chronic non-specific low back pain: a single-blinded randomized controlled trial. *J Bodyw Mov Ther*. 2020;24(1):19–24.

Camacho PM, Petak SM, Binkley N, *et al.* American Association of Clinical Endocrinologists/American College of Endocrinology Clinical Practice Guidelines for the Diagnosis and Treatment of Postmenopausal Osteoporosis—2020 Update. *Endocr Pract*. 2020;26(Suppl 1):1–46.

Centers for Disease Control and Prevention. *Check for Safety: A Home Fall Prevention Checklist for Older Adults*; 2015. www.cdc.gov/steadi/pdf/check_for_safety_brochure-a.pdf

Cheatham CL, Canipe LG 3rd, Millsap G, *et al.* Six-month intervention with wild blueberries improved speed of processing in mild cognitive decline: a double-blind, placebo-controlled, randomized clinical trial [published online ahead of print, 2022 Sep 6]. *Nutr Neurosci*. 2022;1–15.

Chen X, Maguire B, Brodaty H, O'Leary F. Dietary patterns and cognitive health in older adults: a systematic review [published correction appears in *J Alzheimers Dis*. 2019;69(2):595–596]. *J Alzheimers Dis*. 2019;67(2):583–619.

Cheng HY, Carol S, Wu B, Cheng YF. Effect of acupressure on postpartum low back pain, salivary cortisol, physical limitations, and depression: a randomized controlled pilot study. *J Tradit Chin Med*. 2020;40(1):128–136.

Chételat G, Lutz A, Klimecki O, *et al.* Effect of an 18-month meditation training on regional brain volume and perfusion in older adults: the age-well randomized clinical trial. *JAMA Neurol*. 2022;79(11):1165–1174.

Chey SW, Chey WD, Jackson K, Eswaran S. Exploratory comparative effectiveness trial of green kiwifruit, psyllium, or prunes in US patients with chronic constipation. *Am J Gastroenterol*. 2021;116(6):1304–1312.

Chou R, Deyo R, Friedly J, *et al.* Nonpharmacologic therapies for low back pain: a systematic review for an American College of Physicians clinical practice guideline. *Ann Intern Med*. 2017;166(7):493–505.

Coenen P, Parry S, Willenberg L, *et al.* Associations of prolonged standing with musculoskeletal symptoms—a systematic review of laboratory studies. *Gait & Posture*. 2017;58:310–318.

Coles-Brennan C, Sulley A, Young G. Management of digital eye strain. *Clin Exp Optom*. 2019;102(1):18–29.

Cook SD, Kester MA, Brunet ME. Shock absorption characteristics of running shoes. *Am J Sports Med*. 1985;13(4):248–253.

Cramer H, Klose P, Teut M, *et al.* Cupping for patients with chronic pain: a systematic review and meta-analysis. *J Pain*. 2020;21(9–10):943–956.

Doğan İG, Gürşen C, Akbayrak T, *et al.* Abdominal massage in functional chronic constipation: a randomized placebo-controlled trial. *Phys Ther*. 2022;102(7):pzac058.

Du S, Hu L, Dong J, *et al.* Self-management program for chronic low back pain: a systematic review and meta-analysis. *Patient Educ Couns*. 2017;100(1):37–49.

Durmuş İskender M, Çalışkan N. Effect of acupressure and abdominal massage on constipation in patients with total knee arthroplasty: a randomized controlled study. *Clin Nurs Res*. 2022;31(3):453–462.

Dymond A, Mealing S, McMaster J, Holmes H, Owen L. Indoor air quality at home—an economic analysis. *Int J Environ Res Public Health*. 2021;18(4):1679.

Ebrahimi H, Mardani A, Basirinezhad MH, Hamidzadeh A, Eskandari F. The effects of lavender and chamomile essential oil inhalation aromatherapy on depression, anxiety and stress in older community-dwelling people: a randomized controlled trial. *Explore (NY)*. 2022;18(3):272–278.

Efe Ertürk N, Taşcı S. The effects of peppermint oil on nausea, vomiting and retching in cancer patients undergoing chemotherapy: an open label quasi-randomized controlled pilot study. *Complement Ther Med*. 2021;56:102587.

Eyre HA, Siddarth P, Acevedo B, *et al.* A randomized controlled trial of Kundalini yoga in mild cognitive impairment. *Int Psychogeriatr*. 2017;29(4):557–567.

Fan Z, Di A, Huang F, *et al.* The effectiveness and safety of Tuina for tension-type headache: a systematic review and meta-analysis. *Complement Ther Clin Pract*. 2021;43:101293.

Flexner LM, Hertling D. The temporomandibular joint. In: Brody LT, Hall CM. *Therapeutic Exercise: Moving Toward Function,* 4th ed. Baltimore, MD: Wolters Kluwer; 2018.

FootCareMD, American Orthopaedic Foot & Ankle Society. How to select athletic shoes; 2023. www.footcaremd.org/resources/how-to-help/how-to-select-athletic-shoes

French SD, Nielsen M, Hall L, *et al.* Essential key messages about diagnosis, imaging, and self-care for people with low back pain: a modified Delphi study of consumer and expert opinions. *Pain.* 2019;160(12):2787–2797.

Gao R, Tao Y, Zhou C, *et al.* Exercise therapy in patients with constipation: a systematic review and meta-analysis of randomized controlled trials. *Scand J Gastroenterol.* 2019;54(2):169–177.

Gaowgzeh RA, Chevidikunnan MF, Al Saif A, El-Gendy S, Karrouf G, Al Senany S. Prevalence of and risk factors for low back pain among dentists. *J Phys Ther Sci.* 2015;27(9):2803–2806.

Ge W, Leson C, Vukovic C. Dry cupping for plantar fasciitis: a randomized controlled trial. *J Phys Ther Sci.* 2017;29(5):859–862.

George SE, Borello-France DF. Perspective on physical therapist management of functional constipation. *Phys Ther.* 2017;97(4):478–493.

Gerber L, Furst G, Shulman B, *et al.* Patient education program to teach energy conservation behaviors to patients with rheumatoid arthritis: a pilot study. *Archives of Physical Medicine and Rehabilitation.* 1987;68(7):442–445.

Ghaderi F, Solhjou N. The effects of lavender aromatherapy on stress and pain perception in children during dental treatment: a randomized clinical trial. *Complement Ther Clin Pract.* 2020;40:101182.

Godley E, Smith MA. Efficacy of acupressure for chronic low back pain: a systematic review. *Complement Ther Clin Pract.* 2020;39:101146.

Gorce P, Jacquier-Bret J. Global prevalence of musculoskeletal disorders among physiotherapists: a systematic review and meta-analysis. *BMC Musculoskelet Disord.* 2023;24(1):265.

Guo D, Ma S, Zhao Y, Dong J, Guo B, Li X. Self-administered acupressure and exercise for patients with osteoarthritis: a randomized controlled trial. *Clin Rehabil.* 2022;36(3):350–358.

Gyer G, Michael J, Inklebarger J. Occupational hand injuries: a current review of the prevalence and proposed prevention strategies for physical therapists and similar healthcare professionals. *J Integr Med.* 2018;16(2):84–89.

Hammond A, Freeman K. The long-term outcomes from a randomized controlled trial of an educational-behavioural joint protection programme for people with rheumatoid arthritis. *Clin Rehabil.* 2004;18(5):520–528.

Harrington KL, Haskvitz EM. Managing a patient's constipation with physical therapy. *Phys Ther.* 2006;86(11):1511–1519.

He Y, Guo X, May BH, *et al.* Clinical evidence for association of acupuncture and acupressure with improved cancer pain: a systematic review and meta-analysis. *JAMA Oncol.* 2020;6(2):271–278.

Ho MH, Chang HCR, Liu MF, Yuan L, Montayre J. Effectiveness of acupoint pressure on older people with constipation in nursing homes: a double-blind quasi-experimental study. *Contemp Nurse.* 2020a;56(5–6):417–427.

Ho RTH, Fong TCT, Chan WC, *et al.* Psychophysiological effects of dance movement therapy and physical exercise on older adults with mild dementia: a randomized controlled trial. *J Gerontol B Psychol Sci Soc Sci.* 2020b;75(3):560–570.

Hochberg MC, Altman RD, April KT, *et al.* American College of Rheumatology 2012 recommendations for the use of nonpharmacologic and pharmacologic therapies in osteoarthritis of the hand, hip, and knee. *Arthritis Care Res (Hoboken).* 2012;64(4):465–474.

Hoult L, Longstaff L, Moss, M. Prolonged low-level exposure to the aroma of peppermint essential oil enhances aspects of cognition and mood in healthy adults. *American Journal of Plant Sciences.* 2019;10:1002–1012.

Hruska B, Pressman SD, Bendinskas K, Gump BB. Do vacations alter the connection between stress and cardiovascular activity? The effects of a planned vacation on the relationship between weekly stress and ambulatory heart rate. *Psychol Health.* 2020;35(8):984–999.

Hsieh SH, Wu CR, Romadlon DS, Hasan F, Chen PY, Chiu HY. The effect of acupressure on relieving cancer-related fatigue: a systematic review and meta-analysis of randomized controlled trials. *Cancer Nurs.* 2021;44(6):e578–e588.

Huang X, Zhao X, Li B, *et al.* Comparative efficacy of various exercise interventions on cognitive function in patients with mild cognitive impairment or dementia: a systematic review and network meta-analysis. *J Sport Health Sci.* 2022;11(2):212–223.

Hughes D, Judge C, Murphy R, *et al.* Association of blood pressure lowering with incident dementia or cognitive impairment: a systematic review and meta-analysis. *JAMA.* 2020;323(19):1934–1944.

Ishiyama Y, Hoshide S, Mizuno H, Kario K. Constipation-induced pressor effects as triggers for cardiovascular events. *J Clin Hypertens (Greenwich).* 2019;21(3):421–425.

Iversen MD, Westby MD. Arthritis. In: O'Sullivan SB, Schmitz TJ, Fulk GD. *Physical Rehabilitation,* 6th ed. Philadelphia, PA: FA Davis; 2014.

Jang H, Kim S, Kim B, Kim M, Jung J, Won CW. Functional constipation is associated with a decline in word recognition 2 years later in community-dwelling older adults: the Korean frailty and aging cohort study. *Ann Geriatr Med Res.* 2022;26(3):241–247.

Járomi M, Kukla A, Szilágyi B, *et al.* Back School programme for nurses has reduced low back pain levels: a randomised controlled trial. *J Clin Nurs*. 2018;27(5–6):e895–e902.

Jodaki K, Abdi K, Mousavi MS, *et al.* Effect of rosa damascene aromatherapy on anxiety and sleep quality in cardiac patients: a randomized controlled trial. *Complement Ther Clin Pract*. 2021;42:101299.

Kaddoumi A, Denney TS Jr, Deshpande G, *et al.* Extra-virgin olive oil enhances the blood-brain barrier function in mild cognitive impairment: a randomized controlled trial. *Nutrients*. 2022;14(23):5102.

Kalkdijk J, Broens P, Ten Broek R, *et al.* Functional constipation in patients with hemorrhoids: a systematic review and meta-analysis. *Eur J Gastroenterol Hepatol*. 2022;34(8):813–822.

Kanwar A, Thakur M, Wazzan M, *et al.* Clothing and shoes of personnel as potential vectors for transfer of health care-associated pathogens to the community. *Am J Infect Control*. 2019;47(5):577–579.

Kivimäki M, Jokela M, Nyberg ST, *et al.* Long working hours and risk of coronary heart disease and stroke: a systematic review and meta-analysis of published and unpublished data for 603,838 individuals. *Lancet*. 2015;386(10005):1739–1746.

Kling HE, Moore KJ, Brannan D, Caban-Martinez AJ. Walking meeting effects on productivity and mood among white-collar workers: evidence from the walking meeting pilot study. *J Occup Environ Med*. 2021;63(2):e75–e79.

Koch M, Fitzpatrick AL, Rapp SR, *et al.* Alcohol consumption and risk of dementia and cognitive decline among older adults with or without mild cognitive impairment. *JAMA Netw Open*. 2019;2(9):e1910319.

Kolberg E, Hjetland GJ, Thun E, *et al.* The effects of bright light treatment on affective symptoms in people with dementia: a 24-week cluster randomized controlled trial. *BMC Psychiatry*. 2021;21(1):377.

Kongsted A, Ris I, Kjaer P, Hartvigsen J. Self-management at the core of back pain care: 10 key points for clinicians. *Braz J Phys Ther*. 2021;25(4):396–406.

Koyama T, Nagata N, Nishiura K, Miura N, Kawai T, Yamamoto H. Prune juice containing sorbitol, pectin, and polyphenol ameliorates subjective complaints and hard feces while normalizing stool in chronic constipation: a randomized placebo-controlled trial. *Am J Gastroenterol*. 2022;117(10):1714–1717.

Kreye G, Wasl M, Dietz A, *et al.* Aromatherapy in palliative care: a single-institute retrospective analysis evaluating the effect of lemon oil pads against nausea and vomiting in advanced cancer patients. *Cancers (Basel)*. 2022;14(9):2131.

Kühn L, MacIntyre UE, Kotzé C, Becker PJ, Wenhold FAM. Twelve weeks of additional fish intake improves the cognition of cognitively intact, resource-limited elderly people: a randomized control trial. *J Nutr Health Aging*. 2022;26(2):119–126.

Lanier VM, Lang CE, van Dillen LR. Motor skill training in musculoskeletal pain: a case report in chronic low back pain. *Disabil Rehabil*. 2019;41(17):2071–2079.

Lauche R, Wübbeling K, Lüdtke R, *et al.* Randomized controlled pilot study: pain intensity and pressure pain thresholds in patients with neck and low back pain before and after traditional East Asian "gua sha" therapy. *Am J Chin Med*. 2012;40(5):905–917.

Lavé A, Gondar R, Demetriades AK, Meling TR. Ergonomics and musculoskeletal disorders in neurosurgery: a systematic review. *Acta Neurochir (Wien)*. 2020;162(9):2213–2220.

Lebel ED, Finnegan CJ, Ouyang Z, Jackson RB. Methane and NO*x* emissions from natural gas stoves, cooktops, and ovens in residential homes [published correction appears in *Environ Sci Technol*. 2022 May 17;56(10):6791]. *Environ Sci Technol*. 2022;56(4):2529–2539.

Letafatkar A, Rabiei P, Alamooti G, Bertozzi L, Farivar N, Afshari M. Effect of therapeutic exercise routine on pain, disability, posture, and health status in dentists with chronic neck pain: a randomized controlled trial. *Int Arch Occup Environ Health*. 2020;93(3):281–290.

Li J, Yuan M, Liu Y, Zhao Y, Wang J, Guo W. Incidence of constipation in stroke patients: a systematic review and meta-analysis. *Medicine (Baltimore)*. 2017;96(25):e7225.

Li R, Chen X, Zhao Y. Potential triggering factors associated with aneurysmal subarachnoid hemorrhage: a large single-center retrospective study. *J Clin Hypertens (Greenwich)*. 2022;24(7):861–869.

Lim YZ, Chou L, Au RT, *et al.* People with low back pain want clear, consistent and personalised information on prognosis, treatment options and self-management strategies: a systematic review. *J Physiother*. 2019;65(3):124–135.

Lindberg JE, Quinn MM, Gore RJ, *et al.* Assessment of home care aides' respiratory exposure to total volatile organic compounds and chlorine during simulated bathroom cleaning: an experimental design with conventional and "green" products. *J Occup Environ Hyg*. 2021;18(6):276–287.

Liu DM, Wang L, Huang LJ. Tai chi improves cognitive function of dementia patients: a systematic review and meta-analysis. *Altern Ther Health Med*. 2023;29(1):90–96.

Liu-Ambrose T, Davis JC, Best JR, *et al.* Effect of a home-based exercise program on subsequent falls among community-dwelling high-risk older adults after a fall: a randomized clinical trial [published correction appears in *JAMA*. 2019 Jul 9;322(2):174]. *JAMA*. 2019;321(21):2092–2100.

Luger T, Maher CG, Rieger MA, Steinhilber B. Work-break schedules for preventing musculoskeletal symptoms and disorders in healthy workers. *Cochrane Database Syst Rev*. 2019;7(7):CD012886.

Marcum ZA, Hanlon JT, Murray MD. Improving medication adherence and health outcomes in older adults: an evidence-based review of randomized controlled trials. *Drugs Aging*. 2017;34(3):191–201.

Masiero S, Boniolo A, Wassermann L, Machiedo H, Volante D, Punzi L. Effects of an educational-behavioral joint protection program on people with moderate to severe rheumatoid arthritis: a randomized controlled trial. *Clin Rheumatol*. 2007;26(12):2043–2050.

Mathiowetz VG, Finlayson ML, Matuska KM, *et al.* Randomized controlled trial of an energy conservation course for persons with multiple sclerosis. *Multiple Sclerosis*. 2005;11(5):592–601.

McCurry SM, Pike KC, Vitiello MV, Logsdon RG, Larson EB, Teri L. Increasing walking and bright light exposure to improve sleep in community-dwelling persons with Alzheimer's disease: results of a randomized, controlled trial. *J Am Geriatr Soc*. 2011;59(8):1393–1402.

McGill SM. *Low Back Disorders*, 3rd ed. Champaign, IL: Human Kinetics; 2016.

McLean L, Tingley M, Scott RN, Rickards J. Computer terminal work and the benefit of microbreaks. *Appl Ergon*. 2001;32(3):225–237.

Meesters JAJ, Nijkamp MM, Schuur AG, te Biesebeek JD. *Cleaning Products Fact Sheet: Default Parameters for Estimating Consumer Exposure: Updated Version 2018*. Bilthoven, Netherlands: National Institute for Public Health and the Environment; 2018.

Meesters JAJ, te Biesebeek JD, ter Burg W. *Air Fresheners Fact Sheet: Default Parameters for Estimating Consumer Exposure: Version 2021*. Bilthoven, Netherlands: National Institute for Public Health and the Environment; 2022.

Meng F, Duan PB, Zhu J, *et al.* Effect of gua sha therapy on perimenopausal syndrome: a randomized controlled trial. *Menopause*. 2017;24(3):299–307.

Meng XD, Guo HR, Zhang QY, *et al.* The effectiveness of cupping therapy on chronic fatigue syndrome: a single-blind randomized controlled trial. *Complement Ther Clin Pract*. 2020;40:101210.

Milhem M, Kalichman L, Ezra D, Alperovitch-Najenson D. Work-related musculoskeletal disorders among physical therapists: a comprehensive narrative review. *Int J Occup Med Environ Health*. 2016;29(5):735–747.

Modi RM, Hinton A, Pinkhas D, *et al.* Implementation of a defecation posture modification device: impact on bowel movement patterns in healthy subjects. *J Clin Gastroenterol*. 2019;53(3):216–219.

Mohammadi S, Roostayi MM, Naimi SS, Baghban AA. The effects of cupping therapy as a new approach in the physiotherapeutic management of carpal tunnel syndrome. *Physiother Res Int*. 2019;24(3):e1770.

Montero-Odasso M, van der Velde N, Martin FC, *et al.* World guidelines for falls prevention and management for older adults: a global initiative. *Age Ageing*. 2022;51(9):afac205.

Montero-Odasso MM, Kamkar N, Pieruccini-Faria F, *et al.* Evaluation of clinical practice guidelines on fall prevention and management for older adults: a systematic review. *JAMA Netw Open*. 2021;4(12):e2138911.

Moss M, Hewitt S, Moss L, Wesnes K. Modulation of cognitive performance and mood by aromas of peppermint and ylang-ylang. *Int J Neurosci*. 2008;118(1):59–77.

Müller-Lissner S, Bassotti G, Coffin B, *et al.* Opioid-induced constipation and bowel dysfunction: a clinical guideline. *Pain Med*. 2017;18(10):1837–1863.

Murphy SL, Harris RE, Keshavarzi NR, Zick SM. Self-administered acupressure for chronic low back pain: a randomized controlled pilot trial. *Pain Med*. 2019;20(12):2588–2597.

Murphy SL, Smith DM, Lyden AK. Type of activity pacing instruction affects physical activity variability in adults with symptomatic knee or hip osteoarthritis. *J Phys Act Health*. 2012;9(3):360–366.

Nakase T, Tatewaki Y, Thyreau B, *et al.* Impact of constipation on progression of Alzheimer's disease: a retrospective study. *CNS Neurosci Ther*. 2022;28(12):1964–1973.

Nassif MS, Costa ICP, Ribeiro PM, Moura CC, Oliveira PE. Integrative and complementary practices to control nausea and vomiting in pregnant women: a systematic review. *Rev Esc Enferm USP*. 2022;56:e20210515.

National Institute for Occupational Safety and Health. Back belts: do they prevent injury? Centers for Disease Control and Prevention; 2023. www.cdc.gov/niosh/docs/94-127/default.html

Ngandu T, Lehtisalo J, Solomon A, *et al.* A 2 year multidomain intervention of diet, exercise, cognitive training, and vascular risk monitoring versus control to prevent cognitive decline in at-risk elderly people (FINGER): a randomised controlled trial. *Lancet*. 2015;385(9984):2255–2263.

Ni CH, Hou WH, Kao CC, *et al.* The anxiolytic effect of aromatherapy on patients awaiting ambulatory surgery: a randomized controlled trial. *Evid Based Complement Alternat Med*. 2013:927419.

Pach D, Piper M, Lotz F, *et al.* Effectiveness and cost-effectiveness of tuina for chronic neck pain: a randomized controlled trial comparing tuina with a no-intervention waiting list. *J Altern Complement Med.* 2018;24(3):231–237.

Palacio A, Garay D, Langer B, Taylor J, Wood BA, Tamariz L. Motivational interviewing improves medication adherence: a systematic review and meta-analysis. *J Gen Intern Med.* 2016;31(8):929–940.

Park AE, Zahiri HR, Hallbeck MS, *et al.* Intraoperative "micro breaks" with targeted stretching enhance surgeon physical function and mental focus: a multicenter cohort study. *Ann Surg.* 2017;265(2):340–346.

Penninkilampi R, Casey AN, Singh MF, Brodaty H. The association between social engagement, loneliness, and risk of dementia: a systematic review and meta-analysis. *J Alzheimers Dis.* 2018;66(4):1619–1633.

Peters R, Ee N, Peters J, Booth A, Mudway I, Anstey KJ. Air pollution and dementia: a systematic review. *J Alzheimers Dis.* 2019;70(S1):S145–S163.

Peters R, Xu Y, Fitzgerald O, *et al.* Blood pressure lowering and prevention of dementia: an individual patient data meta-analysis. *Eur Heart J.* 2022;43(48):4980–4990.

Qaseem A, Wilt TJ, McLean RM, *et al.* Noninvasive treatments for acute, subacute, and chronic low back pain: a clinical practice guideline from the American College of Physicians. *Ann Intern Med.* 2017;166(7):514–530.

Riemersma-van der Lek RF, Swaab DF, Twisk J, Hol EM, Hoogendijk WJ, Van Someren EJ. Effect of bright light and melatonin on cognitive and noncognitive function in elderly residents of group care facilities: a randomized controlled trial. *JAMA.* 2008;299(22):2642–2655.

Rivera AS, Akanbi M, O'Dwyer LC, McHugh M. Shift work and long work hours and their association with chronic health conditions: a systematic review of systematic reviews with meta-analyses. *PLoS One.* 2020;15(4):e0231037.

Rocabado M, Iglarsh ZA. *Musculoskeletal Approach to Maxillofacial Pain.* Philadelphia, PA: JB Lippincott; 1991.

Roelofs PD, Bierma-Zeinstra SM, van Poppel MN, *et al.* Lumbar supports to prevent recurrent low back pain among home care workers: a randomized trial. *Ann Intern Med.* 2007;147(10):685–692.

Rowe G, Jacobs K. Efficacy of body mechanics education on posture while computing in middle school children. *Work.* 2002;18(3):295–303.

Sadler K, Arnold F, Dean S. Chronic constipation in adults. *Am Fam Physician.* 2022;106(3):299–306.

Saha FJ, Brummer G, Lauche R, *et al.* Gua sha therapy for chronic low back pain: a randomized controlled trial. *Complement Ther Clin Pract.* 2019;34:64–69.

Saha FJ, Schumann S, Cramer H, *et al.* The effects of cupping massage in patients with chronic neck pain: a randomised controlled trial. *Complement Med Res.* 2017;24(1):26–32.

Sajedi SM, Abbasi F, Asnaashari M, Jafarian AA. Comparative efficacy of low-level laser acupuncture and cupping for treatment of patients with myofascial pain dysfunction syndrome: a double-blinded, randomized clinical trial: comparison of the effects of LLL acupuncture and cupping. *Galen Med J.* 2022;11:1–13.

Salemi MM, Gomes VMDSA, Bezerra LMR, *et al.* Effect of dry cupping therapy on pain and functional disability in persistent non-specific low back pain: a randomized controlled clinical trial. *J Acupunct Meridian Stud.* 2021;14(6):219–230.

Salonen H, Salthammer T, Morawska L. Human exposure to ozone in school and office indoor environments. *Environ Int.* 2018;119:503–514.

Sheng Y, Duan Z, Qu Q, Chen W, Yu B. Kinesio taping in treatment of chronic non-specific low back pain: a systematic review and meta-analysis. *J Rehabil Med.* 2019;51(10):734–740.

Sheon RP. A joint-protection guide for nonarticular rheumatic disorders. *Postgrad Med.* 1985;77(5):329–338.

Sheon RP, Orr PM. Appendix B: Joint protection guide for rheumatic disorders. In: Sheon RP, Moskowitz RW, Goldberg VM. *Soft Tissue Rheumatic Pain: Recognition, Management and Prevention*, 3rd ed. Baltimore, MD: Williams & Wilkins; 1996.

Shi X, Chen R, Huo L, *et al.* Evaluation of nanoparticles emitted from printers in a clean chamber, a copy center and office rooms: health risks of indoor air quality. *J Nanosci Nanotechnol.* 2015;15(12):9554–9564.

Silva CA, Motta ME. The use of abdominal muscle training, breathing exercises and abdominal massage to treat paediatric chronic functional constipation. *Colorectal Dis.* 2013;15(5):e250–e255.

Simsek Kücükkelepce D, Timur Tashan S. The effects of health belief model-based education and acupressure for coping with premenstrual syndrome on premenstrual symptoms and quality of life: a randomized-controlled trial. *Perspect Psychiatr Care.* 2021;57(1):189–197.

Singh P, Tuck C, Gibson PR, Chey WD. The role of food in the treatment of bowel disorders: focus on irritable bowel syndrome and functional constipation. *Am J Gastroenterol.* 2022;117(6):947–957.

Snook SH. Self-care guidelines for the management of nonspecific low back pain. *J Occup Rehabil.* 2004;14(4):243–253.

Stocchi F, Torti M. Constipation in Parkinson's disease. *Int Rev Neurobiol.* 2017;134:811–826.

Stoerkel E, Bellanti D, Paat C, *et al.* Effectiveness of a self-care toolkit for surgical breast cancer patients in a military treatment facility. *J Altern Complement Med.* 2018;24(9–10):916–925.

Styck AC, George DR. Evaluating the impact of community gardening on sense of purpose for persons living with dementia: a cluster-randomized pilot study. *J Alzheimers Dis Rep.* 2022;6(1):359–367.

Sundbøll J, Szépligeti SK, Adelborg K, Szentkúti P, Gregersen H, Sørensen HT. Constipation and risk of cardiovascular diseases: a Danish population-based matched cohort study. *BMJ Open.* 2020;10(9):e037080.

Suri P, Rainville J, de Schepper E, Martha J, Hartigan C, Hunter DJ. Do physical activities trigger flare-ups during an acute low back pain episode? A longitudinal case-crossover feasibility study. *Spine (Phila Pa 1976).* 2018;43(6):427–433.

Suri P, Saunders KW, Von Korff M. Prevalence and characteristics of flare-ups of chronic nonspecific back pain in primary care: a telephone survey. *Clin J Pain.* 2012;28(7):573–580.

Tan D, Hodges PW, Costa N, Ferreira M, Setchell J. Impact of flare-ups on the lives of individuals with low back pain: a qualitative investigation. *Musculoskelet Sci Pract.* 2019;43:52–57.

Tang T, Hurraß J, Gminski R, Mersch-Sundermann V. Fine and ultrafine particles emitted from laser printers as indoor air contaminants in German offices. *Environ Sci Pollut Res Int.* 2012;19(9):3840–3849.

Tara F, Bahrami-Taghanaki H, Amini Ghalandarabad M, *et al.* The effect of acupressure on the severity of nausea, vomiting, and retching in pregnant women: a randomized controlled trial. Wirkung der Akupressur auf den Schweregrad von Übelkeit, Erbrechen und Würgereiz bei Schwangeren: eine randomisierte kontrollierte Studie. *Complement Med Res.* 2020;27(4):252–259.

Thosar SS, Bielko SL, Mather KJ, *et al.* Effect of prolonged sitting and breaks in sitting time on endothelial function. *Medicine and Science in Sports and Exercise.* 2015;47(4):843–849.

Toomingas A, Hagberg M, Heiden M, Richter H, Westergren KE, Tornqvist EW. Risk factors, incidence and persistence of symptoms from the eyes among professional computer users. *Work.* 2014;47(3):291–301.

Unno K, Noda S, Kawasaki Y, *et al.* Reduced stress and improved sleep quality caused by green tea are associated with a reduced caffeine content. *Nutrients.* 2017;9(7):777.

Valls-Pedret C, Sala-Vila A, Serra-Mir M, *et al.* Mediterranean diet and age-related cognitive decline: a randomized clinical trial [published correction appears in *JAMA Intern Med.* 2018 Dec 1;178(12):1731–1732]. *JAMA Intern Med.* 2015;175(7):1094–1103.

van Dillen LR, Lanier VM, Steger-May K, *et al.* Effect of motor skill training in functional activities vs strength and flexibility exercise on function in people with chronic low back pain: a randomized clinical trial [published correction appears in *JAMA Neurol.* 2021 Jan 19]. *JAMA Neurol.* 2021;78(4):385–395.

van Duijvenbode IC, Jellema P, van Poppel MN, van Tulder MW. Lumbar supports for prevention and treatment of low back pain. *Cochrane Database Syst Rev.* 2008;2008(2):CD001823.

Vardoulakis S, Giagloglou E, Steinle S, *et al.* Indoor exposure to selected air pollutants in the home environment: a systematic review. *Int J Environ Res Public Health.* 2020;17(23):8972.

Velloso M, Jardim JR. Functionality of patients with chronic obstructive pulmonary disease: energy conservation techniques. *J Bras Pneumol.* 2006;32(6):580–586.

Venes D, ed. *Taber's Cyclopedic Medical Dictionary,* 24th ed. Philadelphia, PA: FA Davis; 2021.

Vincent HK, Vincent KR. ACSM information on... selecting running shoes. American College of Sports Medicine; 2014. www.acsm.org/docs/default-source/files-for-resource-library/running-shoes.pdf

Virtanen M, Ferrie JE, Gimeno D, *et al.* Long working hours and sleep disturbances: the Whitehall II prospective cohort study. *Sleep.* 2009a;32(6):737–745.

Virtanen M, Ferrie JE, Singh-Manoux A, *et al.* Long working hours and symptoms of anxiety and depression: a 5-year follow-up of the Whitehall II study. *Psychol Med.* 2011;41(12):2485–2494.

Virtanen M, Singh-Manoux A, Ferrie JE, *et al.* Long working hours and cognitive function: the Whitehall II Study. *Am J Epidemiol.* 2009b;169(5):596–605.

Vlak MH, Rinkel GJ, Greebe P, van der Bom JG, Algra A. Trigger factors and their attributable risk for rupture of intracranial aneurysms: a case-crossover study. *Stroke.* 2011;42(7):1878–1882.

Waits A, Tang YR, Cheng HM, Tai CJ, Chien LY. Acupressure effect on sleep quality: a systematic review and meta-analysis. *Sleep Med Rev.* 2018;37:24–34.

Wang X, Wu J, Ye M, Wang L, Zheng G. Effect of Baduanjin exercise on the cognitive function of middle-aged and older adults: a systematic review and meta-analysis. *Complement Ther Med.* 2021;59:102727.

Wang Y, Zhang Q, Li F, Li Q, Jin Y. Effects of tai chi and qigong on cognition in neurological disorders: a systematic review and meta-analysis. *Geriatr Nurs.* 2022;46:166–177.

Weatherford BM, Irwin CK. OrthoInfo, American Academy of Orthopedic Surgeons. 2023a. Athletic shoes. https://orthoinfo.aaos.org/en/staying-healthy/athletic-shoes

Weatherford BM, Irwin CK. OrthoInfo, American Academy of Orthopedic Surgeons. Shoes: Finding the right fit. 2023b. https://orthoinfo.aaos.org/en/staying-healthy/shoes-finding-the-right-fit

Winters JN, Sommer NZ, Romanelli MR, Marschik C, Hulcher L, Cutler BJ. Stretching and strength training to improve postural ergonomics and endurance in the operating room. *Plast Reconstr Surg Glob Open*. 2020;8(5):e2810.

Xiang Y, He JY, Tian HH, Cao BY, Li R. Evidence of efficacy of acupuncture in the management of low back pain: a systematic review and meta-analysis of randomised placebo- or sham-controlled trials. *Acupunct Med*. 2020;38(1):15–24.

Xu H, Zhao C, Guo G, *et al.* The effectiveness of tuina in relieving pain, negative emotions, and disability in knee osteoarthritis: a randomized controlled trial [published online ahead of print, 2022 Aug 23]. *Pain Med*. 2022;pnac127.

Xu H, Zhao C, Guo G, *et al.* The effectiveness of tuina in relieving pain, negative emotions, and disability in knee osteoarthritis: a randomized controlled trial. *Pain Med*. 2023;24(3):244–257.

Yen HY, Chiu HL. Virtual reality exergames for improving older adults' cognition and depression: a systematic review and meta-analysis of randomized control trials. *J Am Med Dir Assoc*. 2021;22(5):995–1002.

Yildirim D, Kocatepe V, Talu GK. The efficacy of acupressure in managing opioid-induced constipation in patients with cancer: a single-blind randomized controlled trial. *Support Care Cancer*. 2022;30(6):5201–5210.

Young GR. Energy conservation, occupational therapy, and the treatment of post-polio sequelae. *Orthopedics*. 1991;14(11):1233–1239.

Yuan QL, Guo TM, Liu L, Sun F, Zhang YG. Traditional Chinese medicine for neck pain and low back pain: a systematic review and meta-analysis. *PLoS One*. 2015;10(2):e0117146.

Zhang C, Jiang J, Tian F, *et al.* Meta-analysis of randomized controlled trials of the effects of probiotics on functional constipation in adults. *Clin Nutr*. 2020;39(10):2960–2969.

Zhang YR, Xu W, Zhang W, *et al.* Modifiable risk factors for incident dementia and cognitive impairment: an umbrella review of evidence. *J Affect Disord*. 2022;314:160–167.

Zhou TY, Yuan XM, Ma XJ. Can an outdoor multisurface terrain enhance the effects of fall prevention exercise in older adults? A randomized controlled trial. *Int J Environ Res Public Health*. 2020;17(19):7023.

Zhou Y, Su Y, Xu W, Wang W, Yao S. Constipation increases disability and decreases dopamine levels in the nigrostriatal system through gastric inflammatory factors in Parkinson's disease. *Curr Neurovasc Res*. 2019;16(3):241–249.

Zivkovic V, Lazovic M, Vlajkovic M, *et al.* Diaphragmatic breathing exercises and pelvic floor retraining in children with dysfunctional voiding. *Eur J Phys Rehabil Med*. 2012;48(3):413–421.

Zulauf N, Dröge J, Klingelhöfer D, Braun M, Oremek GM, Groneberg DA. Indoor air pollution in cars: an update on novel insights. *Int J Environ Res Public Health*. 2019;16(13):2441.

Additional Reading

Avila L, da Silva MD, Neves ML, *et al.* Effectiveness of cognitive functional therapy versus core exercises and manual therapy in patients with chronic low back pain after spinal surgery: randomized controlled trial [published online ahead of print, 2023 Aug 7]. *Phys Ther*. 2023;pzad105.

Bellew JW, Michlovitz SL, Nolan TP. *Michlovitz's Modalities for Therapeutic Intervention*, 6th ed. Philadelphia, PA: F.A. Davis Company; 2016.

Benjamin PJ. *Tappan's Handbook of Massage Therapy: Blending Art with Science*, 6th ed. Boston, MA: Pearson; 2016.

Bonakdar RA, Sukiennik AW, eds. *Integrative Pain Management*. New York, NY: Oxford University Press; 2016.

Butler DS, Moseley GL. *Explain Pain*, 2nd ed. Adelaide, Australia: Noigroup Publications; 2013.

Cameron MH. *Physical Agents in Rehabilitation: An Evidence-Based Approach to Practice*, 5th ed. St Louis, MO: Elsevier.

Chirali IZ. *Traditional Chinese Medicine Cupping Therapy*, 3rd ed. New York, NY: Churchill Livingstone Elsevier; 2014.

Chopra S, Kodali RT, McHugh GA, Conaghan PG, Kingsbury SR. Home-based health care interventions for people aged 75 years and above with chronic, noninflammatory musculoskeletal pain: a scoping review. *J Geriatr Phys Ther*. 2023;46(1):3–14.

Daley D, Payne LP, Galper J, *et al.* Clinical guidance to optimize work participation after injury or illness: the role of physical therapists. *J Orthop Sports Phys Ther*. 2021;51(8):CPG1–CPG102.

Davis CM. *Integrative Therapies in Rehabilitation: Evidence for Efficacy in Therapy, Prevention, and*

Wellness. Thorofare, NJ: SLACK Incorporated; 2017.

Donnelly JM, Fernandez-de-las-Penas C, Finnegan M, Freeman JL. *Travell, Simons, & Simons' Myofascial Pain and Dysfunction: The Trigger Point Manual,* 3rd ed. Philadelphia, PA: Wolters Kluwer; 2019.

Duran AT, Friel CP, Serafini MA, Ensari I, Cheung YK, Diaz KM. Breaking up prolonged sitting to improve cardiometabolic risk: dose-response analysis of a randomized crossover trial. *Med Sci Sports Exerc*. 2023;55(5):847–855.

Gubner J, Smith AK, Allison TA. Transforming undergraduate student perceptions of dementia through music and filmmaking. *J Am Geriatr Soc*. 2020 May;68(5):1083–1089.

Huntsman JL, Bulaj G. Health education via "empowerment" digital marketing of consumer products and services: promoting therapeutic benefits of self-care for depression and chronic pain. *Front. Public Health*. 2023;10:949518.

International Association for the Study of Pain. Multidisciplinary Pain Center: Development Manual. 2021. www.iasp-pain.org/resources/toolkits/pain-management-center

Moseley GL, Nicholas MK, Hodges PW. A randomized controlled trial of intensive neurophysiology education in chronic low back pain. *Clin J Pain*. 2004;20(5):324–330.

Mulligan BR. *Manual Therapy: NAGS, SNAGS, MWMS etc.,* 5th ed. Wellington, New Zealand: Plane View Service, Ltd; 2006.

Mulligan BR. *Self-Treatments for Back, Neck, and Limbs,* 3rd ed. Wellington, New Zealand: Plane View Service, Ltd; 2012.

Nachemson A. The lumbar spine: an orthopaedic challenge. *Spine*. 1976;1(1):59–71.

Nielsen A. *Gua Sha: A Traditional Technique for Modern Practice*, 2nd ed. New York, NY: Churchill Livingstone Elsevier; 2013.

Pritchard S. *Tui Na: A Manual of Chinese Massage Therapy*. London, United Kingdom: Singing Dragon; 2015.

Wilke HJ, Neef P, Caimi M, Hoogland T, Claes LE. New in vivo measurements of pressures in the intervertebral disc in daily life. *Spine (Phila Pa 1976)*. 1999;24(8):755–762.

Conclusion

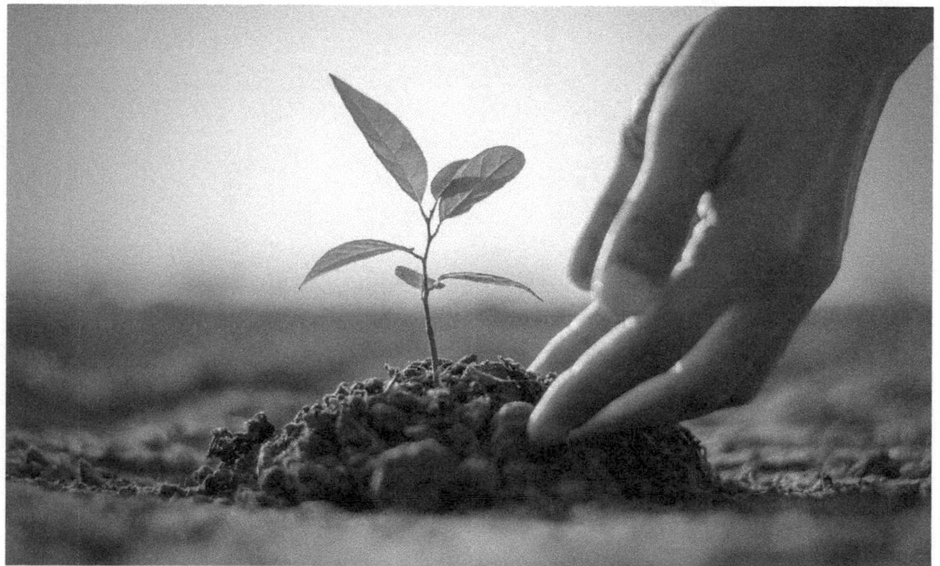

Plant the seeds and watch them grow

Dear Reader,

Even after all these pages, we have actually come to the beginning of this journey. I consider it the beginning, since we all have many seeds to plant to help our patients/clients feel better and enjoy a quality life.

If you wish, please reach out to say hello, share a comment, or provide feedback. Let's stay professionally connected.

Wishing everyone good health and happiness,

Ziya "Z" Altug, PT, DPT, MS

www.linkedin.com/in/zaltug

APPENDICES

Appendices Highlights

- Appendix A: Sample Clinical Practice Guidelines
- Appendix B: Designing Effective Home Exercise Programs
- Appendix C: Sample Exercise Selection Guide

Lifestyle Matters*: Anger is a journey with no destination.*

APPENDIX A

Sample Clinical Practice Guidelines

The following Clinical Practice Guidelines may be used to improve clinical care.

Breast Cancer-Related Lymphedema

- Davies C, Levenhagen K, Ryans K, Perdomo M, Gilchrist L. Interventions for breast cancer-related lymphedema: clinical practice guideline from the Academy of Oncologic Physical Therapy of APTA. *Phys Ther.* 2020;100(7):1163–1179.

Children with Developmental Coordination Disorder

- Dannemiller L, Mueller M, Leitner A, Iverson E, Kaplan SL. Physical therapy management of children with developmental coordination disorder: an evidence-based clinical practice guideline from the Academy of Pediatric Physical Therapy of the American Physical Therapy Association. *Pediatr Phys Ther.* 2020;32(4):278–313.

Chronic Insomnia Disorder

- Edinger JD, Arnedt JT, Bertisch SM, *et al.* Behavioral and psychological treatments for chronic insomnia disorder in adults: an American Academy of Sleep Medicine clinical practice guideline. *J Clin Sleep Med.* 2021;17(2):255–262.
- Qaseem A, Kansagara D, Forciea MA, Cooke M, Denberg TD. Clinical Guidelines Committee of the American College of Physicians. Management of chronic insomnia disorder in adults: a clinical practice

guideline from the American College of Physicians. *Ann Intern Med.* 2016;165(2):125–133.

Depression

- American Psychological Association. Clinical practice guideline for the treatment of depression across three age cohorts; 2019. www.apa.org/depression-guideline/guideline.pdf

Fall Prevention

- Montero-Odasso MM, Kamkar N, Pieruccini-Faria F, *et al.* Evaluation of clinical practice guidelines on fall prevention and management for older adults: a systematic review. *JAMA Netw Open*. 2021;4(12):e2138911.
- Schoberer D, Breimaier HE, Zuschnegg J, Findling T, Schaffer S, Archan T. Fall prevention in hospitals and nursing homes: clinical practice guideline. *Worldviews Evid Based Nurs*. 2022;19(2):86–93.

Headache

- ACOG Committee on Clinical Practice Guidelines—Obstetrics. Headaches in pregnancy and postpartum: ACOG clinical practice guideline no. 3 [published correction appears in *Obstet Gynecol*. 2022 Aug 1;140(2):344]. *Obstet Gynecol*. 2022;139(5):944–972. www.acog.org
- *VA/DoD Clinical Practice Guideline. The Primary Care Management of Headache Work Group*. Washington, DC: U.S. Government Printing Office; 2020. www.healthquality.va.gov

Heart Failure

- Shoemaker MJ, Dias KJ, Lefebvre KM, Heick JD, Collins SM. Physical therapist clinical practice guideline for the management of individuals with heart failure. *Phys Ther*. 2020;100(1):14–43.

High Blood Pressure in Adults

- Whelton PK, Carey RM, Aronow WS, *et al.* 2017 ACC/AHA/AAPA/ABC/ACPM/AGS/APhA/ASH/ASPC/NMA/PCNA Guideline for the prevention, detection, evaluation, and management of high blood pressure in adults: a report of the American College of Cardiology/American Heart Association Task Force on Clinical Practice Guidelines [published correction appears in *J Am Coll Cardiol.* 2018 May 15;71(19):2275–2279]. *J Am Coll Cardiol.* 2018;71(19):e127–e248.

Opioids and Chronic Pain

- Dowell D, Ragan KR, Jones CM, Baldwin GT, Chou R. CDC clinical practice guideline for prescribing opioids for pain: United States, 2022. *MMWR Recomm Rep.* 2022;71(3):1–95. www.cdc.gov
- Sandbrink F, Murphy JL, Johansson M, *et al.* The use of opioids in the management of chronic pain: synopsis of the 2022 U.S. Department of Veterans Affairs and U.S. Department of Defense clinical practice guideline. *Ann Intern Med.* 2023;176(3):388–397.
- *VA/DoD Clinical Practice Guideline. Use of Opioids in the Management of Chronic Pain Work Group.* Washington, DC: U.S. Government Printing Office; 2022. www.healthquality.va.gov

Orthopedics

- American Academy of Orthopaedic Surgeons. Management of Carpal Tunnel Syndrome: Evidence-Based Clinical Practice Guideline; 2016. www.aaos.org
- American Academy of Orthopaedic Surgeons. Management of Osteoarthritis of the Knee (Non-Arthroplasty): Appropriate Use Criteria; 2022. www.aaos.org
- American Academy of Orthopaedic Surgeons. Management of Rotator Cuff Pathology: Appropriate Use Criteria; 2020. www.aaos.org
- Arundale AJH, Bizzini M, Dix C, *et al.* Exercise-based knee and anterior cruciate ligament injury prevention. *J Orthop Sports Phys Ther.* 2023;53(1):CPG1–CPG34.
- Blanpied PR, Gross AR, Elliott JM, *et al.* Neck pain: revision 2017. *J Orthop Sports Phys Ther.* 2017;47(7):A1–A83.
- Cibulka MT, Bloom NJ, Enseki KR, Macdonald CW, Woehrle J, McDonough

CM. Hip pain and mobility deficits—hip osteoarthritis: revision 2017. *J Orthop Sports Phys Ther*. 2017;47(6):A1–A37.

- Daley D, Payne LP, Galper J, *et al.* Clinical guidance to optimize work participation after injury or illness: the role of physical therapists. *J Orthop Sports Phys Ther*. 2021;51(8):CPG1–CPG102.
- Dyer JO, Doiron-Cadrin P, Lafrance S, *et al.* Diagnosing, managing, and supporting return to work of adults with rotator cuff disorders: clinical practice guideline methods. *J Orthop Sports Phys Ther*. 2022;52(10):665–674.
- Enseki KR, Bloom NJ, Harris-Hayes M, *et al.* Hip pain and movement dysfunction associated with nonarthritic hip joint pain: a revision. *J Orthop Sports Phys Ther*. 2023 Jul;53(7):CPG1–CPG70.
- George SZ, Fritz JM, Silfies SP, *et al.* Interventions for the management of acute and chronic low back pain: revision 2021. *J Orthop Sports Phys Ther*. 2021;51(11):CPG1–CPG60.
- Lucado AM, Day JM, Vincent JI, *et al.* Lateral elbow pain and muscle function impairments. *J Orthop Sports Phys Ther*. 2022;52(12):CPG1–CPG111.
- Martin RL, Cibulka MT, Bolgla LA, *et al.* Hamstring strain injury in athletes. *J Orthop Sports Phys Ther*. 2022;52(3):CPG1–CPG44.
- Martin RL, Davenport TE, Reischl SF, *et al.* Heel pain-plantar fasciitis: revision 2014. *J Orthop Sports Phys Ther*. 2014;44(11):A1–A33.
- Martin RL, Davenport TE, Fraser JJ, *et al.* Ankle stability and movement coordination impairments: lateral ankle ligament sprains: revision 2021. *J Orthop Sports Phys Ther*. 2021;51(4):CPG1–CPG80.
- Michener LA, Heitzman J, Abbruzzese LD, *et al.* Physical therapist management of glenohumeral joint osteoarthritis: a clinical practice guideline from the American Physical Therapy Association. *Phys Ther*. 2023 Jun 5;103(6):pzad041.
- VA/DoD Clinical Practice Guideline. The Diagnosis and Treatment of Low Back Pain. Washington, DC: U.S. Government Printing Office; 2022. www.healthquality.va.gov
- van Doormaal MCM, Meerhoff GA, Vliet Vlieland TPM, Peter WF. A clinical practice guideline for physical therapy in patients with hip or knee osteoarthritis. *Musculoskeletal Care*. 2020;18(4):575–595.

Osteoporosis

- Camacho PM, Petak SM, Binkley N, *et al.* American Association of Clinical Endocrinologists/American College of Endocrinology clinical practice guidelines for the diagnosis and treatment of postmenopausal osteoporosis—2020 update. *Endocr Pract*. 2020;26(Suppl 1):1–46.

- Hartley GW, Roach KE, Nithman RW, *et al.* Physical therapist management of patients with suspected or confirmed osteoporosis: a clinical practice guideline from the Academy of Geriatric Physical Therapy. *J Geriatr Phys Ther.* 2022;44(2):e106–e119.

Parkinson's

- Osborne JA, Botkin R, Colon-Semenza C, *et al.* Physical therapist management of Parkinson disease: a clinical practice guideline from the American Physical Therapy Association [published correction appears in *Phys Ther.* 2022 Aug 1;102(8)]. *Phys Ther.* 2022;102(4):pzab302.

Rheumatoid Arthritis

- England BR, Smith BJ, Baker NA, *et al.* 2022 American College of Rheumatology Guideline for Exercise, Rehabilitation, Diet, and Additional Integrative Interventions for Rheumatoid Arthritis. *Arthritis Rheumatol.* 2023 May 25. Epub ahead of print.
- Peter WF, Swart NM, Meerhoff GA, Vliet Vlieland TPM. Clinical practice guideline for physical therapist management of people with rheumatoid arthritis. *Phys Ther.* 2021;101(8):pzab127.

Sports Medicine (Consensus Statements)

- Burke LM, Slater GJ, Matthews JJ, Langan-Evans C, Horswill CA. ACSM expert consensus statement on weight loss in weight-category sports. *Curr Sports Med Rep.* 2021;20(4):199–217.
- Castellani JW, Eglin CM, Ikäheimo TM, Montgomery H, Paal P, Tipton MJ. ACSM expert consensus statement: injury prevention and exercise performance during cold-weather exercise. *Curr Sports Med Rep.* 2021;20(11):594–607.
- Roberts WO, Armstrong LE, Sawka MN, Yeargin SW, Heled Y, O'Connor FG. ACSM expert consensus statement on exertional heat illness: recognition, management, and return to activity. *Curr Sports Med Rep.* 2021;20(9):470–484.

Stroke

- VA/DoD Clinical Practice Guideline. The Management of Stroke Rehabilitation Work Group. Washington, DC: U.S. Government Printing Office; 2019. www.healthquality.va.gov

Substance Use Disorder

- VA/DoD Clinical Practice Guideline. The Management of Substance Use Disorder Work Group. Washington, DC: U.S. Government Printing Office; 2019. www.healthquality.va.gov

APPENDIX B

Designing Effective Home Exercise Programs

This appendix aims to provide healthcare providers and health/fitness professionals with some basic guidelines for designing effective home exercise programs. Home exercise programs may be used for fall prevention (Liu-Ambrose *et al.* 2019), home fitness for older adults (Chaabene *et al.* 2021), knee osteoarthritis (Anwer *et al.* 2016), low back pain (Quentin *et al.* 2021), osteoporosis (Zhang *et al.* 2022), improved quality of life in cancer survivors (Kim *et al.* 2019), and other conditions.

What is the Purpose of a Home Exercise Program?

- Adjunct to a clinic program
- Part of a self-care and self-management program
- Improve function in daily activities
- Empower the patient/client to manage their condition
- Maintain results after therapy is completed
- Educate and inform the person to prevent reoccurrence

What are Some Types of Home Exercise Programs?

Home exercise programs may be designed for aerobic, strength, flexibility, balance, coordination, agility, sport-specific (such as running, throwing, or jumping), and task-specific needs (such as sitting to standing, reaching, or carrying).

Are There Any Strategies I May Use to Improve Home Exercise Program Compliance?

The following are some considerations (Conn *et al.* 2013; Montayre *et al.* 2020; Palazzo *et al.* 2016):

- Make sure the program addresses the person's specific problem (pain, strength, balance).
- Don't give too many exercises. From a clinical perspective, it's recommended you discuss the number of exercises with your patient/client and see if they think it's realistic.
- Provide periodic feedback about the program.
- Use new technologies to keep individuals engaged. For example, some people may want their home program sent as an email attachment or provided as a video or spreadsheet program.
- Determine how the person learns:
  - Is the person an auditory learner (learn by hearing)?
  - Is the person a visual learner (learn by seeing)?
  - Is the person a kinesthetic learner (learn by doing)?
- Determine if there are there any barriers that may play a role. For example:
  - language (you may need to provide the program in the person's native language)
  - cultural (a person may not want to engage in a particular type of exercise)
  - education (the ability to read and write)
  - transportation (getting to therapy or exercise location, bad weather)
  - seasonal allergies (a person may need to avoid outdoor exercise during certain times)
  - financial limitations (a person may not be able to purchase fitness equipment or memberships)
  - visual impairment (a person may need large print to see the home program)
  - hearing impairment (a person may need closed captions for videos or printed handouts for recorded content).
- Is the home program culturally relevant?
  - For example, include photos or examples from different cultures or the person's culture.
  - Try to use the individual's native language.
- Is the home program age-specific?
  - Use photos or images that are specific to the age group.
- Tell the person why the exercises are important. The following are some examples:
  - So you can raise your arm higher.
  - So you can climb the stairs.
  - So you can get out of a chair.
  - So you have less pain with daily activities.
  - So you have less swelling in your feet to get your shoes on.

  - So you have increased stamina for walking.
  - So you can gradually discontinue assistive devices.
  - So you can rely less on pain medications.
- What teaching and coaching cues does the person respond to?
  - Demonstration: show
  - Sound: verbal commands
  - Visual: provide photo or video
  - Tactile: manual cues
- Provide variable routines to prevent boredom. A simple long-term strategy may be to provide several varieties of programs:
  - Program A: bodyweight exercises
  - Program B: elastic or dumbbell exercises
  - Program C: fitness center-based exercises
- Teach the person how to modify their routine and how to progress the program (such as sets, reps, intensity, and days per week).
- Teach the person how to include the program in home and work environments.
- Teach the person how to modify the program in case of a flare-up. For example, if the person experiences a flare-up, should they:
  - reduce the intensity by 50 percent
  - discontinue the exercises for several days
  - contact the therapist or physician?
- Teach the person when to stop performing the exercises. For example, should the person stop performing their exercises after:
  - they reach their goal of...
  - 3 months
  - pain level 0–2/10?

  Or, are these lifelong exercises?
- Teach the person how to track their home program. For example, they could use an app or calendar (traditional wall calendar or a computer-based one).
- Recommend the person creates a reward system for themselves. For example, for every month a person sticks to their program with 80 percent compliance, they can reward themselves with a small gift.

What are Various Ways to Provide Home Exercise Programs to Patients/Clients?

- Create paper handouts of exercises with home instructions.
- Create a booklet of exercises with home instructions.
- Create a paper wall-hanging calendar or app-based calendar with exercises.

- Provide an image display stand with exercises for easy use in the kitchen or at work.
- Provide exercise photos from a web-based exercise platform.
- Send exercise images via an email or text, so the person has access via their smartphone.
- Create and send a spreadsheet for helping individuals track exercises and progress (such as an Excel sheet).
- Send prerecorded exercise videos from a web-based platform.
- Using the patient/client's phone, create individualized exercise videos of them while they are exercising in the clinic or studio.

References

Anwer S, Alghadir A, Brismée JM. Effect of home exercise program in patients with knee osteoarthritis: a systematic review and meta-analysis. *J Geriatr Phys Ther*. 2016;39(1):38–48.

Chaabene H, Prieske O, Herz M, *et al.* Home-based exercise programmes improve physical fitness of healthy older adults: a PRISMA-compliant systematic review and meta-analysis with relevance for COVID-19. *Ageing Res Rev*. 2021;67:101265.

Conn VS, Chan K, Banks J, Ruppar TM, Scharff J. Cultural relevance of physical activity intervention research with underrepresented populations. *Int Q Community Health Educ*. 2013;34(4):391–414.

Kim JY, Lee MK, Lee DH, *et al.* Effects of a 12-week home-based exercise program on quality of life, psychological health, and the level of physical activity in colorectal cancer survivors: a randomized controlled trial. *Support Care Cancer*. 2019;27(8):2933–2940.

Liu-Ambrose T, Davis JC, Best JR, *et al.* Effect of a home-based exercise program on subsequent falls among community-dwelling high-risk older adults after a fall: a randomized clinical trial [published correction appears in *JAMA*. 2019 Jul 9;322(2):174]. *JAMA*. 2019;321(21):2092–2100.

Montayre J, Neville S, Dunn I, Shrestha-Ranjit J, Wright-St Clair V. What makes community-based physical activity programs for culturally and linguistically diverse older adults effective? A systematic review. *Australas J Ageing*. 2020;39(4):331–340.

Palazzo C, Klinger E, Dorner V, *et al.* Barriers to home-based exercise program adherence with chronic low back pain: patient expectations regarding new technologies. *Ann Phys Rehabil Med*. 2016;59(2):107–113.

Quentin C, Bagheri R, Ugbolue UC, *et al.* Effect of home exercise training in patients with nonspecific low-back pain: a systematic review and meta-analysis. *Int J Environ Res Public Health*. 2021;18(16):8430.

Zhang F, Wang Z, Su H, *et al.* Effect of a home-based resistance exercise program in elderly participants with osteoporosis: a randomized controlled trial [published online ahead of print, 2022 Jun 15]. *Osteoporos Int*. 2022;10.1007/s00198-022-06456-1.

APPENDIX C

Sample Exercise Selection Guide

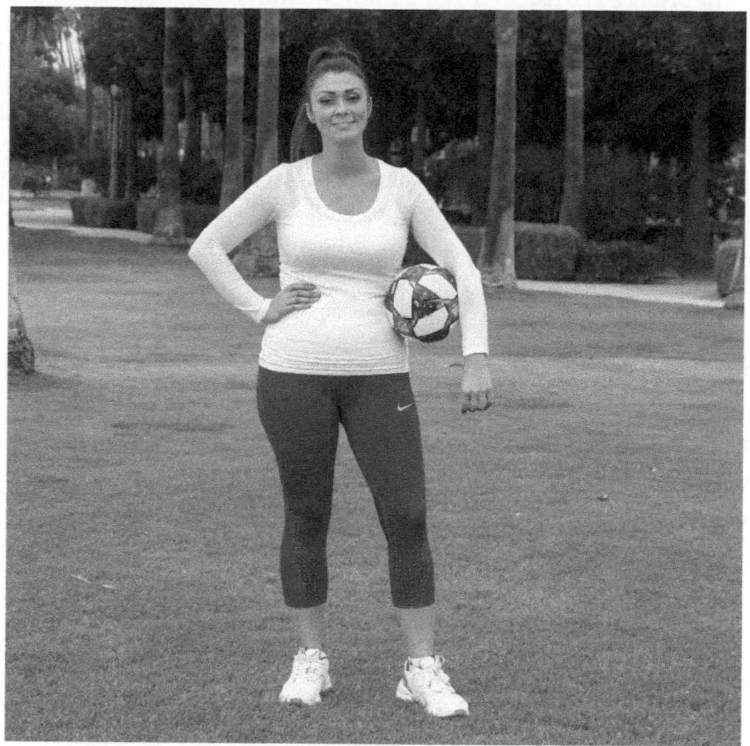

Happiness with fun and sustainable physical activity

Appendix C Highlights

- Warm-Up and Mobility Training Exercises
- Strength Training Exercises
- Flexibility Training Exercises
- Balance Training Exercise
- Aerobic Training Exercises
- Sports-Related Activities
- Function-Related Activities

Introduction

A customized exercise program for each patient/client is based on physical examination findings, equipment availability, and the patient's/client's preferences and needs. Also, program designs will vary, since every practitioner has a personalized approach to therapeutic exercise prescriptions.

Due to space limitations, many other excellent and practical exercises for various disorders are not included in this appendix. This appendix provides sample warm-up and mobility, strengthening, flexibility, balance, and aerobic exercises that may be considered for patients/clients to improve overall function and quality of life.

The sample exercises in this appendix are available to download from https://library.jkp.com/redeem using the code TTMJUJG.

A Word of Caution

Patients/clients should not use this book to perform the following exercises indiscriminately. Practitioners should prescribe and modify the exercises as needed according to the person's:

- medical history, such as pain level, osteoporosis, or total hip surgery
- goals, such as pain reduction, core strengthening, or fall prevention
- preferences, such as if the person wants to exercise in a gym or use bodyweight, elastic, or dumbbell resistance
- tolerances, such as if the person is unaccustomed to exercise or they exercise regularly.

Warm-Up and Mobility Training Exercises

The following are sample warm-up exercises to prepare for more intense activity or sport. These exercises may also be used to improve overall mobility.

Note: Photos and adapted descriptions have been used with permission from the book *Integrative Healing: Developing Wellness in the Mind and Body* (Cedar Fort, Inc., 2018) by Z. Altug.

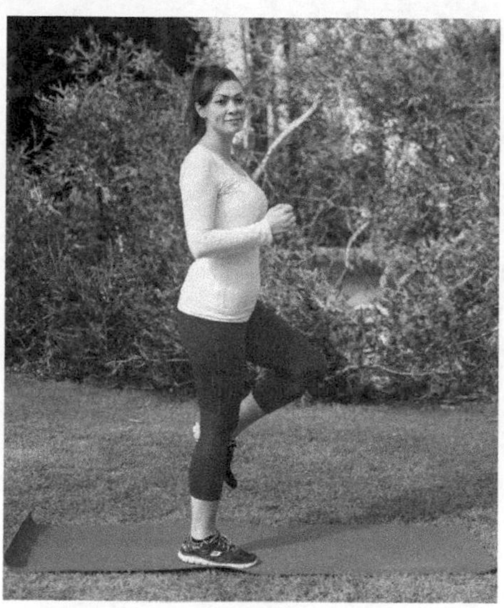

Slow march in place (and may be used for dynamic balance training)

Using an alternate arm and leg motion, march in place.

Perform .... sets and .... reps.

Perform .... per day .... days per week.

Notes: ....

....

....

....

....

....

....

Using an alternate arm motion, reach overhead.

Using an alternate arm motion, punch straight ahead.

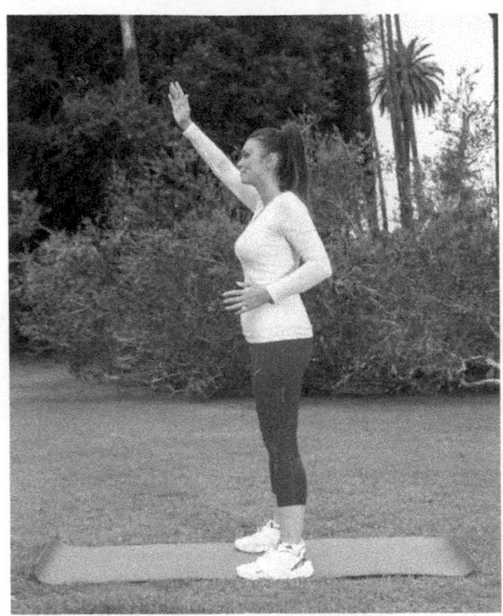

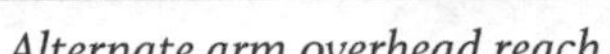

Alternate arm overhead reach

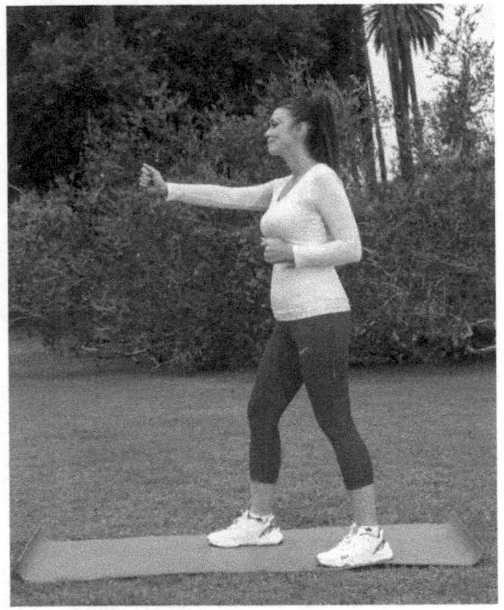

Boxing movements

Perform .... sets and .... reps.

Perform .... per day .... days per week.

Notes: ....

....

....

....

....

....

....

....

....

....

....

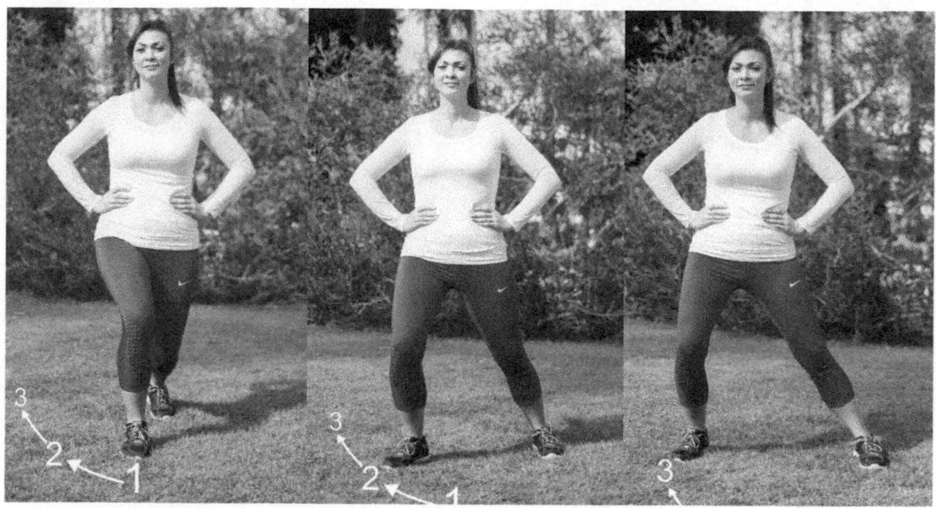

Multidirectional stepping (and may be used for dynamic balance training)

1. Stand with your hands on your hips.
2. Step straight forward with your right foot (position 1) and return to the starting position.
3. Step diagonally forward with your right foot (position 2) and return to the starting position.
4. Step sideways with your right foot (position 3) and return to the starting position.
5. Repeat the entire three-step sequence on the left side. Completing the three-step sequence on both sides is considered one set.

Perform .... sets and .... reps.

Perform .... per day .... days per week.

Notes: ....

....

....

....

....

....

....

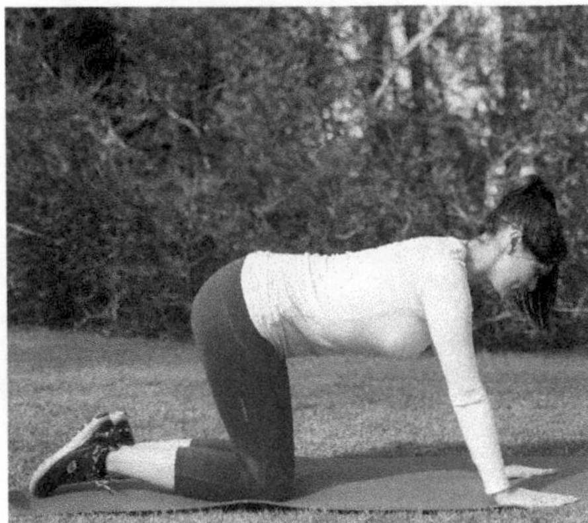

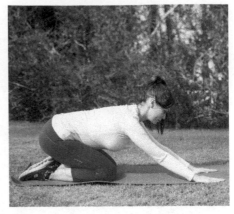

Gentle heel sits

1. Start in a hands-and-knees position with your hands shoulder-width apart and knees hip-width apart.
2. Slowly bring your hips toward your heels, going only as far as is comfortable without overstretching your knees or lower back.

Perform .... sets and .... reps.

Perform .... per day .... days per week.

Notes: ....

....

....

....

....

....

....

....

....

....

Strength Training Exercises

The following are sample strengthening exercises to improve "core" strength, improve posture, and enhance function in daily activities.

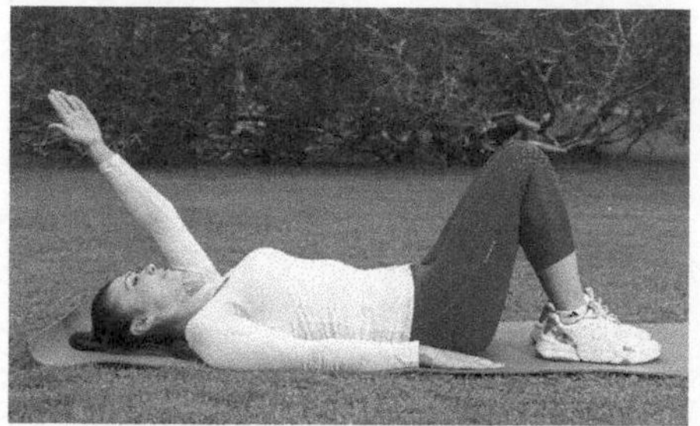

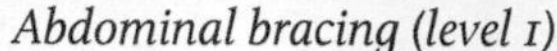

Abdominal bracing (level 1)

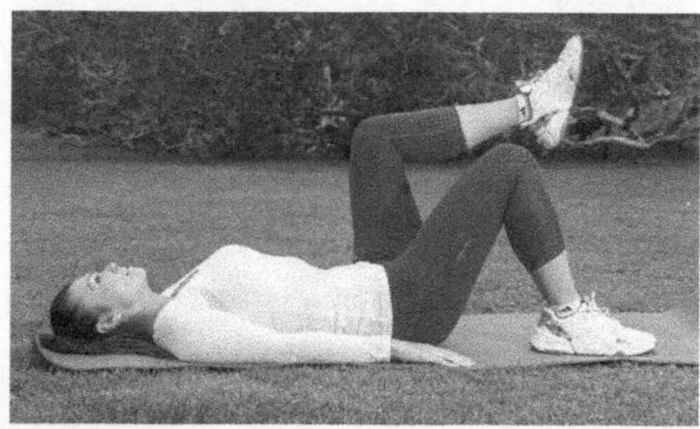

Abdominal bracing (level 2)

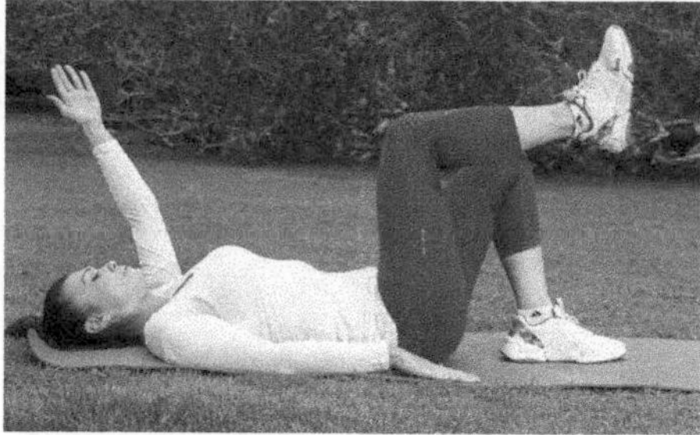

Abdominal bracing (level 3)

1. Lie on your back, with your feet flat on the floor and your knees bent.
2. Level 1—Tighten your abdominal muscles (without holding your breath for levels 1–3) as you alternate moving your arms up and down.
3. Level 2—Tighten your abdominal muscles as you alternate lifting your bent legs up and down from the floor.
4. Level 3—Tighten your abdominal muscles as you alternate moving your opposite arm and leg up and down. Completing the right and left arm/leg sequence is considered one set.

Perform .... sets and .... reps.

Perform .... per day .... days per week.

Notes: ....

....

....

....

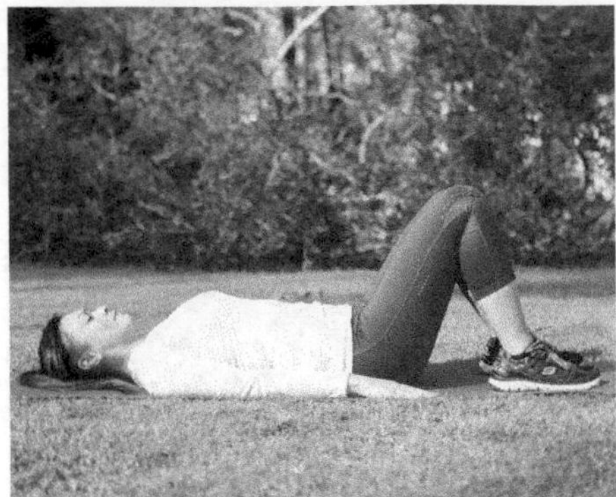

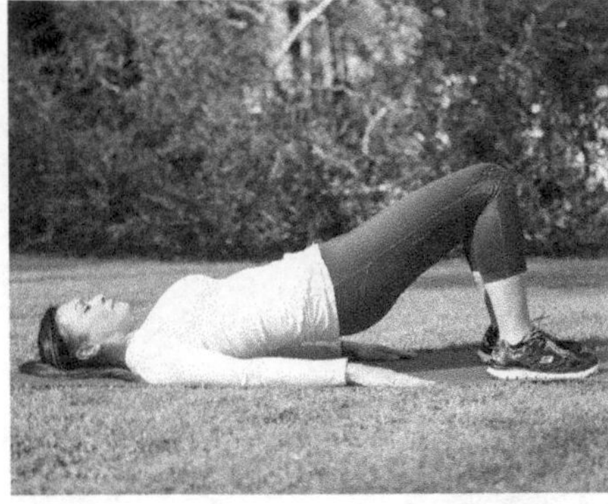

Bridging

1. Lie on your back, with your feet flat on the floor and your knees bent.
2. Moderately brace or tighten your abdominals (without holding your breath) and slightly raise your hips while preserving the natural curve in your lower back.

Perform .... sets and .... reps.

Perform .... per day .... days per week.

Notes: ....

....

....

....

....

....

....

....

....

....

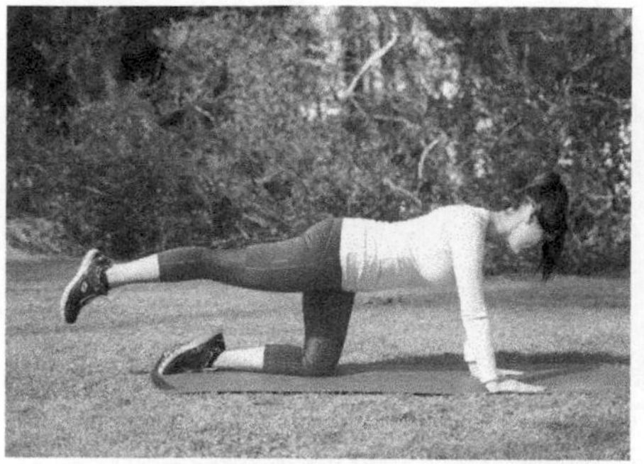

Bird dog (level 1)

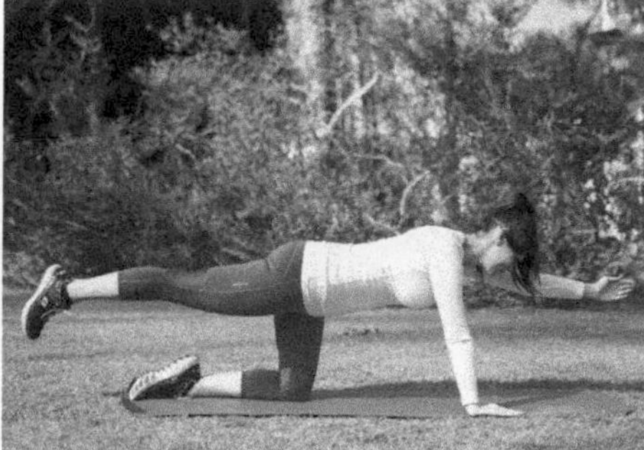

Bird dog (level 2)

1. Level 1—Start in a hands-and-knees position, with your hands shoulder-width and knees hip-width apart. Find the pain-free natural curve in your lower back and neck as you perform this exercise. Stiffen your core muscles just enough to maintain your neck and back curves while still being able to breathe freely. Raise your right and left leg alternately so that they are parallel to the floor.
2. Level 2—Start as described in Level 1 and then simultaneously raise your right leg and left arm, thumb pointing to the ceiling and arm approximately 3–5 inches away from your head, without losing your spine curve or tilting your hips.
3. Slowly return to the starting position, repeating with the opposite leg and arm. Completing the arm/leg sequence on both sides is considered one set.

Perform .... sets and .... reps.

Perform .... per day .... days per week.

Notes: ....

....

....

....

....

....

....

....

....

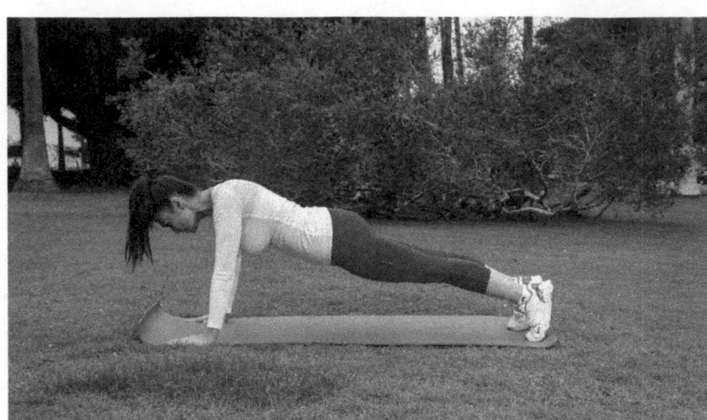

Floor front plank

1. Start in a hands-and-knees position, with your hands shoulder-width and knees hip-width apart.
2. From this position, lift your knees to assume a push-up position by keeping your core muscles tight (without holding your breath) and hold for .... seconds.

Perform .... sets and .... reps.

Perform .... per day .... days per week.

Notes: ....

....

....

....

....

....

....

....

....

....

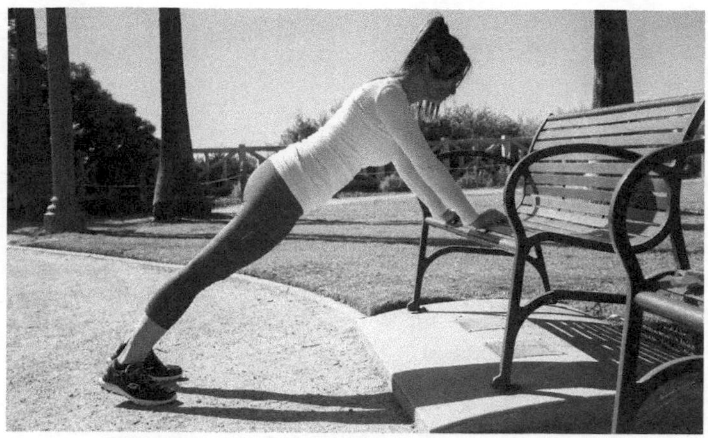

Elevated front plank

1. Place your hands on a sturdy, immovable surface like a wall, your bed, or a couch.
2. From this position, assume an incline push-up position by keeping your core muscles tight (without holding your breath) and hold for .... seconds.

Perform .... sets and .... reps.

Perform .... per day .... days per week.

Notes: ....

....

....

....

....

....

....

....

....

....

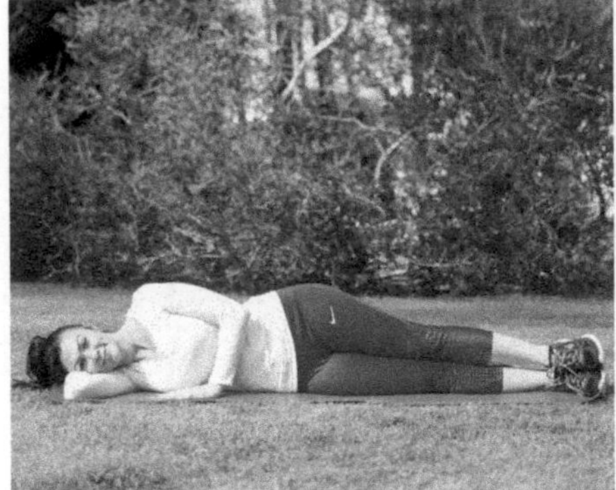
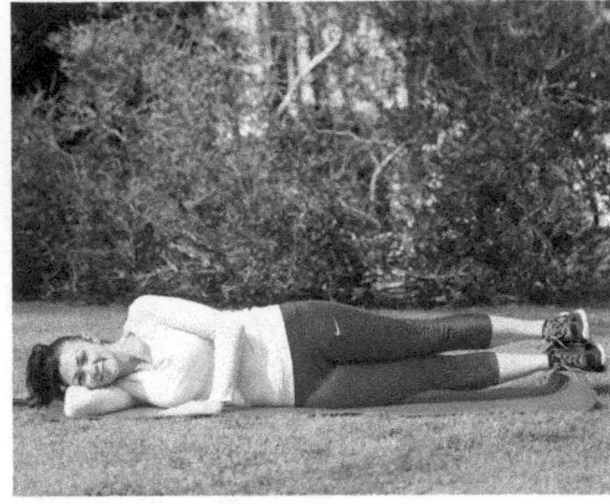

Side leg lift or modified side plank

1. Start by lying on your right side with your right arm under your head for support. Keep your body straight through the shoulder, hip, and knees. Preserve the natural curve in your lower back and neck as you perform this exercise.
2. Place your left hand on the floor in front of your chest for support.
3. Slowly lift both legs together so the outside part of your right knee is approximately 1–2 inches off the floor.
4. Hold this position for .... seconds (without holding your breath), and then relax for .... seconds by lowering both legs. Raising and lowering both legs is considered one repetition.
5. Repeat on the other side.

Perform .... sets and .... reps.

Perform .... per day .... days per week.

Notes: ....

....

....

....

....

....

....

....

....

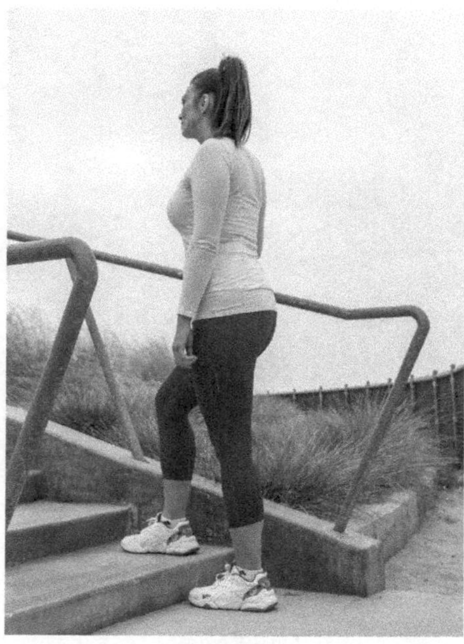

Step-ups

1. Hold on to a rail and perform repeated stepping up and down on the step with your right leg for a designated number of repetitions.
2. Repeat on the other side.

Perform . . . . sets and . . . . reps.

Perform . . . . per day . . . . days per week.

Notes: . . . .

. . . .

. . . .

. . . .

. . . .

. . . .

. . . .

. . . .

. . . .

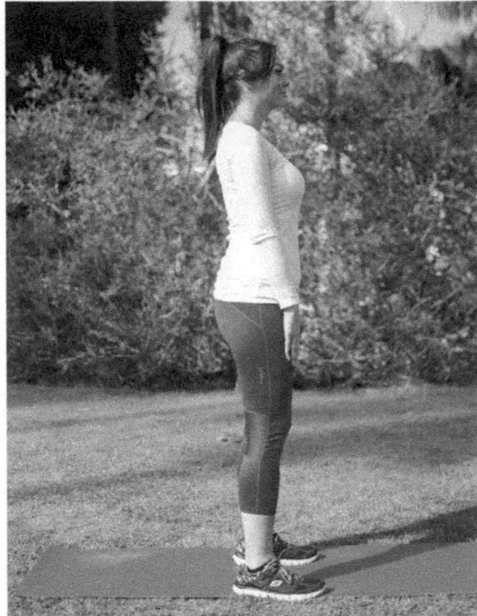

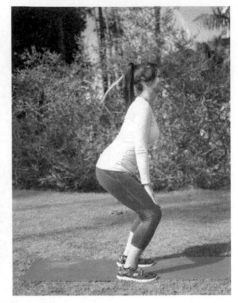

Partial squat

1. Stand with your feet shoulder-width apart and hands on the fronts of your thighs.
2. Slowly bend your hips and knees as you slide both hands until your fingertips are just above your kneecaps. Be mindful of bringing your hips back and knees at or slightly behind your toes as you squat. Keep your shoulders down and back, and your knees slightly out. Preserve the natural curve in your lower back and neck as you perform this exercise. Do not squat any lower than your ability to maintain your natural lower back and neck curves. This will vary from person to person.

Perform .... sets and .... reps.

Perform .... per day .... days per week.

Notes: ....

....

....

....

....

....

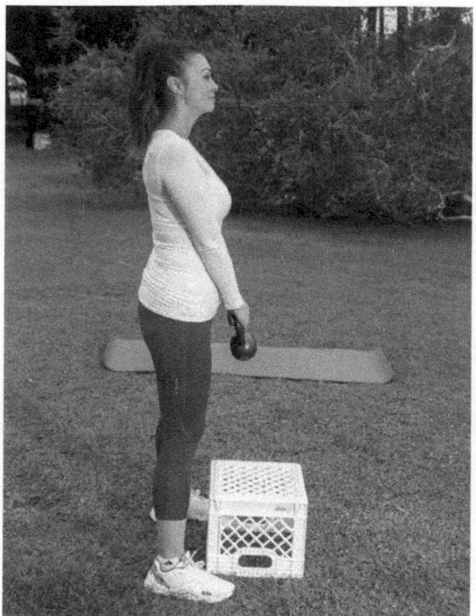

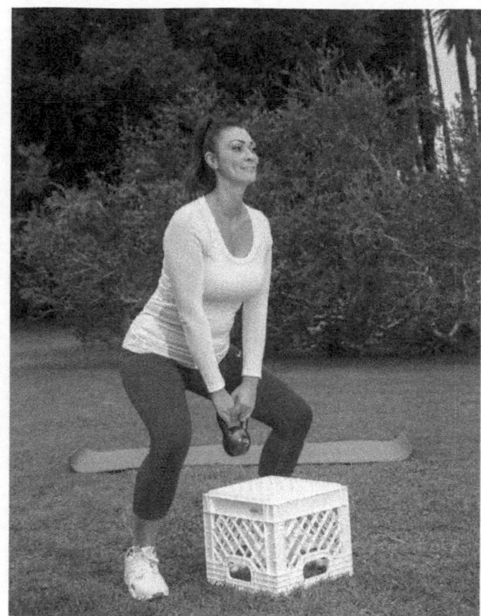

Low kettlebell squat (with elevated finishing position)

1. Choose a weight based on your fitness level and place a box or crate in front of you.
2. Stand with your feet shoulder-width apart as you hold a kettlebell with both hands just in front of your body with your arms hanging straight down.
3. Slowly bend your hips and knees, keeping the knees at or slightly behind your toes as you bring the kettlebell as close as possible to the top of the box in front of you without losing the natural curve in your lower back. As you squat, keep your shoulders down and back and your knees out. Do not squat any lower than your ability to maintain your natural lower back and neck curves. This will vary from person to person.

Perform .... sets and .... reps.

Perform .... per day .... days per week.

Notes: ....

....

....

....

....

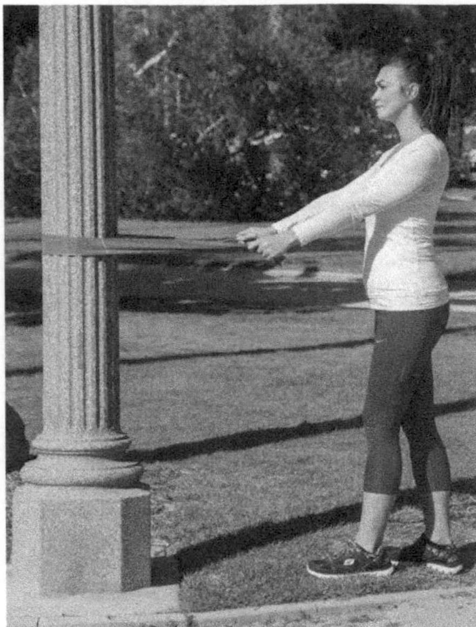

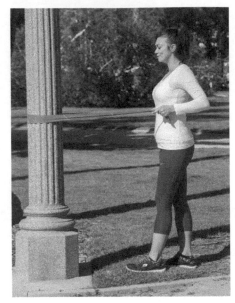

Elastic high pulls

1. Start in a standing or seated position with good posture.
2. Place an elastic band around a sturdy object, such as the knob of a securely shut door, a rail, or a post, and step back just enough so the band has some tension.
3. Pull or "row" the band from an arms-outstretched position to the elbows-by-your-sides position.

Perform .... sets and .... reps.

Perform .... per day .... days per week.

Notes: ....

....

....

....

....

....

....

....

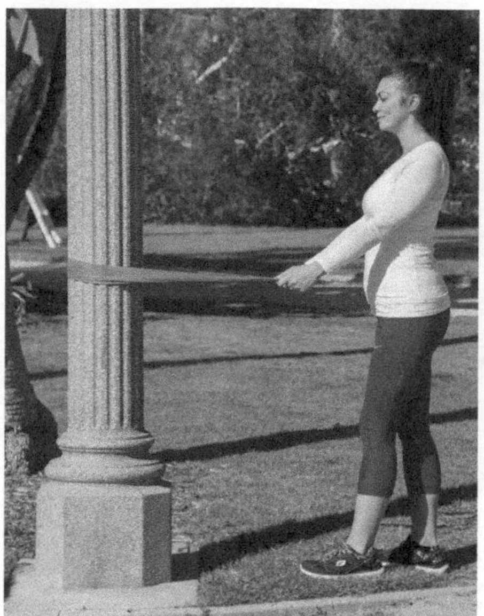
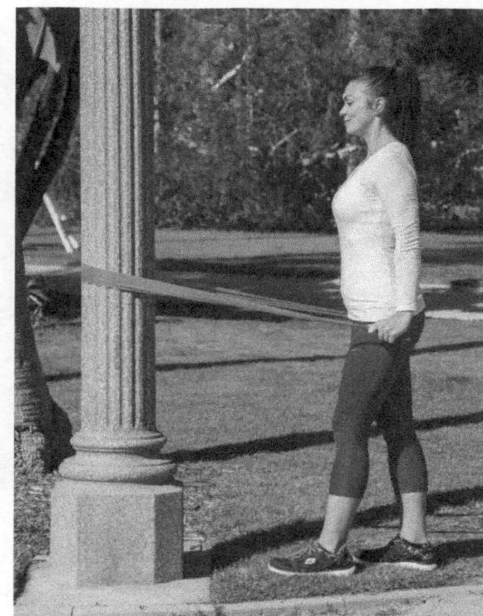

Elastic low pulls

1. Start in a standing or seated position with good posture.
2. Place an elastic band around a sturdy object, such as the knob of a securely shut door, a rail, or a post, and step back just enough so the band has some tension.
3. Pull the band from an arms-outstretched position to the hands-by-your-hips position.

Perform .... sets and .... reps.

Perform .... per day .... days per week.

Notes: ....

....

....

....

....

....

....

....

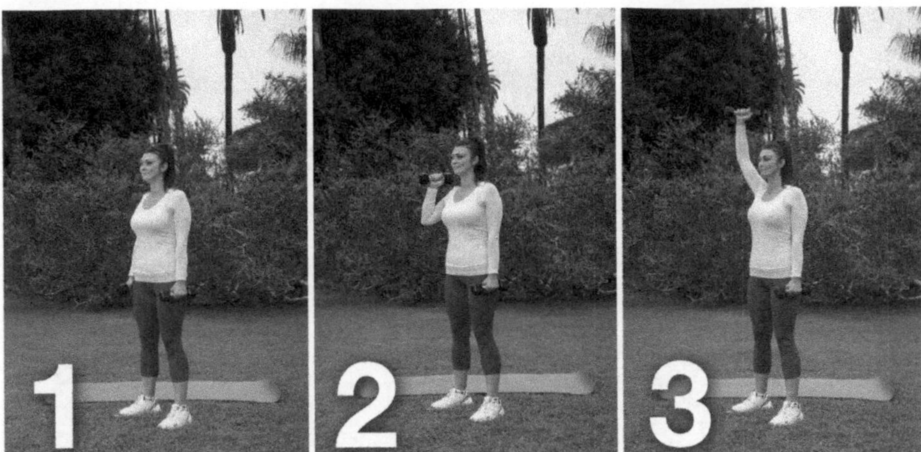

Dumbbell curl and press

1. Stand with your feet approximately shoulder-width apart while holding a dumbbell in each hand that is appropriate for your fitness level.
2. Bend the right arm so the weight is just above shoulder height.
3. Straighten the right arm so the weight is above your head.
4. Slowly lower the weight and repeat the same sequence with the left arm.

Perform .... sets and .... reps.

Perform .... per day .... days per week.

Notes: ....

....

....

....

....

....

....

....

....

....

....

Flexibility Training Exercises

The following are sample flexibility and stretching exercises to improve mobility in daily activities and reduce muscle tension and tightness.

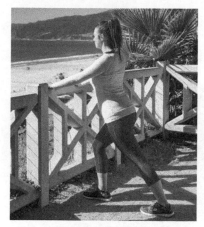

Calf stretch

1. Stand with your feet hip-width apart. Preserve the natural curve in your lower back and neck as you perform this exercise.
2. Place both hands, at about chest height, on a wall or elevated surface in front of you.
3. Position your right leg in front of you with your right knee slightly bent for support.
4. Step back with your left leg, keeping your left knee straight and left foot pointed forward.
5. Lean slightly with your hips and torso until you feel a gentle stretch in your left calf, heel cord, and a little in front of your left hip. Hold the gentle stretch position for .... seconds. Relax for .... seconds.
6. Repeat on the other side.

Perform .... sets and .... reps.

Perform .... per day .... days per week.

Notes: ....

....

....

....

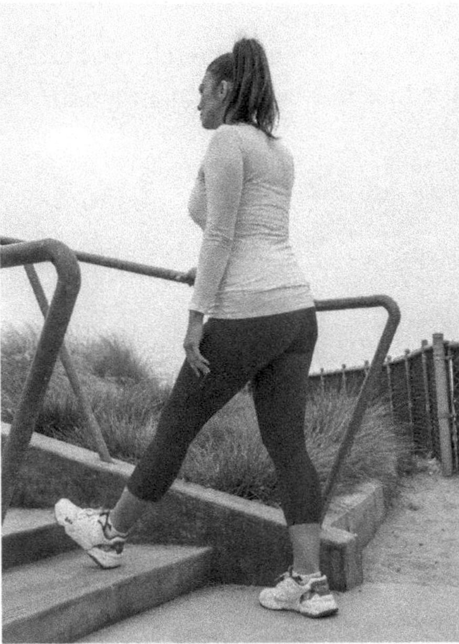

Hamstring stretch

1. Hold on to a rail and place the heel of your left foot on the bottom step of a staircase so you feel a gentle stretch at the back of your left leg.
2. Hold the stretch position for .... seconds. Relax for .... seconds.
3. Repeat on the other side.

Perform .... sets and .... reps.

Perform .... per day .... days per week.

Notes: ....

....

....

....

....

....

....

....

....

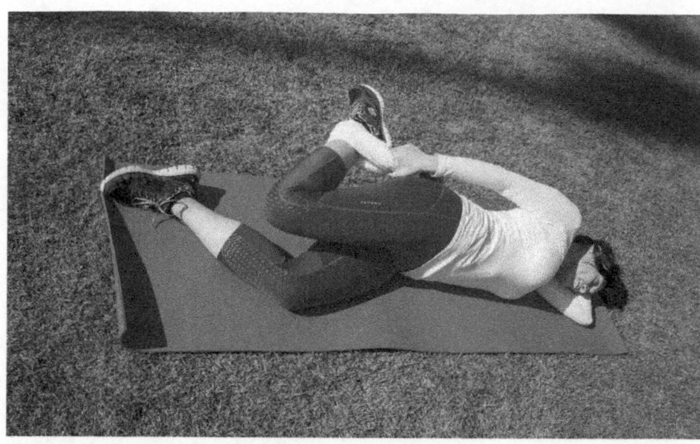

Modified quad stretch

1. Lie on your left side with both knees bent comfortably. Preserve the natural curve in your lower back and neck as you perform this exercise.
2. Using your right hand, grip your right ankle and bring the heel of your right foot toward the back of your hip (or buttocks). Feel the stretch in the front of your right thigh muscles from your knee to the front of your hip. Hold the gentle stretch position for ...... seconds. Relax for ...... seconds.
3. If you have difficulty reaching your ankle, use a towel as an extension (as shown in the photo) to avoid straining your lower back and/or shoulder.
4. Repeat on the other side.

Perform .... sets and .... reps.

Perform .... per day .... days per week.

Notes: ....

....

....

....

....

....

....

....

....

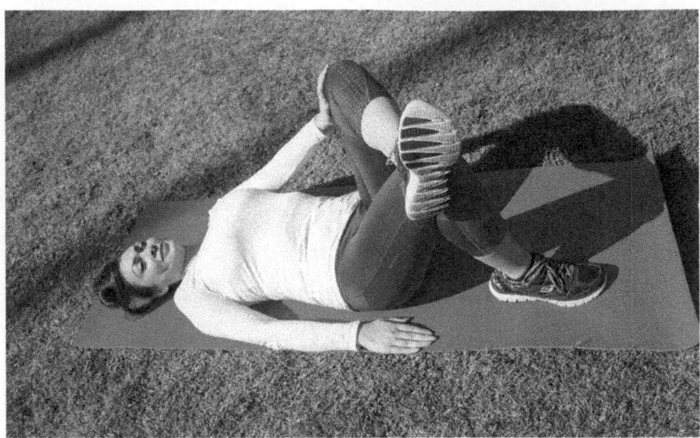

Inner hip stretch

1. Lie on your back with both knees bent comfortably and your feet on the floor.
2. Slowly bend your left hip and knee so the outer part of your left ankle rests on top of your right thigh.
3. Place your left hand on the inner part of your left knee, and very gently apply a force away from you until you feel a gentle stretch in the inner part of your left hip. Hold the gentle stretch position for .... seconds. Relax for .... seconds.
4. Repeat on the other side.

Perform .... sets and .... reps.

Perform .... per day .... days per week.

Notes: ....

....

....

....

....

....

....

....

....

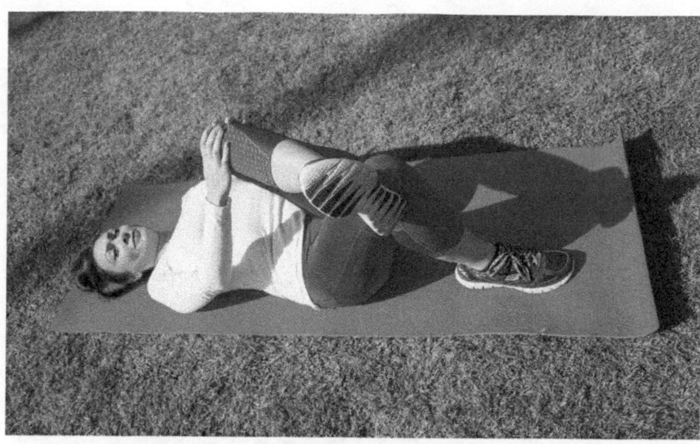

Outer hip stretch

1. Lie on your back with both knees bent comfortably.
2. Slowly bend your left hip and knee so the outer part of your left ankle rests on top of your right thigh.
3. Place both your hands on the outer part of your left knee, and very gently apply a force toward you until you feel a gentle stretch in the outer part of your left hip. Hold the gentle stretch position for .... seconds. Relax for .... seconds.
4. Repeat on the other side.

Perform .... sets and .... reps.

Perform .... per day .... days per week.

Notes: ....

....

....

....

....

....

....

....

....

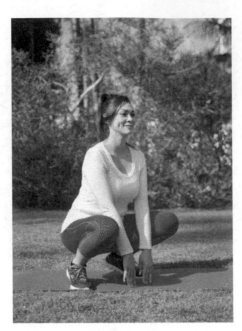

Squat stretch

1. Stand with your legs shoulder-width apart.
2. Slowly squat down as far as you can go comfortably. Place your hands in front of you on the floor for support.
3. Hold the gentle stretch position for .... seconds. Relax for .... seconds.

Perform .... sets and .... reps.

Perform .... per day .... days per week.

Notes: ....

....

....

....

....

....

....

....

....

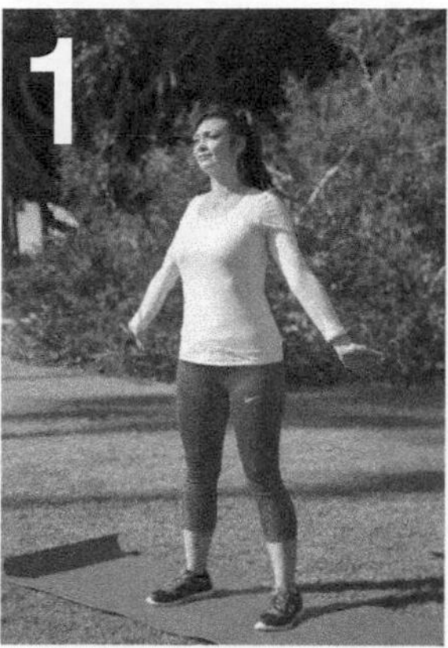

Chest, shoulder stretch ("yawn" stretch)

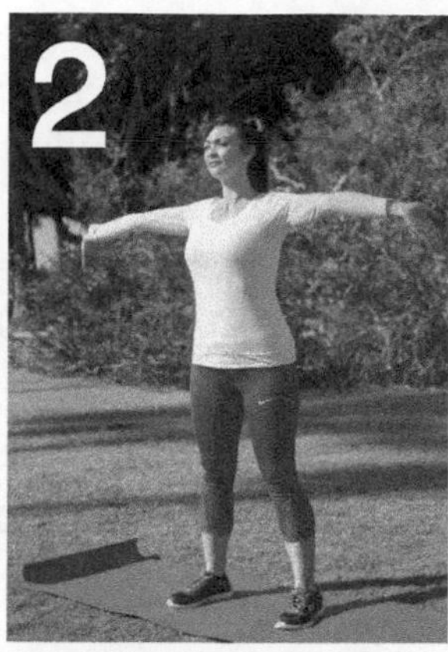

Chest, shoulder stretch ("yawn" stretch)

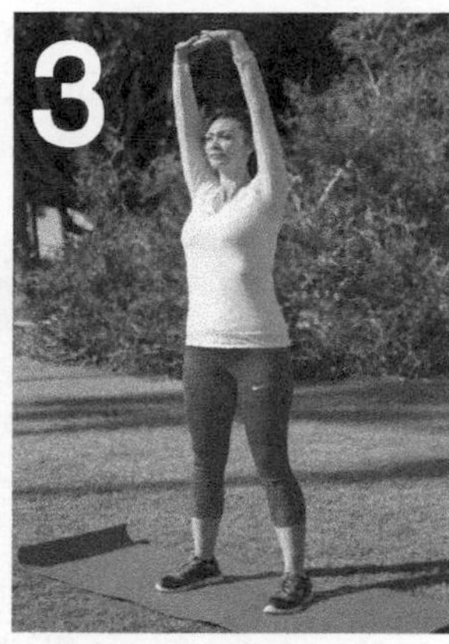

Upper back stretch ("yawn" stretch)

1. Stand with your feet shoulder-width apart, with your hands by your sides and thumbs facing forward.
2. Rotate your thumbs away from the sides of your body, bend your palms away from the inner part of your wrist, and draw your shoulders slightly back to feel a stretch in your forearms, shoulders, and chest (see photo 1). Hold the gentle stretch position for .... seconds.
3. Bring your arms up to shoulder level, bend your palms away from the inner parts of the wrists (with the palms facing away from you), and draw your shoulders slightly back to feel a stretch in your forearms, shoulders, and chest (see photo 2). Hold the gentle stretch position for .... seconds.
4. Raise both arms overhead with your palms facing the ceiling or sky and fingers pointing toward the middle of your body to feel a stretch in your upper back (see photo 3). Hold the gentle stretch position for .... seconds.

Perform .... sets and .... reps.

Perform .... per day .... days per week.

Notes: ....

....

....

....

....

....

Balance Training Exercise

The following is a sample balance exercise that may be a part of a fall prevention program and improve mobility in the community (due to less fear of falling).

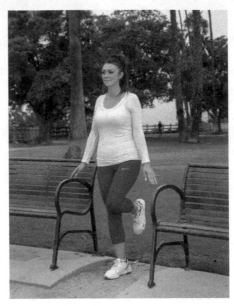

Single leg balance (for static balance)

1. Stand with your feet hip-width apart near two sturdy objects (such as walls or chairs) for support. Keep your eyes open throughout the exercise.
2. Slowly lift your left foot off the ground to about mid-calf level, without touching your right leg.
3. Hold this position in a safe and steady manner for .... seconds, depending on your ability.
4. Repeat by standing on the left leg and lifting your right foot off the ground.

Perform .... sets and .... reps.

Perform .... per day .... days per week.

Notes: ....

....

....

....

....

Aerobic Training Exercises

The following are sample aerobic exercises to improve endurance for daily activities.

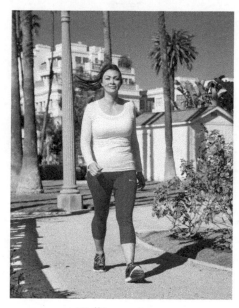

Walking program

Outdoor walking provides fresh air, sunshine, and natural bright light for a better mood. It also promotes relaxation by being in nature.

Perform .... minutes.

Perform .... per day .... days per week.

Notes: ....

....

....

....

....

....

....

....

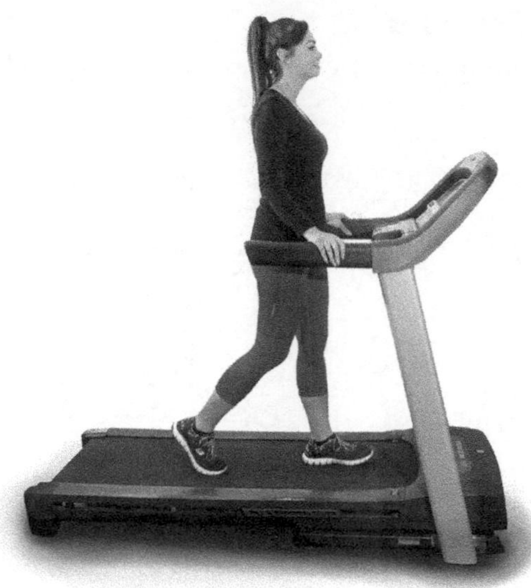

Treadmill program

A treadmill program facilitates exercise during severe weather and for those with seasonal allergies.

Perform .... minutes.

Perform .... per day .... days per week.

Notes: ....

....

....

....

....

....

....

....

....

....

....

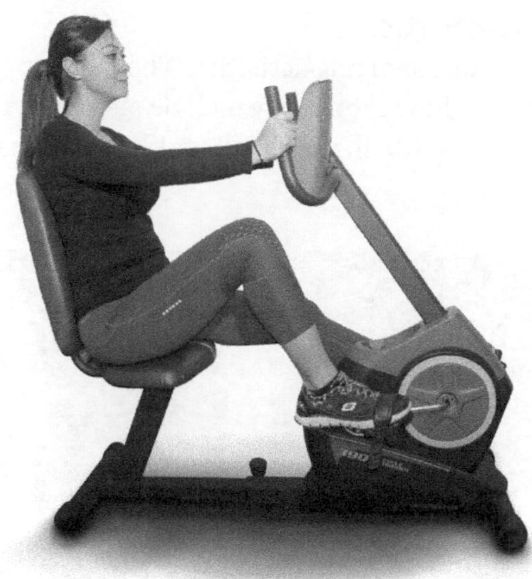

Stationary bike program

A stationary bike program facilitates exercise during severe weather and for those with seasonal allergies.

Perform .... minutes.

Perform .... per day .... days per week.

Notes: ....
....
....
....
....
....
....
....
....
....
....

Sports-Related Activities

The following are sample sporting activities. The key is to help patients/clients find sports they enjoy. These sports may include pickleball, racquetball, badminton, tennis, basketball, softball, volleyball, golf, and football (soccer), to name just a few.

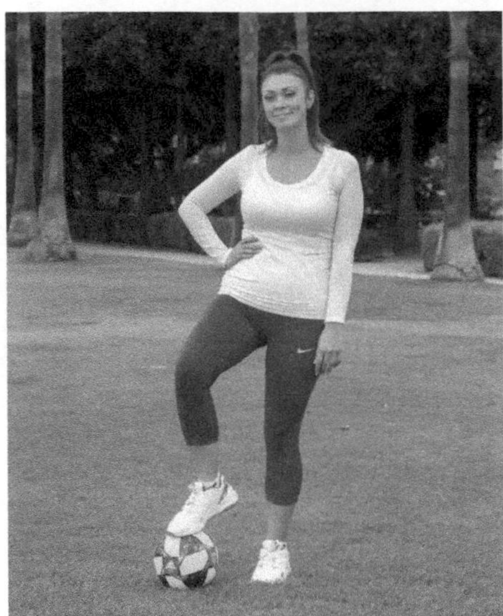

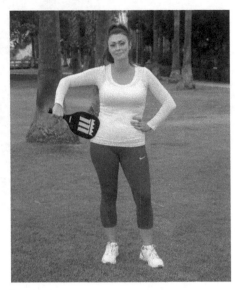

Sports-related activities

Try new and fun sporting activities to give yourself a challenge and make social connections.

Sport: ....

Perform .... minutes.

Perform .... days per week.

Notes: ....

....

....

....

....

....

Function-Related Activities

The following is a sample functional activity to ensure that the patient/client performs activities of daily living with greater ease. Other examples of functional activities may include stairclimbing, getting down to and back up from the floor, kneeling, lifting, and carrying items (such as groceries), to name just a few.

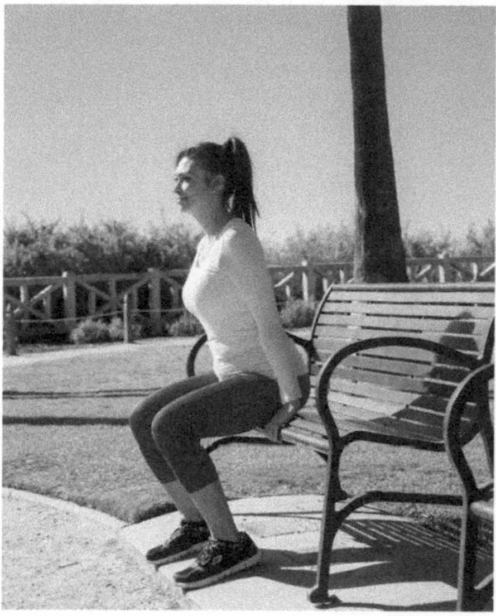

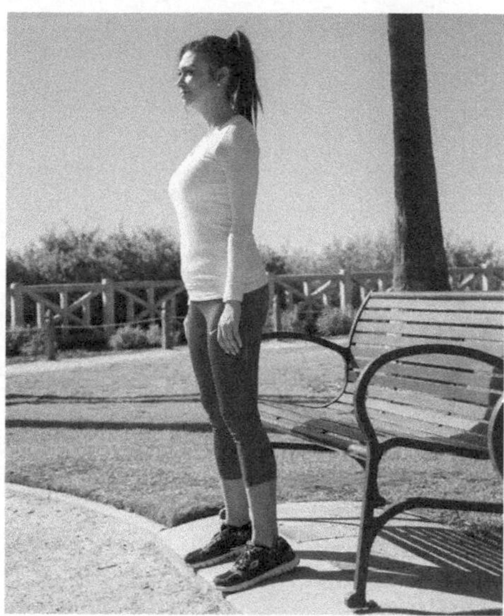

Sit to stand

1. Sit near the edge of a sturdy chair (if needed, place the back of the chair against a wall so it does not slide back) or bench with your feet approximately shoulder-width apart.
2. Lean forward slightly and stand up. Ideally, try not to use your hands for a push-off.
3. Slowly sit back down.

Perform .... sets and .... reps.

Perform .... per day .... days per week.

Notes: ....

....

....

....

....

Additional Reading

American College of Sports Medicine. *ACSM's Guidelines for Exercise Testing and Prescription*, 11th ed. Philadelphia, PA: Wolters Kluwer; 2022.

Brody LT, Hall CM. *Therapeutic Exercise: Moving Toward Function*, 4th ed. Philadelphia, PA: Wolters Kluwer; 2018.

Collings TJ, Bourne MN, Barrett RS, *et al.* Gluteal muscle forces during hip-focused injury prevention and rehabilitation exercises. *Med Sci Sports Exerc.* 2023;55(4):650–660.

Kisner C, Colby LA, Borstad J. *Therapeutic Exercise: Foundations and Techniques*, 7th ed. Philadelphia, PA: FA Davis; 2018.

McGill SM. *Low Back Disorders*, 3rd ed. Champaign, IL: Human Kinetics; 2016.

Subject Index

Sub-headings in *italics* indicate figures.

Author Index